Thermodynamics in Bioenergetics

Jean-Louis Burgot

University of Rennes 1-France
Rennes, France

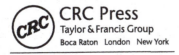

CRC Press
Taylor & Francis Group
Boca Raton London New York

CRC Press is an imprint of the
Taylor & Francis Group, an **informa** business

A SCIENCE PUBLISHERS BOOK

Cover credit: Cover illustration reproduced by kind courtesy of Jean-Louis Burgot

CRC Press
Taylor & Francis Group
6000 Broken Sound Parkway NW, Suite 300
Boca Raton, FL 33487-2742

First issued in paperback 2021

© 2020 by Taylor & Francis Group, LLC
CRC Press is an imprint of Taylor & Francis Group, an Informa business

No claim to original U.S. Government works

Version Date: 20190423

ISBN 13: 978-0-367-77668-8 (pbk)
ISBN 13: 978-1-138-49092-5 (hbk)

Library of Congress Cataloging-in-Publication Data
Names: Burgot, Jean-Louis, author.
Title: Thermodynamics in bioenergetics / Jean-Louis Burgot (University of Rennes 1-France, Rennes, Ile et Vilaine, France).
Description: Boca Raton, FL : CRC Press, 2019.	"A science publishers book."	Includes bibliographical references and index.
Identifiers: LCCN 2019016030	ISBN 9781138490925 (hardback)
Subjects: LCSH: Thermodynamics.	Bioenergetics.	Biochemistry.
Classification: LCC QP517.T48 B87 2019	DDC 572/.436--dc23
LC record available at https://lccn.loc.gov/2019016030

Visit the Taylor & Francis Web site at
http://www.taylorandfrancis.com

and the CRC Press Web site at
http://www.crcpress.com

Preface

Undergraduate biology courses are becoming more and more dependent on mathematics, physics and chemistry. Among the involved physical sciences, there is no need, certainly, to emphasize the part played by thermodynamics! At its origin, thermodynamics was the branch of physics devoted to energy and its transformations. Now, even if its goal remains the same, its realm of applying has considerably grown up to the point that, since for several decades, this science is endowed with a cosmogonic impact! No more!

Energy, the great concept ceaselessly involved in the handling of thermodynamics, can be defined by any property which can be produced from work or which can be converted into work. There are various manifestations of energy as there are different kinds of works. Among them, let us for example mention the thermal, electrical, radiant, potential kinetic ones. It is a well known fact that the conversion of one kind of them into another one together with the "interconversion" energy work are of utmost importance in physics, in chemistry and also in biology. It is also known that if work can be entirely converted into heat, the converse is only partially true, according to the second principle of thermodynamics. In view of all these considerations, heat and work (whatever the kind the latter is) are regarded as being two forms of energy. Hence, it is not surprising that all forms of energy are expressed in work units.

Over the pre-past century, the question to know whether or not living cells obey the laws of physics and chemistry was open. Its negative answer was related to the theory named in the french language as "dogme de la force vitale". Now, we know that physico-chemical laws hold in the biological world and, of course, it is the case of thermodynamics laws. Therefore, we can already assert that living cells, indeed, do possess very powerful systems for transforming energy.

Bioenergetics is the term used to denote the study of energy transformations in living organisms in particular but not only at the cellular level. Bioenergetics is now a study which cannot get away from biochemistry and molecular biology courses, even in the undergraduate ones. But...... there exists a "but"! Beginner students who have chosen to study biological sciences may not be interested in the study of physical sciences. As a result, their background in this realm may be too weak and, therefore, they may quickly exhibit problems of understandings. This is particularly the case with thermodynamics, even with classical thermodynamics. It is true that, at first glance, it appears to be an abstract science. The reason, from the physical standpoint, is that it involves idealized systems which often carry out imaginary experiments! Moreover, from the mathematical one, the symbolism involved in its study is somewhat discouraging because of the fact that it is rather cumbersome with the quasi-systematic presence, notably, of several partial derivatives.

However, for the development of this part of thermodynamics, only a moderate knowledge of mathematics is an essential condition. However, from another standpoint, it is clear that the notion of entropy which is at the heart of thermodynamics complicates its approach more. As for them, statistical thermodynamics and non equilibrium thermodynamics are, both mathematically and physically, more difficult to grasp than the classical one. Some results coming from non equilibrium thermodynamics are only given in this book. It is true that the need for introducing some elements of statistical thermodynamics in it was questionable. Nevertheless, the author has not hesitated: the book does not contain elements of statistical thermodynamics even if its development tremendously confort the theory and results of the classical one. Concerning the introduction of some elements of non equilibrium thermodynamics, there is no doubt. It is, purely and simply, imposed by the fact that living cells are often open systems and because of this fact, it must be known, as we shall see it, that the notion of entropy appears to be endowed with a greater importance than that it has in classical thermodynamics *sensu stricto*.

After these few words concerning thermodynamics, it is now time to give some general considerations on the biological transformations of energy in living organisms. In this book, they are essentially regarded at the cellular level. Actually, the bioenergetics of the cell is one of the central elements in the study of biochemistry as are the basic molecular units intervening in the cellular energy-transforming systems, i.e., the enzymes. The extraordinary biological complexity must firstly be noticed. Its maintenance and its tendency to increase would imply that a kind of energy obeying to thermodynamic principles devoted to them would be defined. Still noteworthy, living organisms possess a very important quality. By some means, they have at their disposal some kinds of information and they can handle them. One of them (and not the least!) is the genetic information. Beyond that, according to the relatively new science of information, the information would actually be also a form of energy. In any case, the information is directly related to the great function of thermodynamics: the entropy. According to some authors, entropy is nothing but a measure of the missing information.

This book is essentially a "book of thermodynamics". Its purpose is to provide the readers, who essentially possess a biological background, with elementary and also with slightly more in depth thermodynamic notions permitting to grasp some thermodynamics aspects of the bioenergetic processes. It does not develop classical thermodynamics in its entirety. Hence, we confined ourselves to mention the items which are directly related to bioenergetics. Nevertheless, and this is not in contradistinction with what has just been said, we did not hesitate to start our recalls of thermodynamics far below the presentation in amount with the exposition of the first and second laws. This is done for the sake of continuity. In the same manner, we have somewhat emphasized the concept of entropy which is puzzling.

The plan of the book is as follows:

– In the first chapters constituting the first part, we develop the necessary basics of thermodynamics together with some other topics which are not obligatorily in the domain of the latter. They are treated, however, because they are of undubitable importance for our purpose and, also, because they are not easily understandable at the sophomore level. We can say that this part is treated in such a way as to introduce and emphasize the notion of Gibbs energy which is the pivotal thermodynamic concept in relation to bioenergetics, as we shall stress it.

– In the following chapters, we recall some developments concerning some points of the chemistry in solutions because, on one hand, they are constantly present in the processes of bioenergetics and, on the other, because they provide interesting examples of processes which are governed by the Gibbs energy rule. The recalled phenomena are the acid-base, redox, complexation and transports in aqueous solutions. Then, we consider rudiments of the thermodynamics of non equilibrium because living cells are open systems. We also recall some properties of enzymes. Of course, we also devote two whole chapters to the Gibbs rule.

– In the third part, we apply these developments to most of the transformations of bioenergetics. Deliberately, we limit ourselves to give explanations justifying the directions of the numerous steps occurring in the way of conversion of energy in cells. Thus, we justify the generation of the cellular energy. The part played by the Gibbs energy in bioenergetics will appear in all its importance in these ways of conversion of energy.

Rennes—December 2018   **Jean-Louis Burgot**

Acknowledgments

I thank Mr. Arsène Lancien who, as usual, has corrected my imperfect English.
To my family…..

Contents

Part II: Some Aspects of Chemical Reactions in Aqueous Solutions

Appendices

Glossary

mathematical

$f()$	function of . Ex : $f(x)$ function of x
$f(x,y....)$	function of x,y ...
$y'(x)$	derivative of $y(x)$ with respect to variable x
dy/dx	idem
$dy, dx...$	differentials of y, x ....
$\Delta y, \Delta x$ ...	changes in y, x....
$(\partial M/\partial N)_{i,j}$	partial derivative of function M with respect to variable N, other variables i and j being held constant
ln	napieran logarithm
log	decadic logarithm
$\delta y, \delta x$	variation of y, x
đ	personal symbolism meaning that the differentials of x, y, W.. etc...are inexact. (Often symbols δ or D are used instead of in literature).

physico-chemical

(In a general manner, a molar quantity is symbolized by a minuscule letter or by a majuscule with the subscript m. Ex molar volume: v or V_m. The exception is a heat quantity which can be indifferently written q or Q, whether it is molar or not)

A	Helmholtz energy (free energy)
A_{ext}	free energy with respect to the environment
A	de Donder's affinity or affinity reaction
a	activity of a species
a	era
B	availability
C	heat capacity
C	general symbol of the "concentration" whatever is its scale of composition
C'	specific (massic) heat capacity?
C_V	heat capacity at constant volume
c_V	molar heat capacity at constant volume
C_P	heat capacity at constant pressure
c_i	molarity
E	global energy
E	electromotive force of an electrochemical cell
E°	standard electromotive force of an electrochemical cell

E_1°, E_2°	standard electrode potentials of redox systems 1,2…
$E_{k;i}$	kinetic energy of the particle i
E.F.M.	electromotive force of an electrochemical cell
F	force (vector)
F	faraday
G	Gibbs energy (free enthalpy)
G°	molar Gibbs energy in the standard state
G_{ext}	free enthalpy with respect to the environment
H	enthalpy
H_T°	standard enthalpy at temperature T
H_0°	standard enthalpy at 0 K
h	hauteur
h	Planck's constant
I	impulsion (vector)
I	ionic strength of the medium
K°	standard equilibrium constant (thermodynamic equilibrium constant)
K	Binding constant (formation)
K_w	ionic product of water
k or k_B	Boltzmann constant
K_a	acid ionization constant
K_b	basic ionization constant
k_c	dissociation constant of a complex
k_{ij}	microscopic dissociation acid constants
k	rate constant
L	displacement (vector)
L	Avogadro number
L	ligand
M	molar mass
M	mass of a compound
m	molality of a substance
m	mass of a particule (molecule or atom) or of a mobile
n	number of moles
n'	numerical density or number of molecules per unit volume
n	number of exchanged electrons in a redox reaction
N	general symbol of a composition
N	number of molecules (particules)
N_A	Avogadro number
p	pressure
P	partition coefficient
p	momentum
P	protein
P	rest phosphate
Q, q	quantity of heat
q_{rev}	heat reversibly exchanged
q_{irr}	heat irreversibly exchanged
Q	reaction quotient
R	perfect gaz constant

S	entropy of the system under study
S'	entropy of its surroundings (reservoir)
S_e	exchanged entropy
s, S	surface
T or T_{kelvin}	absolute temperature
$T_{celsius}$	temperature Celsius scale
t	time
U	internal energy
$U(x_i, y_i, z_i)$	potential energy of the particule i
V	volume
v	speed (vector)
v	speed (module)
v	chemical reaction rate
v	molar volume
v	total rate of a chemical reaction
$v_i^{\cdot}$	molar volume of the pure substance i
x	molar fraction of a substance
X, Y	any variable or quantity
$X_m(i)$	molar extensive property of i
y_i	fraction of species i
W,w	work
W_R	work reversible exchanged during a process including the "p –V work"
W_R^*	work reversible exchanged during a process not taking into account the "p–V work"
$\mathbf{W}_{u.max}$	maximum work
γ	acceleration (vector)
γ	$= C_p/C_V$
γ	activity coefficient
θ	temperature (general symbol)
μ	chemical potential
μ°	standard chemical potential
ρ	volumic mass
Δσ	created entropy
ξ	extent of a chemical reaction
$\Delta Hf°$	standard heat formation of a species from its elements
ν	stoichiometric coefficient of a species
ν	variance of a system
χ	dissociation constant of the half dissociation equilibrium of a complex
Φ	potential function used in thermodynamics of irreversible processes
Λ	exergy

Acronyms

DNA	Desoxyribonucleic acid
RNA	Ribonucleic acid
IUPAC	International Union of Pure and Applied Chemistry
emf	electromotive force

Base Physical Quantities and Derived Physical Quantities

According to IUPAC and by convention, physical quantities are organized in a dimensional system built upon seven *base quantities*, each of which is regarded as having its own dimension. These base quantities and the symbols used to denote them are as follows:

physical quantity	*symbol for the quantity*	*SI unit*	*name of the unit*
length	l	m	meter
mass	m	kg	kilogram
time	t	s	second
electric current	I	A	ampere
thermodynamic temperature	T	K	Kelvin
amount of substance	n	mol	mol
luminous intensity	I_v	cd	candela

All other physical quantities are called derived quantities and are regarded as having dimensions derived algebraically from the seven base quantities by multiplication and division. Their derivation is given as they are introduced bit by bit in the book.

Part I
Fundamentals of Classical Thermodynamics

Chapter 1

Some Recallings of Physics

This first chapter is devoted to some recallings of physics, especially to the notions of pressure, work, heat and temperature since they are recurrent in thermodynamics. Although the methods of classical thermodynamics are independent of any theory concerning the existence of atoms and of molecules, it is now well-admitted that some kind of work, pressure and temperature are manifestations of the movements of these "particles". This is the reason why these notions are tackled now.

1) An approach to a perfect gas

A fluid, defined as being a perfect gas, is an hypothetical one, the properties of which are:
- its structure is discontinuous. It is constituted of independent particules (atoms and molecules) which may be considered as "point-particules" but which, however, are endowed with the mass m;
- all its molecules are moving;
- all the collisions of its molecules with the walls of their container are elastic;
- there exists no "interaction" between the particules. Only the contact-forces developing during the impacts exist;
- it contains a huge number of particules, whatever the volume of the container is. This is the reason why statistical methods must be used to grasp classical thermodynamics in more detail. This is the objective of statistical thermodynamics.

These hypotheses imply that the perfect gas molecules only possess a kinetic energy because they are moving, possess no energy of another kind and there are no interactions between them. Defining the system under study as being constituted by the whole gases, *its internal energy U is only of kinetic kind.*

Actually, a perfect gas is only a theoretical model. However, the behavior of a dilute gas tends to be that of a perfect gas. This is because, then, the average distance between the molecules is great with respect to the range of interactions due to the intermolecular forces.

The conclusions to which this concept leads are of utmost importance. We shall come back several times to it. The concept of perfect gas is far-reaching.

Exercise 1:

Calculate the number of molecules of a perfect gas present in a container of a volume $V = \mu^3$ (1 micrometer power 3) under the normal pressure $p = 1$ atm at the temperature $t = 0°C$, knowing that:
- *the quantities p, V, T and the number of moles n of the gas are related to each other by the equation of perfect gases (R is a constant named perfect gas constant $R = 8,314\ J\,K^{-1}$):*

  $pV = nRT$

- *the number of "true" molecules in one mole is the Avogadro number: N_A (N_A = 6,022 10^{23}). It is known that 1 mole occupies a volume of 22,4 L in the above conditions of pressure and temperature.*

Answ:

The number of moles of the sample n is proportional to the volume V, all the other quantities of the equation being constant. The values of the quantities p, T and of course R being the same as those given, it is clear that, since 22,4 L are occupied by 1 mole, the volume 1 μ^3 = 1 (10^{-5})^3 L is occupied by:

$1.10^{-15}/22,4$ *moles*

Given one mole contains 6,022 10^{23} molecules, the sample contains:

1.10^{-15} *6,022* $10^{23}/22,4$ = *2,68* 10^7 *molecules*

Remark: although the numerical value and the unity of R does not directly intervene in the above calculation, its unity is the joule Kelvin^{-1}. The exercise has not been formulated in coherent units.

2) Elastic collisions

In order to later study the notion of pressure from the microphysical standpoint, we tackle those of elastic collisions and of impulsion.

One speaks of elastic collision when the molecule participating in the process retains its kinetic energy. Most of the time, molecules do not collide with the walls of the container along a direction normal to them. As a result, the incidence angle is equal to that of reflexion and the speed exhibits a change in its direction. One can split up the speed **v** of a molecule into its three components v_x, v_y, v_z parallel to the three orthogonal axes of space and since speeds are vectors:

$$v^2 = v_x^2 + v_y^2 + v_z^2$$

However, there always exists a component of the speed normal to the wall. Let this direction be that of the axis x. During the elastic impact, the speed of this component changes its sign but not its direction. It passes from $+v_x$ before it to $-v_x$ after. As a result, the component of the momentum also changes from $+mv_x$ to $-mv_x$. The absolute value of the change in the momentum is equal to 2 mv_x.

3) Kinetic theory of perfect gases—A molecular view of pressure

It is particularly interesting to study the notion of pressure from the microphysical standpoint, that is to say by considering that the pressure exerted on a surface is due to the collisions of the molecules of the gas with the latter. This standpoint is, of course, out of the scope of classical thermodynamics. It is on the same basic lines as statistical thermodynamics since it takes into account the occurrence of atoms and molecules. Besides, both theories of thermodynamics are in mutual agreement. This is one of the reasons why this point deserves some attention.

Let us recall that pressure is defined as a force divided by the area to which it applies perpendicularly. The SI unit of pressure is the pascal (Pa). 1 pascal is equal to 1 newton per meter-square (1 Pa = 1 N m^{-2}). In base units: 1 Pa = 1 kg m^{-1} s^{-2}. [Other pressure units are frequently encountered. They are the bar (1 bar = 10^5 Pa), the atmosphere (1 atm = 101325 Pa), the torr (1 Torr = 133,322 Pa), and the mercury millimeter (1 mm Hg = 133,322 Pa)].

We have already said that a perfect gas can be considered as being a very dilute gas. Its molecules do not interact with each other. They are moving freely in the container where the gas is located. In usual conditions, molecules exhibit speeds of the order of 100 m s^{-1}. The origin of the pressure exerted by a gas is the continuous striking of the gas molecules on the wall of the container. The higher the kinetic energy, the higher the pressure.

Let us consider an element of the wall of area s and take the x axis normal to it (see Figure 1). Suppose that collisions are perfectly elastic. We know (see above) that, after the collision, the molecule has gained the momentum equal to $-2\,mv_x$. Let us suppose, now, that all the molecules have the same speed **v**. If there are v collisions (on the element) in a time unity, this element leads to the momentum change $-2\,v\,mv_x$ of the gas. According to Newton's law,

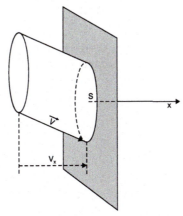

Figure 1. A collision of a molecule with an element of the wall.

the force **F** exerted by the element of the wall is equal to the momentum increase of the gas by time unit. One can temporarily write for its value on the x axis:

$$\mathbf{F} = -2v\,mv_x/\Delta t$$

Conversely, the force exerted on the wall element is $\mathbf{F'} = 2v\,mv_x/\Delta t$. It is normal to the element and opposite to the previous one. v is calculated by noticing that the molecules which strike the element by time unit ($\Delta t = 1$) are those contained in the oblique cylinder of section s and of generatrice **v**, that is to say of volume sv_x (v_x in modulus). If there are n' molecules in the unit-volume, one obtains (n' is the numerical density):

$$v = n's\,v_x$$

$$\mathbf{F'} = 2\,n's\,v_x\,mv_x/1$$

$$\mathbf{F'} = 2\,n'\,mv_x^2\,s$$

and the pressure:

$$p = 2\,n'\,mv_x^2 \qquad \text{in modulus}$$

Actually, all the molecules do not have the same speed **v**. The pressure p is due to the average effect of molecules possessing different speeds. In order to take this fact into account, the term v_x^2 must be replaced by its average value $\overline{v_x^2}$. Moreover, since only the half number of molecules (those with a positive v_x) contribute to the collisions, the number n' must be divided by 2. Hence:

$$p = n'\,m\overline{v_x^2}$$

Moreover, since the gas is isotropic,

$$\overline{v_x^2} = \overline{v_y^2} = \overline{v_z^2} = 1//3\,(\overline{v_x^2} + \overline{v_y^2} + \overline{v_z^2})$$

$$= 1/3\,\overline{v^2}$$

Finally, given the fact that (with N being the number of molecules and V the volume of the container):

n' = N/V

$$p = N \, m \, \bar{v^2}/3 \, V \tag{1}$$

or, after multiplication of the numerator and of the denominator by 2:

$$p = (2/3 \, V) \, (N \, m \, \bar{v^2}/2)$$

The second term (between braces) is the kinetic energy E_k of the whole molecules. This is also, given the working hypothesis, the internal energy U of the system (constituted by the gas molecules):

$$U = N \, m \, \bar{v^2}/2$$

and:

$$pV = (2/3)U$$

or

$$pV = (2/3)E_k$$

In Equation (1), the term $\bar{v^2}$ is named the *mean square of the velocities of the molecules*. Its root mean square is called *mean quadratic speed.* It is an indication of the speed of the molecules.

Exercise 2:

Several iron balls fall vertically at the same speed v = 1,5 m s^{-1} on a plane of area s = 6 m². All have the same mass m = 3 g. On an average, there are 200 balls which fall per m³. Calculate the pressure on the surface.

Answ:

Let us suppose that the x axis is the vertical one. We use the relation F' = 2v m v$_x$/Δt. It remains to calculate the number of balls striking the surface in the period of time Δt. If we choose Δt = 1s, v is equal to the volume V of the cylinder of height vx and cross section s. As a result:

F' = 200. 2 mv$_x$(v$_x$ s)/Δt (in modulus)

m = 3 10^{-3} kg, v$_x$ = 1,5 m s^{-1}, Δt = 1s

F' = 200 . 2. 3 10^{-3}. 1,5 (1,5. s)/1

p = F'/s

p = 200. 2. 3 10^{-3}. 1,5. 1,5

p = 2,7 Pa

Exercise 3:

Calculate the mean quadratic speed of molecules of diazote N$_2$ (M = 28 g mol^{-1}) in normal conditions. Recall that normal conditions are such that one mole of a perfect gas occupies a volume of 22,4 L at 0°C under the pressure of one atmosphere.

Answ:

RT = pV

1,9872 . 4,18 . 273,15 = 101 325 . V

According to the kinetic theory of gases, the kinetic energy E_k is:

$E_k = (3/2) \cdot 1,9872 \cdot 4,18 \cdot 273,15$

and also:

$E_k = (1/2) \cdot M \cdot \bar{c}^2 = (1/2) \cdot 28 \cdot 10^{-3} \cdot \bar{c}^2$

Hence:

$\bar{c} = 490$ m/s

4) The kinetic theory of heat and of temperature

According to the kinetic theory, heat must be identified with a mechanical motion of atoms or particles. Temperature and pressure are nothing else than an expression of the molecular agitation. Whereas pressure is the mean force per unit surface due to the repeated impacts on the walls of the container, according to the kinetic energy, temperature measures the mean kinetic energy of translation of the molecules. An increase of the temperature of a body is equivalent to an increase of the mean kinetic energy of translation of its molecules. This can be formalized by the general relation:

$T = f(E_k)$

If the conditions are those which governed the setting up of the above relation which expresses the pressure (perfect gases), the relation $T = f(E_k)$ exists explicitly. It is (1), from which one obtains:

$pV = (2/3) E_k$

$pV = nRT$

and hence:

$T = (2/3) E_k/nR$

5) Temperature measurement

The temperature measurement is based on the principle that two materials in thermal contact possess the same temperature at equilibrium (principle zero of thermodynamics).

Undoubtedly, the earliest conception of temperature was based on the purely physiological sensations of cold and hot. Given the weakness of such a physiological process, one, later, used the dilation of some liquids such as alcohol, mercury, etc. contained in a glass tube. The temperature θ was marked off by the height h. Then, two fixed points permitted to define a relation of the kind $h = a\theta + b$ (a and b constants) which could be used to measure the temperature θ through the value of h. Celsius choose the values 0°C and 100°C, corresponding to the fusion and ebullition temperatures of water under 1 atmosphere pressure, as fixed points. A centesimal scale was built, based on a simple cross multiplication. The height of water in the tube at 100°C being h_{100}, that at 0°C h_0, and that found in the measurement h, the temperature was given by:

$\theta = 100 \, [(h - h_0)/(h_{100} - h_0)]$

Now, the definition of temperature is set up in terms of measurements of volumes of gases. It is founded on the perfect gas law:

$p V = nRT$ (2)

(p,V, T are the pressure, volume and absolute temperature of the gas. n is the number of moles of the gas and R is a constant named perfect gas constant R = 8,314 J K^{-1}).

It is an operational definition involving, for a constant temperature, a series of measurements of volumes (of gas) at various pressures p and to extrapolate the function pv (pressure-molar volume product v = V/n) to zero pressure. At zero pressure, the curve becomes a straight line. This is not a surprise owing to the relation (2), since the more dilute the gas is, the more ideal its behavior. What is important is the fact that this result is found whatever the temperature and the nature of the gas are. Furthermore, the extrapolation of the curve leads to the *same* p-v intercept, whatever the nature of the gas is, obviously for the same temperature (Figure 2).

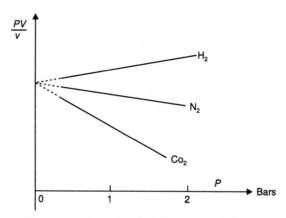

Figure 2. Limiting values of the term PV/n of different gases at the same temperature.

The product pV is a thermometric measurement independent of the nature of the gas. Hence, it is possible to have a universal temperature scale. It is named *absolute temperature scale* and the symbol of this temperature is T. The defined scale is such that:

$$(pv)_0'/(Pv)_0 = T'/T \tag{3}$$

This relation comes from the ratio of the expression (2) written to temperatures T' and T.

T is obligatorily a positive quantity, since all the other terms of relation (2) are positive. Its unit is the degree Kelvin: (K). This way of determination presents a difficulty because it forces to choose a pressure of reference. To overcome it, the triple point of water has been chosen by convention. It is defined by the state of the system for which the equilibria ice-water and water-water vapor occur simultaneously. Its variance is null. As a result, the pressure is imposed by the systems of water. Thus, no intensive variable can be fixed freely. A sole set of values is possible so that the equilibria should exist. This is the case for p = 6 10^{-3} bar and T = 0,01°C. The triple point is endowed with the temperature 273,16 K (degrees Kelvin).

The value 273,16 K comes from the deliberate choice to keep the former centesimal Celsius scale located between the fusion and ebullition points of water. Extrapolation experiments have led to the values:

$$(pv)_0^{100°C}/(pv)_0^{0°C} = 1,3661 \text{ and therefore } T_{100°C}/T_{0°C} = 1,3661$$

Deliberately, it is imposed that:

$$T_{100°C} - T_{0°C} = 100 \text{ K}$$

As a result of the system of the last two equations, it is found:

t (°C) = T (K) – 273,15

This explains the value 273,16 K chosen for the triple point of water.

(Recall that the variance v is given by the relation $v = n + 2 - \phi$ where n is the number of independent constituents here 1 (water), 2 the number of intensive factors playing a part -here pressure and water- and ϕ the number of phases (here 3: vapor, liquid and solid)).

Actually, absolute temperatures can be defined without any consideration of perfect gases. This will be explained when the second law and Carnot' cycle are introduced (see Chapter 11 "entropy"). Let us also mention the fact that the concept of temperature can also be introduced within the framework of statistical thermodynamics.

The thermodynamic temperature is a measure of the kinetic energy (unordered) of the particules constituting the system.

Temperature is an intensive property.

6) Work

From the general standpoint, it can be said that a work is performed when an object is moving against an opposite force. An example of work is that resulting from the expansion of a gas which puts a piston out of a cylinder, permitting, for example, the raising up of weight. The opposite force in this instance is, of course, the weight of the piston. This "p-V" work is most often encountered in thermodynamics. Another example of work is the electrical one. An electric current driven through a resistor, thanks to an appropriate voltage coming from a source of current of an electrochemical cell, may carry out a work, for example indirectly with the help of a motor. There are also works more specifically carried out by living organisms, which however remain true physical works. They are, for example, the chemical work, essentially concerning the biosynthesis of biomolecules, the work of transport and concentration of substances and the mechanical work done by most kinds of cells.

The symbol of work is W or w. The work unit related to the SI system is joule J ($1 \text{ J} = 1 \text{ kg m}^2\text{s}^{-2}$). Formerly (system cgs) the unity was the erg ($1 \text{ erg} = 10^{-7} \text{ J}$).

From the mathematical standpoint, the work W performed by a force **F** is equal to its dot (or scalar) product **and** its displacement **L**:

W = **F . L**

Recall that a dot product (here W) is a scalar whereas the force and the displacement are vectors. In pure scalar terms, the work is given by the expression:

W = F . L cos α   (4)

where α is the angle between F and L. The angle α is defined in such a way that when it is equal to 0 and π radian, the force and the displacement are colinear and:

W = F . L   (α = 0 π radian)

For the same reason:

W = –F L   (α = π radians)

and:

W = 0   (α = π/2 or 3π/2 radians)

Let us write the Equation (4) in differential terms. Consider a very small displacement: the differential dL (see the mathematical appendix II-1). By definition of a differential, it is, in this case, so small that during it the force may be considered as remaining constant. Therefore, the work done dW is given by the relation:

dW = F dL cos α   (5)

For example, let us consider the expansion work ("p-V" work) very often encountered in thermodynamics. This work is due to a change of volume of the system under consideration. It is produced against an external pressure, for example that of the atmosphere. Consider any substance which may be a gas, liquid or even a solid contained in a cylinder of base of area a, equipped with a frictionless piston, Figure 3.

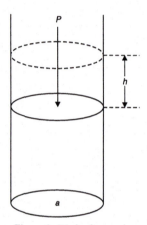

Figure 3. Work of expansion.

A constant pressure p_{ext} coming from the surroundings is exerting on the piston. Before an expansion of the substance inside the cylinder, its initial volume V_i is given by the relation $V_i = L\, a$, where L is the initial height where the piston is at rest. Because of a change in the variables of the system, for example an increase of the temperature, there is a lift of the piston of height dL. But the external pressure p_{ext} operates on the whole surface a of the piston. The total force exerted by the surroundings upon the piston is, therefore:

total force from the surroundings = $p_{ext}\, a$

As a result, the work dW done by the expansion is:

dW = p_{ext} a dL

The product a dL is the change dV in the volume due to the expansion. Hence, the carried out work becomes:

$|dW| = |p_{ext}\, dV|$ (6)

When the pressure p_{ext} does not change with the volume, using differentials is no longer necessary and the work of expansion can be written in terms of variations:

$|\Delta W| = |p_{ext} \Delta V|$ (7)

Three important points must be emphasized now:

- The first one is that the pressure taken into account in these relations is the *pressure developed by the surroundings upon the system under study,* hence the symbol p_{ext} (ext: external). In some cases (see later), it may be the pressure p in the system under consideration itself, but in general, both pressures must not be intermingled. In such an instance, calculations would be false. From a practical viewpoint, in this book and in order to avoid any miscomprehension, all the symbols characterising the surroundings p_{ext}, V_{ext}, T_{ext}, will systematically bring the subscript ext, whereas those characterising the studied system will not bring subscripts, examples p, V, T, etc.

- The second remark is that relations shown above are expressed in absolute values, hence the used symbolism with vertical rods. Actually, there exists two kinds of work. When the displacement is in the same direction as the force, the work is said to be driving. When they have opposite directions, the work is said to be resisting. Hence, a sign must be allocated to a work. According to a convention edicted by IUPAC, a work done on a system (or a work received by a system, both formulations are equivalent) must be positive and, conversely, that done by the system (energy is lost by it) must be negative. That means that in the case of the work of expansion evoked just above, the work performed by the system (opposite to that of pressure) must be negative. Let us consider relations (6) or (7). In the process, where there is expansion,

$$\Delta V > 0$$

and since p_{ext} is always positive, Equations (6) and (7) must be written:

$$dW = -p_{ext} \, dV \tag{8}$$

$$\Delta W = -p_{ext} \, \Delta V \tag{9}$$

Relations (8) and (9) are general. They are, indeed, still valuable when the system receives the "p – V" work from the surroundings. Then, the piston goes down. The volume of the system decreases: $\Delta V < 0$. In this case, using (8) and (9) leads to positive values of dW and ΔW. This is exactly what is demanded by the convention because the system has then received energy.

According to what is preceding, the most general equation permitting the calculation of a work done or received is:

$$W = -\int_{Li}^{Lf} F \cos \alpha \, dL \tag{10}$$

L_i and L_f (i: initial and f: final) are the limits of integration (see the mathematical appendix). Concerning the "p-V work":

$$W = -\int_{Vi}^{Vf} p_{ext} \, dV \tag{11}$$

(For the definition of an integral, see the mathematical appendix II-2).

Exercise 4:

Calculate the work done by a force of 15 N for a displacement of 1,5 m when both form an angle of 30°.

Answ:

With the angle of 30°, the component of the force on the direction of the displacement and the latter have the same direction. The work will be positive. It is given by the relation (1):

$$W = + 15 \,.\, 1,5. \cos 30 = + 19,5 \, J$$

Chapter 2

Some Definitions of Thermodynamics

Here, we recall some definitions. They pertain to all the kinds of thermodynamics, but essentially to classical thermodynamics.

1) Thermodynamic systems

    A thermodynamic system is a part of space and its contents is delimited by a real or by a fictitious closed surface (Figure 4).

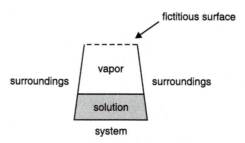

Figure 4. Example of a thermodynamic system with its surroundings.

The surroundings of the system are all but the system. They are the remaining of the Universe! The limits of the system must be perfectly known. Its dimensions, that is to say its volume together with the quantity of matter it contains, must be sufficiently great in order that its quantities can be macroscopically defined.

Several kinds of systems may be distinguished;
- the closed systems: They can only exchange energy (heat and work) and cannot exchange matter with their surroundings;
- the open systems which exchange energy and matter with their surroundings;
- the isolated systems which exchange nothing with their surroundings.

Incidentally, this definition leads, without fail, to the following cosmological question: is Universe an isolated system?

Distinctions between these types of systems are at the heart of the foundations of statistical thermodynamics.

2) Thermodynamic state of a system

    The thermodynamic state of a system is defined by the values of some parameters. Most often (but not obligatorily) in chemistry and biochemistry, the thermodynamic state of a system is defined by four measurable parameters called "state variables". They are:

– its temperature T,
– its composition N,
– its volume V,
– its pressure p.

In less usual conditions, some preceding variables may be replaced by new ones or, alternatively, according to the physico-chemical conditions governing the behavior of the system, some new variables may be added. This is the case when, for example, an intense magnetic field is occurring. To sum up, all the physical properties necessary for the description of the system must be known and taken into account.

3) Extensive and intensive properties

A property is to be extensive when it is additive. It is said to be intensive when it is not additive. An extensive property is one in which the value of the property changes according to the amount of the material which is present. As examples of extensive properties, let us mention the following physico-chemical ones such as the mass, volume, etc., and as intensive properties the temperature, pressure, concentrations of its components expressed, for example, in mol l^{-1} and so forth.

4) Transformation

A transformation is a process the result of which is evidenced by a change in the value of at least one of the variables defining the state of the system. This definition encompasses a cyclic process at the end of which the system is returned to its initial state.

5) Thermodynamic equilibrium

A system is in thermodynamic equilibrium when the values of the variables characterising the system do not change with time. The thermodynamic equilibrium entails that thermal, mechanical and chemical equilibria are simultaneously reached. This means that the temperature, pressure and concentrations must be identical in all the parts of the system. The state of thermodynamic equilibrium must not be confused with a stationary state (see Chapter 24, Open systems—some rudiments of non-equilibrium thermodynamics).

6) Reservoir

A reservoir is a very great device of constant volume which cannot perform any work by itself even with the help of non-changing surroundings such as catalysts and inert electrodes. It is a body which merely acts as an acceptor or donor of heat. The qualifier "very great" means that the reservoir must be sufficiently great in order that its interactions with other systems, whichever they are, remain negligible. As a result, the temperature, pressure and all the intensive properties change, which would be produced by them, are negligible. Moreover, the temperature and the pressure must be uniform in a reservoir, otherwise temperature and pressure gradients might induce work from it.

The reservoir is an example of ideal system often evoked in the development of the thermodynamics science. It is a theoretical model.

7) Reversible and irreversible processes—Quasi-static processes

A process is said to be reversible if, at every moment of its course, the system is at equilibrium. If it is not the case, it is said to be irreversible. During the course of a reversible process, in the successive states of equilibrium, an infinitely small change in the acting force governing the process may inverse the direction of the process. An excellent example is provided by a galvanic cell, the potential difference of which being quasi-counterbalanced by the elements of the circuitry

As an example, let us again consider the perfect gas law, dividing both sides of (12) by V and symbolising the ratio n/V by ρ, we obtain (ρ is named the gas density):

$$p = R \rho T \tag{14}$$

Equation (14) is exactly of the same kind as (13), since the three functions p, ρ and T are intensive ones. (It is evident that this is the case for ρ since it is related to a well-specified number of moles). Given Equation (14), two among the three state functions are independent. When two are fixed, the third is also fixed, too. Now, if beyond the two intensive functions already fixed, an extensive one is also specified, the mass of the system is determined. To continue the study of this example, let us fix the volume V of the system. The mass m of the gas is immediately determined since:

$$n = \rho V$$

and also:

$$n = m/M$$

M being its molar mass.

3) Generalization

According to the nature of the studied systems, there exist several different state equations. This is the case, for example, of systems constituted by a van der Waals real gas, the dilatation of a simple liquid or solid, an electrochemical cell and so forth.

Equations of state are of the greatest importance since they permit to calculate some properties of systems under different conditions.

Chapter 4

The First Law of Thermodynamics

Before stating the first law of thermodynamics, we must first proceed briefly to an analysis of some thermodynamic concepts such as heat, and work and must distinguish the internal energy from the global energy of the system under study. After that, we shall state it but, in this chapter, we shall confine ourselves to only giving some generalities. Further considerations on the first law will be given in the following ones. In brief, one can say that, essentially, the first law introduces the notion of internal energy.

Before all, it must be noticed that the first law is regarded by some authors as being the Everest of thermodynamics (P. Atkins).

1) Heat

Heat can be considered as being a mode of energy transfer between two bodies. However, it is different for work, which is, nevertheless, another mode of transfer of energy. Instruments (and also our senses) do not provide us with a direct means of knowledge of heat. However, as we shall see, an amount of exchanged heat must be measured by the amount of work which causes the same change of state.

Heat is commonly defined in terms of temperature changes. The method is based on the use of calorimeters which, on absorbing heat, exhibit changes in the temperature of the systems. The equation relating the absorbed heat Q and the corresponding temperature change of the calorimeter (the system) $(T_2 - T_1)$ (T_1 being its initial temperature before the absorption of heat and T_2 its final temperature) is:

$$Q = C (T_2 - T_1) \tag{15}$$

C is the proportionality constant. C is characteristic of the substance within the calorimeter and is proportional to its mass. It is named its *heat capacity.* More about it will be said later.

Let us recall that, historically, heat was treated as a fluid called the calorific fluid. Actually, this interpretation must be discarded because this fluid does not exist. However, this interpretation remains very useful for a first approach to thermodynamics.

2) Internal energy and global energy

The global energy (total energy) possessed by a system can be regarded as falling into two categories:

– the energy which is determined by the position of the system as a whole in an external force field (magnetic, electric and gravitational) and, also, by its motion,

– the energy which is characteristic of the system itself, that is to say which is independent of any external influence. This energy may include the translational energy of its moving atoms or molecules, the energy of vibration and rotation of its molecules and those of their nuclei and electrons constituting it.

In thermodynamics, the energy of first category is usually ignored. It is the second which is taken into account. It is named *internal energy* U, whereas the *global energy* is symbolized by E*. (According to IUPAC, E is the general symbol of energy and U stands for internal energy). Both total and internal energies are state functions.

If energy changes can be measured, it is not the case for their absolute value. The absolute value of an energy cannot be known. There are other (usual) quantities in physics for which this is the case.

The internal energy is an extensive property.

It is interesting to remark that the notion of energy is one of the most difficult questions of the whole physics. Actually, one cannot know what signifies this concept because we do not possess any image of its fundamental idea. The only comment that can be certainly maintained is that "there exists a quantity named energy which does not change during the numerous transformations that exist in the nature". For some physicists, the concept of energy is, purely and simply, a strange fact.

3) The conservation of energy

In several experiments, J.P. Joule converted known amounts of work into heat and measured the amount of heat thus produced. As a result of these, Joule came to the very important conclusion that the expenditure of a given amount of work, no matter what is its origin, always produced the same quantity of heat. This fact is the basis of the old notion of the *mechanical equivalent of heat*. Historically, it is the constant ratio between the number of ergs of mechanical work done and the number of calories produced by the conversion of this work into heat. The present accepted value is 4,184 joules/calorie. Particularly interesting was the fact that the same proportionality factor was found with several quite different methods of transforming work into heat.

One of the methods used by Joule to convert work into heat consisted in stirring water contained in a calorimeter with a paddle wheel (the rotation of which happened due to the decrease of the height of a mass) and in measuring the increase in temperature of the latter knowing its heat capacity (see Figure 6):

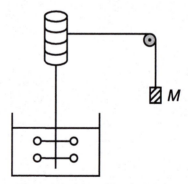

Figure 6. Joule's paddle wheel device.

---

* In literature, there subsists some confusion about the significance of both symbols.

The equivalence between work and heat plus the impossibility of obtaining a perpetual motion of first kind, for long time accepted by scientists, lead to the law of conservation of energy. (*The perpetual motion of first kind would be the production of energy of a particular type without the disappearance of an equivalent amount of energy of another form. It is not possible*).

4) The first law of thermodynamics

The first law of thermodynamics is the law of conservation of energy. It is stated in various forms, perhaps the most important of which are:
– although energy may be converted from one form to another, it cannot be created or destroyed;
– whenever a quantity of one kind of energy is produced, an exactly equivalent amount of another kind (or other kinds) must be used up.

The law of conservation of energy is purely the result of experience.

The first law requires immediately that the total energy of an isolated system is constant, although there may be changes from one form of energy to another in it. The isolated system may be considered, indeed, as being constituted by the system under study itself and by its surroundings. The energy change in the system under consideration (not the isolated system) must be exactly compensated by that of its surroundings, both differing uniquely by their sign (see Figure 7).

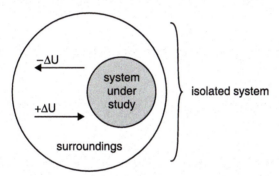

Figure 7. Energy changes in direct and reverse paths.

5) Some consequences of the first law

– The internal energy of the system under consideration must depend on its thermodynamic state. This is an evidence. In other words, the energy must be described by a single-valued function of the thermodynamic variables of the system. Consider any system represented by the point A (Figure 8). The coordinates chosen in this example are the pressure and the volume. (In some cases, their knowledge is sufficient to know the energy of the system). Suppose that there is a transformation from state A to state B, along the path I.

The system is then returned to the initial state A by the path II. The first law of thermodynamics says that the energy change along the path I is equal to that of path II, but opposite in sign, provided the surroundings remain unchanged. If this were not the case, a perpetual motion device would be possible. Imagine, indeed, that the increase of energy along the pass I is greater than the decrease along the path II. In this case, both successive transformations A → B → A would abandon a residuum of energy if the surroundings remain unchanged. This is in contradistinction with the first law. As a result, states A, B… are always the same (for the same conditions of the transformation). Only one single-valued function may characterize them.

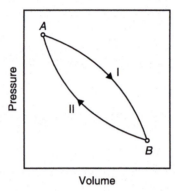

Figure 8. Proof that the energy of a system is described by a single-valued function of the thermodynamic variables of the system.

- The second consequence of the first law is as follows: the change in energy of a system, accompanying a change of its thermodynamic state, depends only on the initial and the final state and is independent of the followed path. To be convinced by this proposition, it is sufficient to consider several paths I,I',I'' from A to B and the different cycles I',II I',II I''',II (Figure 8'). Whatever the paths I,I',I'' are, the corresponding changes in energy are identical, since the path II of the cycle where they are involved is the same.

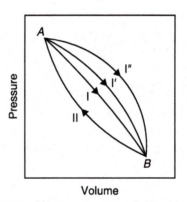

Figure 8'. Proof that the energy of a system is described by a single-valued function.

Chapter 5

Mathematical Counterparts of First Law

In this chapter, we point out some aspects of the first law with the aid of mathematical equations.

1) Mathematical expression of the first law

The first law simply expresses the conservation of energy. The internal energy U of a system only depends on its thermodynamic state. *In other words, the internal energy change $U_f - U_i$ (U_f and U_i: final and initial internal energies) of a system during a transformation is equal to the received energy.* In thermodynamics, most often, the internal energy of systems changes by exchanges of heat and work. Therefore, the mathematical transcription is:

$$U_f - U_i = q + w \tag{16}$$

The heat q received by the system during the process obeys the same convention of signs as the work. When q is positive, the system has actually received heat and conversely. It is the same for the received work. For an infinitesimal transformation, the relation is:

$$dU = đq + đw \tag{17}$$

The symbol đ means that the differential is inexact, as we shall prove it now.

According to the preceding reasonings (see Figures 8: preceding chapter) and as it is shown by relations (16) and (17), internal energy states U_1, U_2 are characterised by a single-valued function of the variables defining them. It is named the internal energy (of the system). One can independently write:

$$dU = đq_I + đw_I$$

$$dU = đq_{II} + đw_{II} \quad \text{idem.}$$

Therefore, it is established that:
- *the received (or given) work and heat are not state functions* (these conclusions are notified in the writing of relation (17) by the use of the symbol d for qualifying as exact the differential dU and as inexact the differentials đq and đw).
- the internal energy U is a state function.
- the internal energy is an extensive property.

From the algebraic standpoint, $-C\Delta T$ is also the heat received by water during the second step. The system being closed and once the come back carried out, the transformation has been cyclic. Hence, we can write:

$$Mgh - C\Delta T = 0$$

whence:

$$|Mgh| = |C\Delta T|$$

This expresses the conservation of the energy.

To come back to its initial state, the calorimeter must give the quantity of heat $q = -C\Delta T$. (This value is obligatorily negative, since it is given by the system).

Chapter 6

Enthalpy and Heat Capacity

This chapter is essentially devoted to the definition of *enthalpy* and to the principles of the determination of its change accompanying a chemical reaction, carried out at constant pressure. It is a very important thermodynamic function. Let us only recall that enthalpy is one of the two components of one of the auxiliary thermodynamic functions, that is to say: the Gibbs energy. We have already presented the latter as being the pivotal thermodynamic function for our purpose. We shall explain it repeatedly in the next chapters.

In fact, most biochemical and chemical reactions are carried out at constant pressure (most often at atmospheric pressure) and temperature. The question is: does the heat absorbed during a process carried out in these conditions, depend or not on the followed pathway (from the initial to the final state)? This is the same question as the one to know if it is only dependent on its initial and final states as it is the case with the internal energy. We demonstrate here that it is also the case. The introduction of a new function, the *enthalpy*, permits to explain this point. As it will be seen, the introduction of enthalpy induces the notion of *useful work*. It also leads to many predictions of numerical values of thermodynamic functions accompanying a process.

Another thermodynamic quantity, named the *heat capacity,* is defined in this chapter. It relates heat quantities (including enthalpy changes) developed during a process to the temperature changes of the participating system.

1) Enthalpy

   1-1) Definition

      The function enthalpy H is defined in terms of the following variables U, p and V by the relation:

$$H = U + pV \tag{22}$$

      U, p and V are the internal energy, the pressure and the volume of the system. Hence, the enthalpy is a property of the system. According to what has been already specified in Chapter 2, the enthalpy unit derived from the SI system is joule J. (The term *heat content*— which is no longer recommended by IUPAC whatever the function it would represent—must not be used for the enthalpy, as it has been the case in the past).

   1-2) Some properties of the function enthalpy

      – U, P, V are state functions. As a result, the enthalpy is also a *function of state.*

      – Absolute values of the enthalpy cannot be known since it is the case of the internal energy. Only changes in enthalpies ΔH are measured. According to (22), changes in enthalpies are given by the relation:

Answ:

$$C_{10}H_8(s) + 12O_2(g) \rightarrow 10\ CO_2(g) + 4H_2O(l)$$

$\Delta n = -2$

$AH = -5,1339\ kJ.\ mol^{-1}$

Even in this case, the difference is very weak.

1-3) Enthalpy and useful work

Consider now the changes in enthalpy when the processes can exchange any kind of work, not only that of expansion as above. Let us distinguish the expansion work "$p_{ext}V$" from the sum ΔW^* of other works which simultaneously occur with it during the investigated process. The sum $[\Delta W^* + (-p_{ext}V)]$ is the total work exchanged during the process. The "p-V" work which very often occurs is also generally useless. This is the reason why the work ΔW^* is named "useful work". In the realms of chemistry, it can be, for example, the electrical work. Changes in internal energy and in enthalpy accompanying the process are:

$$dU = đq - p_{ext}\ \Delta V + \delta W^*$$

$$dH = đq - p_{ext}\ dV + đW^* + pdV + Vdp$$

For an isobaric process in mechanical equilibrium (see above: $p_{ext} = p$; $p = $ constant)

$$dH = đq + đW^* \text{ (isobaric process in mechanical equilibrium)}$$

Notice that $đW^*$ is an inexact differential. Therefore, the enthalpy change under isobaric, mechanical equilibrium conditions equals the heat absorbed plus the useful (non expansion) work:

$$\Delta H_p = Q_p + W^*_p$$

1-4) Enthalpy changes in steady-flow systems

The function enthalpy is interesting to take into account in the study of steady-flow systems. This point will be treated briefly in the part devoted to the thermodynamics of non-equilibrium systems (see Chapter 24).

2) Heat capacity

2-1) Definition

The notion of heat capacity C of a system has already be mentioned in Chapter 2. It can be considered as being the proportionality constant of the following equation:

$$Q = C(T_2 - T_1)$$

where Q is the heat quantity given to the system for an increase of its absolute temperature from T_1 to T_2. C is proportional to the mass of the system. For 1 g of it, its value is called the *specific heat*. The heat capacity for 1 mole of material is named the *molar heat capacity*.

Actually, it has been found that the value of a heat capacity depends on the temperature. This is the reason why, for its definition, it is necessary to consider a small temperature interval (a differential). Hence, a better definition is:

$$C = đq/dT$$

But, đq being an inexact differential, C depends on the path under which the heat is supplied, according to this definition. This is no longer the case when the heat is supplied under constant volume or constant pressure. Therefore, one defines two kinds of heat capacities, one at constant volume C_V and the other at constant pressure C_P:

$$C_V = (đq/dT)_V \quad \text{and} \quad C_P = (đq/dT)_P$$

- If we have a substance which absorbs heat at constant volume, we know that (see:

$$đq_V = dq_V$$

$$đq_V = dU_V$$

and:

$$C_V = (dU/dT)_V$$

In this condition, the value of the heat capacity at constant volume is perfectly defined.

- If the material absorbs heat at constant pressure, one knows that (see above)

$$đq_P = dq_P$$

and according to (24):

$$dH_P = dq_P$$

In this condition, the value of the heat capacity at constant pressure is perfectly defined.

2-2) Relations between C_P and C_V

Several equations connect the values of C_P and C_V. We do not give them in this book because they are not of interest for our purpose. (They are obtained by the handling of some partial derivatives).

2-3) Few considerations concerning the values of the heat capacities

There is much to say upon heat capacities. We confine ourselves to saying that:
- it is impossible to predict numerical values of heat capacities without going out of the realm of classical thermodynamics, whatever the phase (solid, liquid, gas) under which the material is.
- most of them are determined calorimetrically. However, statistical thermodynamics may bring aid in some cases because it permits their determination from spectroscopic data. Below is an example of determination of a reactional enthalpy.

100 ml of a 0,3 mol L^{-1} solution of adenosine triphosphate is put into a Dewar flask together with an ATPase. The other conditions of the process are: pH = 7, pMg = 3, T = 298 K, ionic strength = 0,25 mol L^{-1}. During the process, the temperature increase is 1,65 K. The biochemical reaction constituting the process is the hydrolysis of ATP into adenosine diphosphate ADP and phosphate P:

ATP + H_2O → ADP + P   (see Chapter 32 for precisions)

The heat capacity of the Dewar is 562,4 JK^{-1}. Calculate the enthalpy change of the reaction. (ATPase is an enzyme, that is to say a catalyst—see Chapter 32. It does not intervene in the thermal effect. Other conditions are those of the biochemical standard state—see Chapter 21—they must not be taken into account in the following calculations). What is the enthalpy of the reaction?

Probably, the most often used calorimeters are the bomb calorimeters. The material, previously sealed in a strong metal vessel, reacts under constant volume conditions. Owing to this fact, it is evident that these calorimeters permit to measure heat effects at constant volume, that is to say the internal energies. But they are also used to determine enthalpies. This is done after necessary corrections of the effect measured at constant volume in a first step. Most of the time, this kind of apparatus is used to obtain heats of combustion. The strong metal vessel (the bomb) is immersed in a water jacket. It is filled with an excess of dioxygen and ignited. The increase of temperature of the water jacket is noted. Then the apparatus is calibrated by using a substance whose enthalpy of combustion is known or by electrical heating.

Biochemical reactions, most often, occur under constant pressure. For this reason, we briefly mention here how thermal effects at constant pressure can be also measured. We confine ourselves to only give the principle of their measurements, either by batch calorimetry or by scanning calorimetry.

- In batch calorimetry, the reactants are mixed together in the calorimeter and the temperature increase (or decrease) is measured either with a thermometer or with a thermocouple or with a thermistance. The reaction can be initiated by adding a small amount of an enzyme which catalyses the reaction under study, without changing the thermal effect. The enthalpy is calculated through the equations (T_1 and T_2 being the initial and final temperatures of the calorimeter):

$$dH = dq_p$$

$$dH = C_p dT$$

$$\Delta H = \int_{T1}^{T2} C_p dT$$

The heat capacity of the system itself is calculated in another experiment by putting a known account of heat into the system through an electrical heater and measuring the temperature change. (It is a well-known fact that an enthalpy value accompanying a process changes with the temperature. In principle, it is the case in the last determination. But here, it is not necessary to rectify the found value in order to take into account the increase or the decrease of the temperature of the system since changes in enthalpies are, indeed, negligible for very weak changes in temperatures. In such measurements, the temperature variation is of the order of 2°C).

- Scanning calorimetry consists in the measurement of heat capacities as a function of temperatures. The principle of the method is the following one. Heat is added to the system in successive and very small amounts through electrical heating and temperature changes are registered. Heat capacities are calculated for each amount of heat added. The diagram given by the calorimeter is the diagram C_p/T. It presents peaks whose surfaces are proportional to the enthalpies of the processes.

3) Standard states and standard reactions in chemical systems

Reactional enthalpies depend on the temperature, pressure, the amounts of reactants and products and also, when they are solids, on the crystalline form under which they react. From a practical standpoint, one of the objectives of thermochemistry is to give the possibility of calculation of reactional heats of chemical reactions (included virtual ones) from tabulated data. Therefore, at the beginning, it is necessary to collect all the data in order to build the tables. To easily handle this first level of data later, it is judicious to determine and to group them for reactional conditions as close as possible to those prevailing for the determination of the same kind of data for other compounds. For this reason, it is necessary to define the *standard state* of a system.

By convention, the standard states adopted for the determination of heats of reactions are:

Table 1. Standard states and conventions for heats of reaction.

standard state of a solid	the most stable form at 1 bar pressure
standard state of liquid	the most stable form at 1 bar pressure
standard state of a gas	zero pressure

The following precisions must be given:

- In principle, no temperature is recommended in the definition of a standard state. Every temperature can be chosen. However, for historical reasons, heats of reactions are generally quoted at 298 K (25°C);
- the standard states of the components of a solution are defined as the states for which their activity is equal to unity. The notion of activity is rather complicated to grasp (see Chapter 19—Activity-Ideal Solution-Standard States);
- Sometimes, it may be more convenient to adopt other standard states than those cited. In such occurrence, they must be specified. For example, when a solid may react in a crystalline form or in another, the reaction under study may involve the least stable and not the most stable. Therefore, the form under which it reacts must be specified if it is not that which is conventionally adopted. For example, the standard state adopted for carbon is usually graphite. If it is diamond which takes part in the reaction under study, this must be specified and taken into account.

Standard reactions are those occurring between reactants and products in their standard states. The most often tabulated standard reactional enthalpies are: heats of formation, combustion, and transition. In thermochemistry, some symbols are written together within the equation of the reaction under study in order to clarify the experimental conditions. The numerical value of the thermodynamic quantity (here the enthalpy) is also given. The equation is then named a *thermochemical equation*. An example is:

$$6C(s) + 3H_2(g) \rightarrow C_6H_6(l) \qquad \Delta_r H_{298K} = + 49{,}0 \text{ kJ mol}^{-1}$$

The symbols s, l, g mean the physical states of the reactants and products (solid, liquid, gaseous), and r means reactional.

4) The biological standard state

Let us already mention that there exists a special convention for the definition of the standard states and, hence, for standard reactions of the biological systems. This point will be studied in full details later because biochemical reactions may also involve ionic equilibria and they have not been considered so far. It is the reason why biological standard states deserve further attention (see Chapter 21 Gibbs Energy Function Changes—Further Comments).

5) Law of constant heat summation—Hess' law

Hess' law states that the heat change at constant pressure or volume in a given chemical reaction is the same whether it takes place in one or in several stages. More precisely, it means that the heat absorbed or evolved in a given chemical reaction is the same whether the reaction is processing through one step or through several other reactions, provided that the global reaction is the exact resultant of the multiple ones. The result of Hess' law is that thermochemical equations can be added or substracted like algebraic equations. Let us, for example, take the case of the heat of formation of carbon dioxide CO_2 from carbon graphite and dioxygen (for the definition and the symbolism of a heat of formation, see below):

Remark: Using the term element to define the standard enthalpies of formation (as it is often noticed in literature) is somewhat misleading. In the example above, indeed, if C can be considered as being the symbol of the element carbon, it is not the case of O_2. The element oxygen is symbolized by O. Some authors prefer to speak from simple compounds (derivatives) rather than from elements.

2) Calculations of standard enthalpies of reactions from heats of formation

Here, the searched for standard enthalpy are those of reaction. They are symbolized by $\Delta_r H°$ (r for reactional). For example, it is that of the following reaction:

$$CH_4(g) \; + \; 2O_2(g) \; \rightarrow \; CO_2(g) \; + \; 2H_2O(l) \tag{31}$$

The adjective standard means that reactants and products are in their standard states (see the previous chapter). The standard enthalpy can be calculated from the heats of reaction of the reactants and products, the heats of formation of $CH_4(g)$, $CO_2(g)$ and $H_2O(l)$ being known (see Table 2). In order to solve the problem, let us use Hess' law. In the first step, some reactions involving the reactants and products of the reaction under study must be chosen. Their standard enthalpies of formation must have been already determined. The chosen reactions are:

$$C_{(graphite)} \; + \; 2\,H_2(g) \; \rightarrow \; CH_4(g) \qquad \Delta_f H° = -74,81 \text{ kJ mol}^{-1}$$
$$C_{(graphite)} \; + \; O_2(g) \; \rightarrow \; CO_2(g) \qquad \Delta_f H° = -393,5 \text{ kJ mol}^{-1}$$
$$2\,H_2(g) \; + \; O_2(g) \; \rightarrow \; 2H_2O(l) \qquad \Delta_f H° = -2.285,83 \text{ kJ mol}^{-1}$$

(Notice the factor 2 of the last equation) By inversion of the direction of the first thermochemical equation, we obtain the system:

$$CH_4(g) \; \rightarrow \; C_{(graphite)} \; + \; 2\,H_2(g) \qquad \Delta_f H° = 74,81 \text{ kJ mol}^{-1}$$
$$C_{(graphite)} \; + \; O_2(g) \; \rightarrow \; CO_2(g) \qquad \Delta_f H° = -393,5 \text{ kJ mol}^{-1}$$
$$2\,H_2(g) \; + \; O_2(g) \; \rightarrow \; 2H_2O(l) \qquad \Delta_f H° = -2.285,83 \text{ kJ mol}^{-1}$$

By summing the three equations, some chemical terms vanish. It remains only Equation (30). Summation of the enthalpies of the last system leads to the value:

$$\Delta_r H° \text{ reaction (30)} \; = -890,3 \text{ kJ mol}^{-1}$$

The above reasoning may be reversed. It allows to obtain the heat of formation of a compound, knowing its heat of reaction and the heats of formation of the other reactants and products.

3) Heats of combustion

Organic compounds, by definition, contain carbon and hydrogen. They burn in dioxygen to yield carbon dioxide and liquid water, even when their molecules already contain oxygen atoms. The heat of combustion is the heat change accompanying the complete combustion of 1 mole of compound at a given temperature under 1 bar pressure. Heats of combustion are usually measured at constant volume in a bomb calorimeter. Some standard heats of combustion are mentioned in Table 3.

Table 3. Some standard heats of combustion of organic compounds at 298 K in kJ mol^{-1} (according to G.M. Barrow "Physical chemistry for the life sciences" McGraw Hill, general bibliography).

methane (g)	−882	D-glucose (s)	$(C_6H_{12}O_6)$	−2802
ethane (g)	−1541	glycerol (l)	$(C_3H_8O_3)$	−1661
propane (g)	−2217,91	glycine (s)	$(C_2H_5NO_2)$	−981
L-fructose (s) $(C_6H_{12}O_6)$	−2827	glycogen (s)	$(C_6H_{10}O_5)x$	−17518 (kJ/kg)
citric acid (s) (anhydride)	−1985	glycylglycine (s)	$(C_4H_8O_3N_2)$	−1969

By convention, the standard states adopted for the determination of heats of reactions are:

Table 1. Standard states and conventions for heats of reaction.

standard state of a solid	the most stable form at 1 bar pressure
standard state of liquid	the most stable form at 1 bar pressure
standard state of a gas	zero pressure

The following precisions must be given:

- In principle, no temperature is recommended in the definition of a standard state. Every temperature can be chosen. However, for historical reasons, heats of reactions are generally quoted at 298 K (25°C);

- the standard states of the components of a solution are defined as the states for which their activity is equal to unity. The notion of activity is rather complicated to grasp (see Chapter 19—Activity-Ideal Solution-Standard States);

- Sometimes, it may be more convenient to adopt other standard states than those cited. In such occurrence, they must be specified. For example, when a solid may react in a crystalline form or in another, the reaction under study may involve the least stable and not the most stable. Therefore, the form under which it reacts must be specified if it is not that which is conventionally adopted. For example, the standard state adopted for carbon is usually graphite. If it is diamond which takes part in the reaction under study, this must be specified and taken into account.

Standard reactions are those occurring between reactants and products in their standard states. The most often tabulated standard reactional enthalpies are: heats of formation, combustion, and transition. In thermochemistry, some symbols are written together within the equation of the reaction under study in order to clarify the experimental conditions. The numerical value of the thermodynamic quantity (here the enthalpy) is also given. The equation is then named a *thermochemical equation*. An example is:

$$6C(s) + 3H_2(g) \rightarrow C_6H_6(l) \qquad \Delta_r H_{298K} = +49,0 \text{ kJ mol}^{-1}$$

The symbols s, l, g mean the physical states of the reactants and products (solid, liquid, gaseous), and r means reactional.

4) The biological standard state

Let us already mention that there exists a special convention for the definition of the standard states and, hence, for standard reactions of the biological systems. This point will be studied in full details later because biochemical reactions may also involve ionic equilibria and they have not been considered so far. It is the reason why biological standard states deserve further attention (see Chapter 21 Gibbs Energy Function Changes—Further Comments).

5) Law of constant heat summation—Hess' law

Hess' law states that the heat change at constant pressure or volume in a given chemical reaction is the same whether it takes place in one or in several stages. More precisely, it means that the heat absorbed or evolved in a given chemical reaction is the same whether the reaction is processing through one step or through several other reactions, provided that the global reaction is the exact resultant of the multiple ones. The result of Hess' law is that thermochemical equations can be added or substracted like algebraic equations. Let us, for example, take the case of the heat of formation of carbon dioxide CO_2 from carbon graphite and dioxygen (for the definition and the symbolism of a heat of formation, see below):

$$C(s, graphite) + O_2(g) \rightarrow CO_2(g) \quad \Delta_f H° = -393,5 \text{ kJ.mol}^{-1} \tag{27}$$

The same result is obtained if we add the enthalpies of the two following reactions in which the carbon monoxide CO intervenes:

$$C(s, graphite) + 1/2 \, O_2(g) \rightarrow CO(g) \quad \Delta_f H° = -110,4 \text{ kJ.mol}^{-1} \tag{28}$$

$$CO(g) + 1/2 \, O_2(g) \rightarrow CO_2(g) \qquad \Delta_f H° = -282,72 \text{ kJ.mol}^{-1} \tag{29}$$

Hess' law results from the first law of thermodynamics. Hess' law exists, of course, because the initial and the final states of the resultant reaction are the same as those of the coupled ones. One consequence of the law is that the heat change accompanying a reaction in a given direction is exactly equal in magnitude, but opposite in sign, to that associated with the same reaction but in the reverse direction. For example, reaction (29), the reverse of (26):

$$CO_2(g) \rightarrow C(s, graphite) + O_2(g) \qquad \Delta_r H° = 393,5 \text{ kJ.mol}^{-1} \tag{30}$$

shows the same enthalpy than (26), but of opposite sign.

Hess' law is very useful because it permits the calculation of heat changes for reactions which cannot be studied directly or even which are purely virtual!

Chapter 8

Thermochemistry (Following)–Heats of Reactions and Bond Energies

In this chapter, we give the principles of determination of heats accompanying some kinds of chemical reactions. Some examples of such calculations are mentioned.

1) Heat of formation

There exist many tables of heats of reactions. They have been established by starting from standard enthalpies of formation of various compounds from their elements in their reference states. The reference state of an element is its most stable state at the specified temperature and under the pressure of 1 bar. Standard enthalpies of formation $\Delta_f H°$ are expressed as enthalpies per mole of the compound (unit: J mol^{-1}).

By convention, the standard formation enthalpies of elements are null in their reference states, whatever the temperature is. We also note that the standard pressure in the reference state of solids is 1 bar, instead of 0 bar for gases. (There exists some confusion in the literature between a reference state and a standard state. We do not enter into this discussion in this book*).

For example, the enthalpy of formation of CO_2 (at 298 K and 1 bar) is determined according to the chemical reaction:

$$C \quad + \quad O_2 \quad \rightarrow \quad CO_2 \qquad \Delta_f H° = -393,5 \text{ kJ mol}^{-1}$$

(graphite,   (gas,   (gas,
298 K, 1 bar)   298 K, 0 bar)   298 K, 0 bar)

(Notice that in agreement with the conventions, it is the graphite which is chosen—carbon form being the most stable—to determine the standard enthalpy of formation of the carbon dioxide). We give in Table 2 some values of heats of formation.

Table 2. Enthalpies of formation (kJ mol^{-1}) of some substances at 298 K (according to P. Atkins, "Physical Chemistry", seventh edition Oxford University Press—general bibliography).

CO_2 (g)	−393,5	CH_3COCH_3(l)	−248,1	$CH_3CHOHCOOH$(s)	−694
H_2O (l)	−285,8	C_2H_5OH(l)	−277,7	$C_6H_{12}O_6$(s) (α-D-glucose)	−1274
H_2O(g)	−241,8	CH_3COOH(l)	−485,8	$C_{12}H_{22}O_{11}$(s) (sucrose)	−2222
CH_4(g)	−74,8	$(COOH)_2$(s)	−827,2	$C_6H_{12}O_6$(s) (β-D-fructose)	−1266

---

* Burgot J-L, "The notion of activity" Springer, general bibliography.

Remark: Using the term element to define the standard enthalpies of formation (as it is often noticed in literature) is somewhat misleading. In the example above, indeed, if C can be considered as being the symbol of the element carbon, it is not the case of O_2. The element oxygen is symbolized by O. Some authors prefer to speak from simple compounds (derivatives) rather than from elements.

2) Calculations of standard enthalpies of reactions from heats of formation

Here, the searched for standard enthalpy are those of reaction. They are symbolized by $\Delta_r H°$ (r for reactional). For example, it is that of the following reaction:

$$CH_4(g) + 2O_2(g) \rightarrow CO_2(g) + 2H_2O(l) \tag{31}$$

The adjective standard means that reactants and products are in their standard states (see the previous chapter). The standard enthalpy can be calculated from the heats of reaction of the reactants and products, the heats of formation of $CH_4(g)$, $CO_2(g)$ and $H_2O(l)$ being known (see Table 2). In order to solve the problem, let us use Hess' law. In the first step, some reactions involving the reactants and products of the reaction under study must be chosen. Their standard enthalpies of formation must have been already determined. The chosen reactions are:

$$C_{(graphite)} + 2H_2(g) \rightarrow CH_4(g) \quad \Delta_f H° = -74{,}81 \text{ kJ mol}^{-1}$$
$$C_{(graphite)} + O_2(g) \rightarrow CO_2(g) \quad \Delta_f H° = -393{,}5 \text{ kJ mol}^{-1}$$
$$2H_2(g) + O_2(g) \rightarrow 2H_2O(l) \quad \Delta_f H° = -2.285{,}83 \text{ kJ mol}^{-1}$$

(Notice the factor 2 of the last equation) By inversion of the direction of the first thermochemical equation, we obtain the system:

$$CH_4(g) \rightarrow C_{(graphite)} + 2H_2(g) \quad \Delta_f H° = 74{,}81 \text{ kJ mol}^{-1}$$
$$C_{(graphite)} + O_2(g) \rightarrow CO_2(g) \quad \Delta_f H° = -393{,}5 \text{ kJ mol}^{-1}$$
$$2H_2(g) + O_2(g) \rightarrow 2H_2O(l) \quad \Delta_f H° = -2.285{,}83 \text{ kJ mol}^{-1}$$

By summing the three equations, some chemical terms vanish. It remains only Equation (30). Summation of the enthalpies of the last system leads to the value:

$$\Delta_r H° \text{ reaction } (30) = -890{,}3 \text{ kJ mol}^{-1}$$

The above reasoning may be reversed. It allows to obtain the heat of formation of a compound, knowing its heat of reaction and the heats of formation of the other reactants and products.

3) Heats of combustion

Organic compounds, by definition, contain carbon and hydrogen. They burn in dioxygen to yield carbon dioxide and liquid water, even when their molecules already contain oxygen atoms. The heat of combustion is the heat change accompanying the complete combustion of 1 mole of compound at a given temperature under 1 bar pressure. Heats of combustion are usually measured at constant volume in a bomb calorimeter. Some standard heats of combustion are mentioned in Table 3.

Table 3. Some standard heats of combustion of organic compounds at 298 K in kJ mol^{-1} (according to G.M. Barrow "Physical chemistry for the life sciences" McGraw Hill, general bibliography).

methane (g)	−882	D-glucose (s)	$(C_6H_{12}O_6)$ −2802
ethane (g)	−1541	glycerol (l)	$(C_3H_8O_3)$ −1661
propane (g)	−2217,91	glycine (s)	$(C_2H_5NO_2)$ −981
L-fructose (s) $(C_6H_{12}O_6)$	−2827	glycogen (s)	$(C_6H_{10}O_5)x$ −17518 (kJ/kg)
citric acid (s) (anhydride)	−1985	glycylglycine (s)	$(C_4H_8O_3N_2)$ −1969

We also give heats of combustion of some cellular fuels in Table 4.

Table 4. Heats of combustion ΔH (KJ mol^{-1}) of some cellular fuels (according to Lehninger A.L. "Bioenergetics", W.A. Benjamin Inc. general bibliography).

D-glucose	−2813
lactic acid	−1363
palmitic acid	−9948
tripalmitin	−31392
glycin	−313,5

4) Heats of hydrogenation

The measurements of enthalpy changes accompanying the hydrogenation of 1 mole of an unsaturated compound is, usually, a convenient way of estimating mesomeric energies in conjugated systems, owing to the quasi-constancy of the heat of hydrogenation of an unsaturated molecule devoid of any conjugation. They may also serve for the determination of some heats of formation and of combustion.

5) Heat of phase changes: Latent heats of vaporization, fusion, etc.

Phase changes are accompanied by changes in enthalpies. They were called formerly latent heats. Such phase changes may be the phenomena of vaporization, fusion or sublimation of a solid, transition from one crystalline modification into another. Latent heats of phases change and the corresponding enthalpies are the differences in the enthalpies of 1 g or 1 mole of the two considered phases at the pressure and temperature at which the phase change takes place. Like other heat changes, phase change enthalpies vary with temperature. The results may be presented under the form of thermochemical equations. We give here the molar enthalpies of some phases' changes related to very usual substances.

- for water:

$H_2O(s) \quad \rightarrow \quad H_2O(l) \qquad \Delta_{fus}H_{273K} = 6,01$ kJ mol^{-1} (fus: fusion)

$H_2O(l) \quad \rightarrow \quad H_2O(g) \qquad \Delta_{vap}H_{273K} = 40,62$ kJ mol^{-1} (vap: vaporization)

- for carbon:

C(diamond) $\quad \rightarrow \quad$ C(graphite) $\quad \Delta_{trs}H_{273K} = -1,89$ kJ mol^{-1} (trs: transition)

- for sulfur:

S(s-rhombic) $\quad \rightarrow \quad$ S(s-monoclinic) $\qquad \Delta_{trs}H_{273K} = 0,12$ kJ mol^{-1}

These kinds of equations are handled in the same manner as those involving the determination of the heats of different reactions. This is the case, particularly, when reactants or products are under an unusual physical state.

6) Heat changes of reactions in solutions

When a reaction takes place in solution, the reactional heat change does vary with respect to the case in which the reactants and products are in the pure state. This is because, generally, the formation of a solution is accompanied by a heat effect. We shall study some reactions in solutions, such as those involving ions. They will be under consideration in Chapters 26, 27, 28, namely, "Acid-base reactions in aqueous solutions", "Redox reactions—redox couples—brief description of an electrochemical cell" and "Other equilibria of interest". Reactions in solutions constitute the vast majority of cases of reactions of biological systems.

7) Bond energies

Chemical reactions involve the break of some bonds and the formation of new ones. Given this result, it is intuitive that there must exist some numerical links between some heats of reactions and bond energies. The question behind this hypothesis is to know if it is possible to approximate the heat of formation of a material by summation of the appropriate bond energies once, of course, its molecular structure is known.

One may consider that two systems of such calculations exist. They are systems of bond energies and of thermochemical groups.

Firstly, it is necessary to distinguish the notions of *bond energy* and of *bond dissociation energy*.
- The *bond dissociation energy* refers to the energy required to break a given bond of a specific compound.
- The *bond energy* is an average value of the bond dissociation energies of a given bond in a series of different compounds possessing the same bond. (The obtained value may have suffered from a few small adjustments for the purpose of matching a great deal of data).

As an example, let us consider the water molecule which possesses two O-H bonds. Consider the dissociation of water according to the two following steps:

$$H_2O(g) \quad \rightarrow \quad H(g) \quad + \quad OH(g) \quad \Delta_r H_{298} = 531,39 \text{ kJ mol}^{-1} \tag{32}$$

$$OH(g) \quad \rightarrow \quad O(g) \quad + \quad H(g) \quad \Delta_r H_{298} = 422,97 \text{ kJ mol}^{-1} \tag{33}$$

In both cases, it is the same bond (the bond O-H) which is under consideration. It appears, however, that the heat of dissociation of the O-H bond depends on the nature of the species from which H atom is separated. In other words, each value given above is a bond dissociation energy. On the opposite side, the average value:

$$(531,39 + 422,97)/2 = 477,18 \text{ kJ mol}^{-1}$$

$$\varepsilon_{OH} = 477 \text{ kJ mol}^{-1}$$

corresponds to the bond energy of OH (ε_{OH}). (Actually, it is the value 462,18 kJ mol^{-1} which is retained after a small adjustment). It is not surprising that values of reactions (31) and (32) differ because the O and H atoms of the O-H bond do not have the same local environment in H_2O and in the radical OH.

– System of bond energies

Let us begin by saying that specific bond energies' values are difficult to determine. They have been obtained by using such techniques as mass spectrometry and UV-visible spectroscopies. On the whole, there are very few accurate values.

Let us now specify that since bond energies refer to a sort of average value of bond dissociation energies and since the latter ones refer to data obtained for substances in gaseous state, they are equal to their so-called *heats of atomization in the ideal gas state into their atomic elements:*

$$O - H(g) \rightarrow O(g) + H(g)$$

From the knowledge of heats of dissociation of various molecules into atoms and of the standard heats of formation of others, it has been possible to derive the mean energies of several bonds. They are given in Table 5. They are also named *bond enthalpies of chemical bonds*.

Table 5. Some bond energies in kJ mol^{-1} (*bond enthalpies of chemical bonds*) (according to S.G. Waley "Mechanisms of organic and enzymic reactions", Oxford at the Clarendon Press, general bibliography).

bond					
H – H	432 ; 436	C-O	350 ; 357	O-H	463 ; 462
C – H	365 ; 410	C-N	292 ; 304	S-S	266 ; 226
C – C	245 ; 345	N-H	391 ; 382	C=O	724 ; 744

An example of calculation of a bond energy is provided by the determination of the bond energy C-H (ε_{C-H}). It has been obtained from the enthalpy of the reaction:

$$CH_4(g) \rightarrow C(g) + 4H(g) \quad \Delta H$$

by setting up:

$$\varepsilon_{C-H} = \Delta H/4$$

Notice that this reaction, in no case, corresponds to a standard reaction of formation since products are not in their standard states nor is the hydrogen atom considered as being an element in terms of standard states. The enthalpy ΔH is obtained through the summation of the following reactions:

$$CH_4(g) + 2O_2(g) \rightarrow CO_2(g) + 2H_2O(l) \quad \Delta H = -889,50 \text{ kJ mol}^{-1}$$

This is the heat of combustion of methane.

$$CO_2(g) \rightarrow C_{(graphite)} + O_2(g) \qquad \Delta H = 393,13 \text{ kJ mol}^{-1}$$

This is the opposite of the heat of formation of carbon dioxide.

$$2H_2O(l) \rightarrow 2H_2(l) + O_2(g) \qquad \Delta H = 571,16 \text{ kJ mol}^{-1}$$

$$2H_2(g) \rightarrow 4H(g) \qquad \Delta H = 870,94 \text{ kJ mol}^{-1}$$

$$C_{(graphite)} = C(g) \qquad \Delta H = 717,70 \text{ kJ mol}^{-1}$$

$$\Sigma \Delta H = 1663,43 \text{ kJ mol}^{-1}$$

and hence:

$$\varepsilon_{C-H} = 416 \text{ kJ mol}^{-1} \text{ (298 K)}$$

(Since the enthalpy values used in these calculations had been previously obtained at 298 K, this is also the case for the obtained value ε_{C-H}).

Using bond energy values permits to estimate heats of reaction in gas phase. The principle of the estimation is the following one. It consists in counting, on one hand, the number of bonds which are broken up (so that the reaction should be carried out) and the involved heat to do it and, on the other hand, to proceed in the inverse manner for the products, however after having changed the sign. The search for value is given by the difference of both summations. Of course, heats are calculated through the bond energies.

As an example, estimate the heat of formation of propane $\Delta_f H$ (C_3H_8 : g), that is to say the heat of the reaction:

$$3C(s) + 4H_2(g) \rightarrow C_3H_8(g)$$

Knowing that the sublimation heat of graphite is 711 kJ mol⁻¹ and that $\varepsilon_{H\text{-}H}$ = 432 kJ mol⁻¹, $\varepsilon_{C\text{-}H}$ = 365 kJ mol⁻¹ and $\varepsilon_{C\text{-}C}$ = 245 kJ mol⁻¹, one can perform the following calculation according to the above principle:

$$\Delta_f H\ (C_3H_8\ g) = -[(8 \times 365) + (2 \times 245)] + [(3 \times 711) + (4 \times 432)]$$

$$\Delta_f H\ (C_3H_8\ g) = 451\ \text{kJ mol}^{-1}$$

8) Other methods of calculation of heats of reactions—Thermochemical groups

Several methods of calculation of heats of formation and of combustion have been devised. Results are not very accurate but they give the order of size of the values of the quantities under study. This possibility may be very interesting either directly or indirectly, especially when some hypotheses on the feasibility of some reactions must be done.

Such is, for example, the case of the combustion of organic substances. In analogous series, there is a change of about 650 kJ mol⁻¹ per methylene group added. Therefore, some approximate rules relating the molecular structure to the heats of combustion have been edicted. Hence, the heat of combustion of a compound may be calculated approximately by Thornton's rule which assumes that it is equal to the factor –219,5 . n kJ mol⁻¹, where n is the number of oxygen atoms required to burn a molecule of the compound.

Recently, more group contribution methods have been proposed. They are based on the fact that molecules are built up of groups called thermochemical groups which are identical from one molecule to the other and which are endowed with a definite value of the quantity under consideration. These methods are not frequently used in the case of heats of reactions. They are more used for the calculation of other thermodynamic quantities, in particular Gibbs energies.

Of course, in these methods, it is necessary to include allowances for various types of sub-structures. It is from this point of view that one can say that these methods are approximate. We shall come back to the methods of determination and of estimation of thermodynamic quantities in Chapter 21.

9) Heat of reaction as a function of temperature—Kirchhoff's rule

So far, only methods of determination of heats of reaction at a fixed temperature were mentioned. It is pertinent now to consider procedures permitting to determine the heat of reaction at constant temperature at one temperature different from that obtained for the same reaction at another one. Such determination is evidently of great practical interest.

The procedure is based on the use of Kirchhoff's equation.

- Actually, we are interested here in the variation of enthalpy with temperature, at constant pressure. The definition of the heat capacity at constant pressure involves these three parameters:

$$(\partial H / \partial T)_p = C_p$$

By integration at constant pressure, one obtains the relation:

$$H = \int C_p\, dT + H_0$$

where H_0 is the integration constant. To perform the integration, it remains to know how C_p vary with the temperature and the heat capacity C_p corresponds to what global system.

Let us consider the reaction:

$$A + B + ... \rightarrow L + M + ...$$

Each species I, reactant or product, does possess its own enthalpy and its own heat capacity, both being related to by the expressions:

$$\overline{H_i} = \int C_{P_i} \, dT + H_{0i}$$

where the indice i stands for A, B, L and M. Actually, symbols are the partial molar enthalpies of the species. At this point of the reasoning, it is sufficient to know that the $\overline{H_i}$ keep all the significance of an enthalpy. Besides, if each of the reactant and product constitutes a distinct phase, the partial molar enthalpies $\overline{H_i}$ are not more or less than the enthalpies H_i in the pure state. Writing the difference between the sum of the enthalpies of the products and of the reactants permits to write:

$$\Delta_r H = [H_{0L} + H_{0M} + .. - H_{0A} - H_{0B} - ...] + [\int C_{PL} \, dT + \int C_{PM} \, dT + ... - \int C_{PA} \, dT - \int C_{PB} \, dT]$$

Symbolising ΔH_0 as the first term in crochets of the right hand of this equality, one obtains:

$$\Delta_r H = \Delta H_0 + [\int C_{PL} \, dT + \int C_{PM} \, dT + ... - \int C_{PA} \, dT - \int C_{PB} \, dT]$$

Taking into account the distributivity property of an integral, that is to say by setting up the relation:

$$\int C_{PL} \, dT + \int C_{PM} \, dT + ... - \int C_{PA} \, dT - \int C_{PB} \, dT = \int [C_{PL} + C_{PM} + ... - C_{PA} - C_{PB} - ...] dT$$

and:

$$\int [C_{PL} + C_{PM} + ... - C_{PA} - C_{PB} - ...] dT = \int_{T0}^{T2} \Delta C_p \, dT$$

we finally obtain:

$$\Delta_r H = \Delta H_0 + \int_{T0}^{T} \Delta C_p \, dT \tag{34}$$

This expression is called the Kirchoff's rule. The problem now is to know the dependence of ΔC_p with the temperature, that is to say that of the heat capacities of the reactants and products with temperature. The heat capacity changes with temperature are usually calculated with the aid of series developments.

As an example, let us find the equation permitting to calculate the change in the enthalpy of formation of carbon dioxide with the temperature. The thermochemical reaction at 298,15 K is:

$$C_{(graphite)} \quad + \quad O_2(g) \quad \rightarrow \quad CO_2(g) \quad \Delta_f H_{298,15} = -393,13 \; kJ \, mol^{-1}$$

The series developments of the involved substances are:

$$C_{p(C)} = -5,2877 + 58,55 \; 10^{-3} \, T - 431,84 \; 10^{-7} \, T^2$$

$$C_{p(O2)} = 25,699 + 12,966 \; 10^{-3} \, T - 38,581 \; 10^{-7} \, T^2$$

$$C_{p(CO2)} = 25,9745 + 43,455 \; 10^{-3} \, T - 148,18 \; 10^{-7} \, T^2$$

The problem is essentially a matter of integration. The integration constant is found by taking into account that at $T = 298,15 \; K \; \Delta_f H = -393,14 \; kJ \, mol^{-1}$. The relation is:

$$\Delta_f H_T - \Delta_f H_{T'} = 5,5636T - 14,032 \; 10^{-3} \, T^2 + (107,413 \; 10^{-7}) \, T^3$$

Another way of carrying out the calculation of the enthalpy changes of reactions is to proceed as in the application of Hess' law (see paragraph 5 preceding chapter). The problem is to imagine the judicious steps.

As another example, let us calculate the enthalpy change ΔH of the transformation:

$$H_2O(-10°C, l, _{surfusion}) \rightarrow H_2O(-10°C, s) \quad \Delta H$$

The three following steps may be imagined:

$$H_2O(-10°C, l, _{surfusion}) \rightarrow H_2O(0°C, l) \quad \Delta H_1$$

$$H_2O(0°C, l) \quad\quad\quad \rightarrow H_2O (0°C, s) \quad \Delta H_2$$

$$H_2O(0°C, s) \quad\quad\quad \rightarrow H_2O(-10°C, s) \quad \Delta H_3$$

Notice that the summation of the latter three thermochemical equations is strictly equivalent to the one under consideration. Their enthalpy changes remain to be added.

$$\Delta H = \Delta H_1 + \Delta H_2 + \Delta H_3$$

ΔH_1 and ΔH_3 are given by the relations:

$$\Delta H_1 = \int_{-10}^{0} C_P(H_2O, l)\, dT \quad\quad \Delta H_3 = \int_{0}^{-10} C_P(H_2O, s)\, dT$$

ΔH_2 is the enthalpy of freezing of water at 0°C. The results are the following ones:

$$\Delta H = -5{,}614 \text{ kJ mol}^{-1}; \Delta H_2 = -6{,}002 \text{ kJ mol}^{-1}; \Delta H_1 = 0{,}754 \text{ kJ mol}^{-1}; \Delta H_3 = -0{,}364 \text{ kJ mol}^{-1}$$

Exercise 1:

Given the following heats of reactions at 25°C:

$$C_2H_4(g) + 3O_2(g) \rightarrow 2CO_2(g) + 2H_2O(l) \quad \Delta H = -1409{,}9 \text{ kJ}$$

$$H_2(g) + 1/2O_2(g) \rightarrow H_2O(l) \quad\quad\quad\quad\quad \Delta H = -285{,}5 \text{ kJ}$$

$$C_2H_6 + 3/2O_2(g) \rightarrow 2CO_2(g) + 3H_2O(l) \quad \Delta H = -1558{,}3 \text{ kJ}$$

determine the heat change of the reaction:

$$C_2H_4(g) + H_2(g) \rightarrow C_2H_6(g) \quad \Delta H ?$$

Answ:

Adding the two first equations and substracting the latter give:

$$\Delta H = -137{,}1 \text{ kJ mol}^{-1}$$

Exercise 2:

The standard heat of formation of glucose $C_6H_{12}O_6(s)$ α-D is −1274 kJ mol^{-1} at 298 K. Standard heats of formation of $CO_2(g)$ and $H_2O(l)$ are −393,51 and −285,84 kJ mol^{-1}, respectively. Calculate the heat ΔH of the following reaction:

$$6 CO_2(g) + 6H_2O(l) \rightarrow C_6H_{12}O_6(s) + 6 O_2(g)$$

Answ:

It is sufficient to decompose the above reaction into the three following ones, to sum them algebraically. The result is $\Delta H = 2802$ kJ mol^{-1}.

$$6H_2(g) + 3O_2(g) \rightarrow 6H_2O(l)$$

$$6C(graphite) + 6O_2(g) \rightarrow 6CO_2(g)$$

$$6C(graphite) + 6H_2(g) + 3O_2(g) \rightarrow C_6H_{12}O_6(s)$$

Remark: this reaction is essential in the phenomenon of respiration (see Chapter 31).

Exercise 3:

The problem is to find the equation permitting to calculate the change in the enthalpy of formation of carbon dioxide with the temperature. The thermochemical reaction at 298,15 K is:

$$C_{(graphite)} + O_2(g) \rightarrow CO_2(g) \quad \Delta_f H_{298,15} = -393,13 \text{ kJ mol}^{-1}$$

The series developments of the involved substances are:

$$C_{p(C)} = -5,2877 + 58,55 \ 10^{-3} \ T - 431,84 \ 10^{-7} \ T^2$$

$$C_{p(O2)} = 25,699 + 12,966 \ 10^{-3} \ T - 38,581 \ 10^{-7} \ T^2$$

$$C_{p(CO2)} = 25,9745 + 43,455 \ 10^{-3} \ T - 148,18 \ 10^{-7} \ T^2$$

Answ:

It is essentially a matter of integration. The integration constant is found by taking into account that at $T = 298,15$ K $\Delta_f H = -393,14$ kJ mol^{-1}. The relation is:

$$\Delta_f H_T - \Delta_f H_{T'} = 5,5636 \ T - 14,032 \ 10^{-3} \ T^2 + (107,413 \ 10^{-7}) \ T^3$$

Exercise 4:

Calculation of the enthalpy change ΔH of the transformation:

$$H_2O(-10°C, l,_{surfusion}) \rightarrow H_2O(-10°C, s) \quad \Delta H$$

Answ:

The three following steps may be imagined:

$$H_2O(-10°C, l,_{surfusion}) \rightarrow H_2O(0°C, l) \quad \Delta H_1$$

$$H_2O(0°C, l) \rightarrow H_2O \ (0°C, s) \quad \Delta H_2$$

$$H_2O(0°C, s) \rightarrow H_2O(-10°C, s) \quad \Delta H_3$$

Notice that the summation of the latter three thermochemical equations is strictly equivalent to the one under consideration. Their enthalpy changes remain to be added.

$$\Delta H = \Delta H_1 + \Delta H_2 + \Delta H_3$$

ΔH_1 and ΔH_3 are given by the relations:

$$\Delta H_1 = \int_{-10}^{0} C_P(H_2O, l)\, dT \qquad \Delta H_3 = \int_{0}^{-10} C_P(H_2O, s)\, dT$$

ΔH_2 is the enthalpy of freezing water at 0°C. Results are the following ones:

$\Delta H = -5{,}614 \ kJ \ mol^{-1}$; $\Delta H_2 = -6{,}002 \ kJ \ mol^{-1}$; $\Delta H_1 = 0{,}754 \ kJ \ mol^{-1}$; $\Delta H_3 = -0{,}364 \ kJ \ mol^{-1}$

Chapter 9

The First Law and the Ideal Gases

Although the fact that in bioenergetics the properties of gases are rarely evoked, it is interesting to apply the first law and its associated relations to the case of ideal gases. Results coming from these considerations are of great aid to introduce the concept of entropy and to begin to grasp its meaning.

1) Ideal gases

- One definition of an ideal gas stipulates that such a gas:
  - obeys the equation of state:

    $$pV = nRT \tag{35}$$

    where p is the pressure of the gas, V and T its volume and absolute temperature, n its number of moles and R the perfect gas constant. In the occurrence, R is the molar perfect gas constant (unit: $JK^{-1}mol^{-1}$). The constant R is related to the boltzmann constant k (or k_B) (unit: JK^{-1}) by the relation:

    $$R = kN_A$$

    where N_A is the Avogadro number (unit: mol^{-1}). (From the historical standpoint, this equation may be considered as the sum of the old laws of Boyle and Charles, not recalled here).
  - possesses an internal energy which is only function of the temperature. This means that it is not dependent on its pressure and volume, that is to say:

    $$(\partial U/\partial V)_T = 0 \tag{36}$$

    $$(\partial U/\partial p)_T = 0 \tag{37}$$

    We shall see that these definitions come from the hypothesis that the "particles" (molecules or atoms) of gas are independent of each other. In other words, they are not in mutual interactions. This explains the fact that the more diluted the gases, the more ideal their character.

- Another definition of a perfect gas

  Any substance, pure or in mixture, whatever its physical state and whatever the medium where it is located, is characterized by a thermodynamic quantity of utmost importance named the *chemical potential* μ (see Chapter 17 Partial molar quantities—chemical potential). One also distinguishes another quantity named *standard chemical potential* $\mu°$ of the substance. A gas is qualified as "perfect" or "ideal" when its chemical potential obeys the following relation:

  $$\mu = \mu° + RT\ln (p/p°) \tag{38}$$

where p is its pressure and p° its pressure in a particular state called *standard state*. It is interesting to already note that definitions (34) and (37) are strictly equivalent, as it can be demonstrated.

2) Dependence of the enthalpy of an ideal gas on pressure and volume

The relation defining the quantity enthalpy is:

$H = E + pV$

Concerning its change with the volume at constant temperature $(\partial H/\partial V)_T$:

$(\partial H/\partial V)_T = (\partial E/\partial V)T + (\partial [pV])/\partial V)_T$

Since relation (34) is obeyed:

$(\partial [pV])/\partial V)_T = (\partial nRT/\partial V)_T$

$(\partial nRT/\partial V)_T = 0$

Moreover, according to (35)

$(\partial E/\partial V)T = 0$

Hence:

$(\partial H/\partial V)_T = 0$ (39)

Concerning now the change with the pressure $(\partial H/\partial p)_T$, it is the same result for the same reason:

$(\partial H/\partial p)_T = 0$ (40)

3) Relationship between C_p and C_v

According to the following relation (see mathematical appendices and Chapter 5):

$dU = (\partial U/\partial V)_T (\partial V/\partial p)_T dp + [(\partial U/\partial V)_T (\partial V/\partial T)_p + (\partial U/\partial T)_V] dT$

at constant pressure:

$dU/dT = (\partial U/\partial V)_T (\partial V/\partial T)_p + (\partial U/\partial T)_V \quad dp = 0$

$(\partial U/\partial T)p = (\partial U/\partial V)_T (\partial V/\partial T)_p + (\partial U/\partial T)_V$ (41)

By definition:

$C_p = [\partial(U + pV)/\partial T)]_p$

$C_p = (\partial U/\partial T)_p + p(\partial V/\partial T)_p$ (42)

Regrouping (40) and (41), one obtains:

$C_p = (\partial V/\partial T)_p [(\partial U/\partial V)_T + p] + (\partial U/\partial T)_V$

By definitions:

$(\partial U/\partial V)_T = 0$

and:

$(\partial U/\partial T)_V = C_v$

$C_p = p\,(\partial V/\partial T)_p + C_v$

Lastly, after relation (1), for $n = 1$:

$C_p = R + C_v$ (43)

4) Thermodynamic changes in expansion processes

We are essentially concerned by isothermal and adiabatic reversible expansion and compression of perfect gases. The results mentioned below have permit to calculate some thermodynamic quantities, in particular the entropy in some conditions.

4-1) Isothermal expansion

Recall that the work received by the system (constituted by the gas) is given by the relation (see Chapter 2 "some definitions of thermodynamics"):

$W = -\int_{V1}^{V2} p_{ext}\, dV$ (44)

where V is the volume of the system (gas) whereas p_{ext} is the pressure of the surroundings.

In a reversible process, as it is the case in a quasi-static transformation, the pressure of the system p and the external one p_{ext} are equal all along the process. As a result, (43) becomes:

$W = -\int_{V1}^{V2} p\, dV$ (45)

Since the perfect gas law is satisfied:

$W = -\int_{V1}^{V2} (nRT/V)\, dV$ (46)

and the process isothermal:

$W = -nRT \ln (V_2/V_1)$

W is the work performed by the system in these conditions. Notice that in agreement with the conventions, it is negative when it is a true expansion ($V_2 > V_1$). The system has effectively performed a work against the surroundings. It is positive when there is a reduction of the volume ($V_2 < V_1$) when it has received work from the surroundings.

Now, concerning the changes of the internal energy ΔU and heat Q of the system accompanying the transformation, they are found by starting from the general expression giving the total differential dU:

$dU = (\partial U/\partial T)_V\, dT + (\partial U/\partial V)_T\, dV$

Since the gas is perfect, $(\partial U/\partial V)_T = 0$ and since the process is isothermal $dT = 0$. As a result:

$\Delta U = 0$

and since according to the first principle:

$\Delta U = Q + W$

$$Q - nRT \ln (V_2/V_1) = 0$$

The heat received by the system (from the surroundings) under these conditions is given by the equation:

$$Q = + nRT \ln (V_2/V_1) \tag{47}$$

It is particularly useful when it comes to calculating the entropy change of the system in these conditions. When there is compression, it can be demonstrated in an analogous way that:

$$W = nRT\ln (V_2/V_1)$$

and

$$Q = -nRT\ln (V_2/V_1)$$

whereas ΔU remains null.

4-2)   Adiabatic expansion

By definition, there is no transfer of heat, đ$Q = 0$ and:

$$dU = dW = đW \qquad \text{(adiabatic process)}$$

Since, as above:

$$dU = (\partial U/\partial T)_V dT + (\partial U/\partial V)_T dV$$

and

$$(\partial U/\partial V)_T = 0 \qquad \text{(perfect gas)}$$

$$dU = (\partial U/\partial T)_V dT$$

$$dU = C_v dT$$

where C_v is the calorific constant at constant volume of the system:

$$C_v dT = dW$$

$$W = \int_{T1}^{T2} C_v dT$$

If C_v is independent of the temperature (it is often the case for a perfect gas if the temperature change $T_2 - T_1$ is not too important):

$$W = C_v (T_2 - T_1)$$

Since, by hypothesis, the process is reversible, the perfect gas law is satisfied and $p = p_{ext}$. Hence

$$dW = -p_{ext} dV$$

$$dW = -pdV$$

$$C_v dT = -pdV$$

C_v is the calorific capacity at constant temperature of the system, that is to say for n gas molecules:

$C_v = n\, c_V$

where c_V is the molar thermal capacity at constant volume. Since the perfect gas law is also satisfied in this case:

$n\, c_V\, dT = -n\, (RT/V)\, dV$

After separation of variables, we find:

$(c_V/T)\, dT = -(R/V)dV$

After integration within limits T_1 and T_2 for which the corresponding values of the volume are T_2 and T_1, we obtain;

$c_V \ln(T_2/T_1) = -R \ln (V_2/V_1)$

This equation can be written in an equivalent manner:

$(T_2/T_1)^{c_V} = (V_2/V_1)^{-R} = (V_1/V_2)^{R}$

$T_2/T_1 = (V_1/V_2)^{R/c_V}$

$T_2 V_2^{\,R/c_V} = T_1 V_1^{\,R/c_V}$

We can equivalently also write:

$TV^{\,R/c_V} = $ constant

$T^{\,c_V/R}\, V = $ constant'

These relations permit to calculate the final temperature from the initial temperature and the observed volumes, by analysing the adiabatic curve. If one measures pressures instead of temperatures, it is possible to use the following equation:

$PV^{\,c_p/c_v} = $ constant ''

The last equation comes from the relation relating cp and cv in the case of perfect gases.

Chapter **10**

The Second Law of Thermodynamics

One way to introduce the second law of thermodynamics is to begin by defining the entropy function. We partly study this concept through an approach based on the theory of thermodynamics of irreversible processes (see Chapter 24) and partly through reasonings of classical thermodynamics. Further, different developments concerning the entropy will be given elsewhere in this book especially in the last chapter with respect to the theory of information.

We begin the chapter by briefly saying why entropy is so important for our purpose. After, we recall the second law of thermodynamics under Clausius' statement and, immediately after, it will be possible to evoke Carnot's theorem and also another statement of the second law.

1) Entropy and bioenergetics

Entropy is a very puzzling function for different reasons. Perhaps is it because it is a non-conservative quantity? Perhaps is it also because it may appear as being only a "simple" mathematical function? Let us also say that it is somewhat difficult to grasp because its value is often related to the rather indefinite concept of order or disorder. Finally, it is a highly puzzling concept because it seems to be related with the very troublesome one of "time's arrow".

In any case, *for our purpose*, it is a very important function because it is a component of the functions of Helmholtz and Gibbs energies (formerly free energy and enthalpy functions). As we shall see, the Gibbs' energy function, indeed, govern the fate of chemical and biochemical reactions in solutions at *constant temperature and pressure, at least for closed systems*. This precisely can be considered and supposed as being the case of the reactions of bioenergetics.

2) Clausius' statement of the second law

Clausius' statement of the second law of thermodynamics is:

"It is impossible to construct a machine that is able to convey heat by a cyclical process from one reservoir (at a lower temperature) to another at a higher temperature unless work is done on the machine by some outside agency". Recall that a cyclical process (or a series of processes constituting the cycle) is a transformation, the result of which is that the system returns exactly to its original thermodynamic state. The term cyclical is introduced to indicate that the machine must function continuously.

In other words, heat cannot spontaneously transfer from a source at lower temperature to another at higher temperature, unless work is given to the system by the surroundings.

The qualifier "spontaneously" is very important. Actually, it is possible that heat can transfer from the lower temperature source to the higher one, but it is at the expense of work provided by the surroundings to the system. It is not a spontaneous transfer.

According to Clausius' statement, the second law is a postulate. It is accepted because deductions from it correspond to the experience. This statement reflects the man's impotence to construct a perpetual-motion machine of the first kind.

There are other statements of the second law (see paragraph 4).

3) Carnot's theorem of heat engines

Heat engines are devices which convert heat into work. If the device is devoted to produce work, it must operate between a hot source (reservoir) at temperature T_2 and a cold source at temperature T_1 (Figure 9). At this point of their description immediately comes in mind the following property which is systematically evoked in physics. In order for any form of energy to be available for the performance of work, it must be associated with a kind of "potential difference". Among familiar examples, let us cite the work that can be done by falling water due to its difference of potential energy at the upper and lower levels. Let us also cite the electrical one due to a difference of potential. The functioning of heat-engines is quite analogous to these machines.

Let us consider that the system is the device performing the work w. It contains a working substance which may be, for example, a perfect gas. It functions between a reservoir at temperature T_2 (the hot source) which is at the exterior and which gives the heat q_2 to the system and a reservoir at temperature T_1 (the cold source) to which it gives back the heat q_1. Notice that Clausius' law is satisfied, meaning that the transfer of heat in this direction is spontaneous.

According to the first law, the work w performed by the system is in these conditions:

$$|w| = |q_2| - |q_1|$$

It is a consequence of the properties of entropy (see Chapter 12 "Calculations involving the function entropy") that the maximum work w_{max} done by the machine is given by the relation:

$$|w_{max}| = q_2 (1 - T_1/T_2)$$

This is Carnot's theorem. Recall that according to the conventions of signs, q_2 is positive (heat given to the system), q_1 is negative (heat given by the machine to the cold source) and w is negative (work carried out by the system). The work is maximum when the transformation is reversible. w_{max} is independent of the working substance.

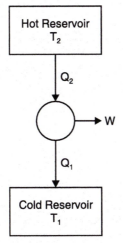

Figure 9. Functioning of a kind of heat engine.

4) Other statements of the second law

We confine ourselves to recall the Kelvin-Planck statement and to an another, more recent one.

According to Kelvin and Planck:

It is impossible to construct a machine that, operating in a cycle, will take heat from a reservoir at constant temperature and convert it into work without accompanying changes in the reservoir or its surroundings.

In other words, it is impossible to carry out a cyclical process in which heat from a reservoir at a fixed temperature has been converted into work. If such a machine could be constructed, it would be a "perpetual-motion" machine of the second kind.

There are other statements. They are all equivalent. It seems that the most "finalized" one is the one appearing in Clausius' famous sentence also concerning the first law:

"die Energie der Welt ist constant, die Entropie der Welt strebt einem Maximum zu".

The entropy of an isolated system (the Universe said with emphasis) tends toward a maximum during an irreversible process or remains constant if the process is reversible. The concept of entropy is further studied in the next chapter.

The part of the previous sentence devoted to the entropy has been developed within the realm of "thermodynamics of irreversible processes".

Chapter 11

The Entropy Function

Now, the second law being stated as a postulate, it is interesting to introduce it in another way. It consists in using the entropy function which must be, firstly, introduced and secondly studied.

1) Notion of balance-sheet

It is interesting to begin with the general notion of balance-sheet. It is directly related to the non-conservative property of entropy (see under).

Let us consider an extensive state quantity X of a system. During the course of an elementary process between times t and t + dt, its change dX is given by the relation:

$$dX = X_{t+dt} - X_t$$

This change may be due to two phenomena:

- one, symbolized by d_eX due to an *exchange* of the quantity X with the surroundings through the partition of the system,
- the other, symbolized by d_iX, due to an *internal creation* of X (that is to say it is exclusively created- or destroyed- within the system).

Both changes are algebraic quantities. The balance-sheet is hence:

$$dX = d_eX + d_iX$$

The term dX_i or ΔX_i is named the "the source of irreversibility term" or "the source term".

- As an example, let us consider the following "macroscopic case". It is a park of 700 animals. During the considered time interval, 70 are brought into it whereas 65 are sold. There are also 12 births and 4 deaths. The balance sheets are: $\Delta X_e = +5$; $\Delta X_i = +8$; $\Delta X = +13$;
- As another example, let us consider that a chemical reactor is working in a stationary state. This means that the values of the different quantities do not change with time. In every second, it enters into the system: 2 g of ethane, 8 g of nitrogen whereas 0,56 g of ethylene, 0.04 g of dihydrogen, 8 g of dinitrogen and 1,4 g of ethane go out the system. Draw up the mass balance-sheets of each species.

Evidently, the occurring chemical reaction is:

$$C_2H_6 \rightarrow C_2H_4 + H_2$$

The mass balance-sheet is

$$C_2H_6 = -0,6 \text{ g}$$

$N_2 = 0$ g

$C_2H_4 = +0,56$

$H_2 = +0,04$

(The chosen system is the contents of the reactor).

2) Conservative and non-conservative quantities

With these few explanations concerning the balance-sheets, it is now possible to specify the notions of conservative and non-conservative quantities.

- A state function X is *conservative* when it can only change through exchanges with the surroundings. In other words:

X is conservative when:

$\delta_i X = 0$ and then $\Delta X = \Delta_e X$

- X is non-conservative when it can change through exchanges with the surroundings and, also, *by internal creation or destruction.*

$\Delta X = \Delta_e X + \Delta_i X$

(It may be possible that in certain conditions, the term $\Delta_i X$ is null even with non-conservative quantities).

As examples, let us mention that:

- the internal energy of a system defined by the relation:

$\Delta U = \Delta W + \Delta Q$

both terms ΔW and ΔQ are exchanged with the surroundings. There is no term involving a source. *The internal energy of a system is conservative;*

- *the heat of a system is not conservative.* For example we know that a heat creation due to friction may occur.

3) Irreversible and reversible processes

The concept of entropy being intimately related to the notions of reversibility and irreversibility, it is judicious to give here a further criterion of reversibility (see Chapter 2).

A process is reversible if one can envisage another experiment which can, at the same time, bring back both the system and its surroundings to their initial state.

For example, in the Joule experiment (see Chapter 4), a paddle-wheel system operated by a falling weight permits to stir a solution contained in an adiabatic vessel and to raise its temperature (Figure 6).

The inverse process is impossible. There does not exist another process which would permit the solution calorimeter to recover its initial temperature and, at the same time, the weights be raised back to their initial heights. The process is irreversible.

4) The need of a common quantitative measure of the tendency of systems to evolve in a given direction

Numerous experiments show the existence of a unique sense of the evolution of processes and the impossibility of some transformations to occur spontaneously. For example, when a hot object is placed in contact with a cold one, heat flows from the former to the latter.

It has been evident for a long time that the changes ΔU and ΔH accompanying a process do not provide an accurate criterion of the spontaneous direction of a natural (spontaneous) process. At best, they only provide an approximate one.

As a result, the need of another thermodynamic law, in order to explain these phenomena, became clear. In 1850, R. Clausius introduced the function *entropy* which plays the required part.

5) The function entropy

For every *closed system*, there exists a *state function* called *entropy*. Like other state functions, the entropy change accompanying a transformation depends only on its initial and final states. (A demonstration of this property is given in Chapter 13). Entropy is an extensive and non-conservative function. Its symbol is S. (In this book, when the symbol S does not bring any subscript, it is the "entropy state-function"). According to the theory entitled "Non-equilibrium thermodynamics", entropy is introduced by the relation:

$$\Delta S = \Delta_e S + \Delta \sigma \tag{48}$$

$\Delta_e S$ is the exchange term. $\Delta \sigma$ is the term of "source", that is to say the *created entropy* in the system under study. By definition, the exchanged entropy $\Delta_e S$ is given by (see Figure 10):

$$\Delta_e S = q_{ext}/T_{ext} \tag{49}$$

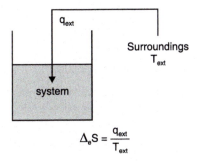

$$\Delta_e S = \frac{q_{ext}}{T_{ext}}$$

Figure 10. Definition of the exchanged entropy.

It is important to already notice that the heat q may be either reversibly exchanged or irreversibly.

By definition, the change in the entropy of the system during a transformation under study, ΔS, is given by the expression:

$$\Delta S = q_{rev}/T_{ext} \tag{50}$$

or, of course, by:

$$dS = dq_{rev}/T_{ext} \tag{51}$$

where q_{rev} is the heat received by the system in a *reversible* way from the surroundings (a reservoir) at the temperature T_{ext}. q_{rev} may be positive or negative according to the fact that the system effectively receives heat from the surroundings or it gives heat to it (Figure 11).

Through examples, let us answer the following two questions:

• What is the received entropy by a vessel initially containing 80 g water at 100°C which has cooled until the temperature of 25°C? (The thermal calorific capacity of water is 4,18 J g^{-1}K^{-1}). The answer is: $q_e = -4,18. 80.(100 - 25) = -25080$ J. $\Delta_e S = -25080/298,15 = -84,12$ JK^{-1}.

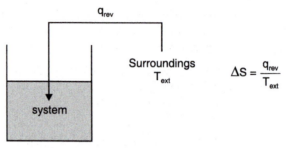

Figure 11. Definition of the function entropy.

- What quantity of entropy has received 1 g of ice when it is placed in an atmosphere of 25°C? (thermal–calorific–capacity of water: 4.18 J $g^{-1}K^{-1}$ and at 0°C, the heat of fusion of ice is 334,4 $Jg^{-1}K^{-1}$).

On one hand, the heat exchanged permits the fusion of ice at 0°C and the rise of the temperature of the system up to 25°C:

q_e' fusion = 334,4.1 J

q_e" for the increase of the temperature = 4,18.25 = 104,5 J

Therefore:

$\Delta_e S$ = + (334,4 + 104,5)/298,15 = + 1,47 J K^{-1}

6) A second, but equivalent, definition of the function entropy

In several cases, the entropy change of the system under study ΔS is defined in terms of the change of its surroundings ΔS' (during the same process). According to Equation (49), when the heat q is exchanged from the reservoir to the system, we can write:

$\Delta S' = -q/T_{ext}$

Hence,

$\Delta_e S = -\Delta S'$

and according to (47):

$\Delta S + \Delta S' = \Delta \sigma$ (52)

This is the other definition of the entropy.

The sum ($\Delta S + \Delta S'$) is the change of the entropy of the system and of its surroundings. Said with emphasis, it is the entropy change of the Universe during the studied process. In any case, it is the change in a system which is considered as being isolated.

As a result, it can be said that the entropy of an isolated system, during a transformation, can only increase or be null. (When the process is reversible, indeed, $\Delta S = -\Delta S'$).

Relation (51) seems to be the most general definition of the entropy and of the second law.

It appears that the quantity entropy does not describe a true property of a system, that is to say a quantity immediately measurable. Hence, entropy appears to be essentially a *mathematical function*.

From this standpoint, the entropy is somewhat similar **to** the internal energy, which is defined in terms of work and heat and is not directly measurable.

7) The second law of thermodynamics

The second law can be summarized by the following relations:

$$\Delta S = \Delta_e S + \Delta\sigma \tag{47}$$

$$\Delta S = q_{rev}/T_{ext} \tag{48}$$

$$\Delta\sigma \geq 0 \qquad\qquad (53) \quad \text{(feasible process)}$$

$$\Delta\sigma < 0 \qquad\qquad (54) \quad \text{(impossible process)}$$

Relation (52) means that entropy can only be created or remain null during a possible transformation. Moreover:

– *when the latter is reversible, $\Delta\sigma = 0$*
– *when it is irreversible, $\Delta\sigma > 0$.*

As it has already been said, there exist other statements of the second law of thermodynamics.

8) Some consequences of the above statement of the second law

– In an isolated system, there is no flow of entropy, $\Delta_e S = 0$. In an isolated system, the entropy may only be null or may increase.
– Entropy is a non-conservative function, as relation (47) shows it.
– It is clear that the entropy unit must be the joule kelvin^{-1}: J K^{-1}.
– According to (47), the entropy change ΔS can be split into two parts: that of the change due to the exchange of heat with the reservoir (in abbreviated form, the "exchanged entropy" $\Delta_e S$) and eventually that of the "created entropy" $\Delta\sigma$.
– *The entropy state function ΔS and that exchanged $\Delta_e S$ must not be confused,* except, of course, when the process is reversible. This is a great source of "miscomprehension". It is in relation with the fact that the exchange of heat in any transformation is not obligatorily carried out reversibly:

$$\Delta_e S = q_e/T_{ext}$$

that is to say with $q_e = q_{irr}$ or q_{rev}.

As a result, $\Delta_e S$ is not a state function. (Notice that, up to the end of this book, the symbol S without any subscript exclusively represents the entropy state function).

– There is another source of misconception of the concept of entropy. It is the confusion between the entropy of the system under study S_{syst} and the entropy of the system under study plus its surroundings. The whole system, by principle, constitutes an isolated system.

In the following lines are given some exercises devoted to the calculation of entropy changes accompanying some processes.

Exercise 1:

What is the received entropy by a vessel initially containing 80 g water at 100°C which has cooled until the temperature of 25°C? (Thermal calorific capacity of water is 4,18 J g^{-1}K^{-1}).

Answ:

$q_e = -4,18 . 80.(100 - 25) = -25080\ J. \Delta_e S = -25080/298,15 = -84,12\ JK^{-1}$.

Exercise 2:

At 0°C, the heat of fusion of ice is 334,4 Jg⁻¹K⁻¹. 1 g of ice is placed in an atmosphere of 25°C. What quantity of entropy has it received? (thermal capacity of water: 4.18 J g⁻¹K⁻¹)

Answ:

On one hand, the heat exchanged permits the fusion of ice at 0°C and the rise of the temperature of the system up to 25°C, on the other:

q_e'*fusion* $= 334,4.1\ J$

q_e''*for the increase of the temperature* $= 4,18.25 = 104,5\ J$

$\Delta_e S = + (334,4 + 104,5)/298,15 = + 1,47\ J K^{-1}$

Exercise 3:

1 g water, taken at 25°C, is in contact with surroundings at 0°C. It solidifies. What entropy has it received?

Answ:

The heat "given" by surroundings to the system "1 g water" is the sum of the heats of cooling of water from 25°C to 0°C without solidification and of the heat of solidification. The heat of cooling $q_e' = (0 - 25).4,18 = -104,5\ J$. *The heat of solidification* q_e' *is* $q_e' = -334,4\ Jg^{-1}K^{-1}$ *(see Exercise 4).*

$\Delta_e S = -(104,5 + 334,4)/273,15 = -1,61\ J.K^{-1}$

Exercise 4:

In the Joule's experiment carried out to discover the mechanical equivalent of the calorie (see Chapter 4), the temperature of 100 g water raises from 25°C up to 35°C, the temperature of the surroundings being at 25°C. What is the entropy received by water taken as the system under study?

Answ:

$\Delta_e S = 0$

The system has not received heat from the surroundings.

9) Come back to the notion of reversibility

  9-1) Equivalence of the reversibility of a transformation and the created entropy

  In this paragraph, we will check that setting up that $\Delta\sigma = 0$ and that the fact that the corresponding transformation is reversible are two equivalent notions.

  Let us consider the transformation A→B and its inverse B→A which brings back the system into its initial state (Figure 12). The followed ways in both directions are identical. It is possible to define them in coordinates P,V.

  Let us set up the entropic balance-sheets of the three transformations AB, BA and ABA:

  $\Delta S_{AB} \rightarrow \Delta S_{eAB} + \Delta\sigma_{AB}$

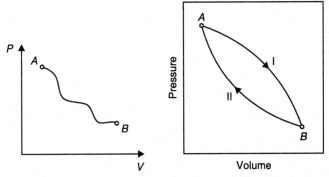

Figure 12. Equivalence null entropy creation/reversibility of the process.

$$\Delta S_{BA} \rightarrow \Delta S_{eBA} + \Delta \sigma_{BA}$$

$$\Delta S_{ABA} \rightarrow \Delta S_{eABA} + \Delta \sigma_{ABA}$$

The first point which may be mentioned is:

$$\Delta S_{ABA} = 0$$

since S is a state function and the transformation ABA is cyclic. Notice that, at this point of the reasoning, the reversible or irreversible character of the transformation has not yet been mentioned. Now, let us just suppose that the transformation AB is reversible. Let us seek the conditions the entropy changes must obey so that it is the case. According to the previous definition (paragraph 7), the reversiblity means, among other things, that after the cyclic transformation, the surroundings must recover its initial state and hence its initial entropy. Since during both transformations (forward and backward) the surroundings only exchange heat with the system, we deduce:

$$\Delta S_{eAB} = -\Delta S_{eBA}$$

Hence, taking now into account the additivity of the entropy function:

$$\Delta S_{ABA} = \Delta \sigma_{AB} + \Delta \sigma_{BA}$$

$$\Delta \sigma_{AB} + \Delta \sigma_{BA} = 0$$

Since according the second law, as it is stated above, the created entropy cannot be anything else but null or positive, therefore we found:

$$\Delta \sigma_{AB} = 0 \text{ and } \Delta \sigma_{BA} = 0$$

The proposition is demonstrated: the result $\Delta \sigma = 0$ is synonymous to reversibility.

9-2) Condition for reversible heat exchanges

In order to determine this condition, let us imagine an isolated system, split into two parts 1 and 2. Each possesses its own constant temperature T_1 and T_2 (Figure 13). Both subsystems can only exchange heat. Let us write the entropic balance-sheets of both subsystems and that of the whole one. For the latter, since it is isolated:

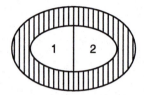

Figure 13. Isolated system with its two subsystems at constant temperatures.

$$\Delta S = \Delta \sigma \quad \text{with} \quad \Delta \sigma \geq 0$$

$\Delta \sigma$ is the entropy possibly created in the whole system. For the subsystem 1, however, system 2 is its surroundings. Let us apply the second law, according to its second definition:

$$\Delta S_1 = q_{2\rightarrow 1}/T_2 = \Delta_e S_{1\rightarrow 2} + \Delta \sigma_1$$

and likewise for the second subsystem:

$$\Delta S_2 = q_{1\rightarrow 2}/T_1 = \Delta_e S_{2\rightarrow 1} + \Delta \sigma_2$$

$$\Delta S = \Delta_e S_{1\rightarrow 2} + \Delta_e S_{2\rightarrow 1} + \Delta \sigma_1 + \Delta \sigma_2$$

The transformation being reversible, the following three relations must be obeyed:

$$\Delta \sigma = 0, \ \Delta \sigma_1 = 0, \ \Delta \sigma_2 = 0$$

Hence:

$$\Delta_e S_{1\rightarrow 2} + \Delta_e S_{2\rightarrow 1} = 0$$

$$q_{2\rightarrow 1}/T_2 + q_{1\rightarrow 2}/T_1 = 0$$

But,

$$-q_{2\rightarrow 1}/T_2 = q_{1\rightarrow 2}/T_1$$

The only way to do that is to put:

$$T_2 = T_1$$

A heat exchange can be reversible if, and only if, both substances are at the same temperature.

Chapter 12

Calculations Involving the Function Entropy

So far, we have just mentioned the calculation of the exchanged entropy but not that of the entropy (the state function) change of the system or of the created entropy. In this chapter, we mention some methods of their evaluation. The first one takes into account the equation called the fundamental equation of thermodynamics. The second mentions a general strategy.

An important fact emerges from the reasonings of this chapter: the entropy is a state function. This property simplifies the calculations.

1) Entropy and internal energy—The combination of first and second laws of thermodynamics

There exists a thermodynamic relation which, in certain conditions, links the changes of internal energy, entropy and volume during a process. It is useful because, among several calculations, it permits the determination of entropy change in a simplified way. It is called the combination of the first and the second laws' relation.

- Recall that in a transformation in which only the "p-V work" intervenes, the exchanged work đW is given by the expression:

$$\text{đ}W = -p_{ext}\, dV \quad \text{(in absolute value)}$$

When, moreover, the transformation is quasi-static (that is to say reversible), the pressure p of the system is systematically equal to the pressure of the surroundings p_{ext} and its temperature T is equal to that of the surroundings T_{ext}:

$$p = p_{ext}$$

$$T = T_{ext}$$

and the exchanged work becomes (reaction reversible process):

$$dW_R = -p\, dV$$

- Now, let us consider some irreversible transformation involving both work and heat and exchanges of them. Its infinitesimal change in internal energy dU is:

$$dU = \text{đ}Q + \text{đ}W \tag{55}$$

Let us consider an identical transformation (same initial and final states) in which the heat and work exchanged are carried out reversibly:

$dU = dQ_R + dW_R$

Given the definition of the entropy:

$dS = dQ_R/T_{ext}$

$dU = TdS - pdV$ (56)

U and V being state functions, it appears that S is also a state function. It also appears that according **to** the properties of total differentials (see appendix mathematics II-4).

$T = (\partial U/\partial S)_V$ and $p = -(\partial U/\partial V)_S$

The entropy S and the volume V are said to be "the natural thermodynamic variables" of the internal energy.

Equation (55) permits to simplify the calculations by comparing the changes in internal energy accompanying a process obtained reversibly or irreversibly, by considering Equations (54) and (55). They must, of course (first principle), lead to an identical dU change (Exercise 2.3). (The internal energy is a state function). Equation (55) is called the fundamental equation for a closed system. It is applicable only when the volume change is the only form of work and when the system is closed. Nevertheless, it is entirely applicable to a system which changes its composition due to internal chemical reactions provided that the latter take place reversibly for the calculation dU remains correct (see Chapter 16).

- Likewise, the enthalpy change dH accompanying a transformation can permit, in some cases, to obtain its entropy value, in particular at constant pressure. This possibility is founded on the relation:

$dH = TdS + Vdp$

obtained by adding the two following equations:

$dH = dU + pdV + Vdp$

$dU = TdS - pdV$

2) General principle of the calculation of the entropy changes of systems

So far, we do not know how to calculate the change ΔS accompanying any transformation. In fact, only the exchanged entropy is always accessible. The created entropy $\Delta\sigma$ is not reachable and, as a consequence, neither is ΔS. However, for reversible systems:

$\Delta\sigma = 0$

and then:

$\Delta S = \Delta_e S$ (reversible processes)

These properties permit to free out the following strategy in order to calculate the entropy change ΔS of a system during the course of any transformation:

The adopted strategy is as follows. Firstly, a transformation "identical" to that studied must be conceived. (By "identical", it is signified that both transformations must have identical initial and final states). The important point is that the conceived identical transformation must be reversible.

Along the course of this one, it is then possible to calculate the received entropy. The received entropy can be identified with that of the system under study, since the process is reversible:

ΔS (system under study) = $\Delta_e S$ ("identical" system but reversibly)

The created entropy is calculated in the last step, by determining the exchanged entropy $\Delta_e S'$ during the process (irreversible) under study, with the aid of the relation:

$\Delta\sigma = \Delta S - \Delta_e S'$

It is, of course, important to notice that finding a reversible pathway between the same initial and final states is always possible.

Exercise 1:

The reaction of formation of water from gaseous dihydrogen and dioxygen, according to the equation (l:liquid):

$$H_2(g) + 1/2O_2(g) \rightarrow H_2O(l)$$

is spontaneous at room temperature but exceedingly slow without the presence of a catalyst. At 298 K, the heat of the irreversible reaction at constant pressure is –285,565 kJ mol⁻¹. The same reaction can be carried out, but in conditions of reversibility, with the aid of an electrochemical cell equipped with a pair of suitable electrodes (see Chapter 27). Under the reversible conditions, the heat of reaction is –48,601 kJ mol⁻¹. Calculate the created entropy when $H_2O(l)$ is formed irreversibly.

Answ:

The exchanged entropy is: –285565/298,15 = –957,8 J mol⁻¹K⁻¹

The entropy of the reaction is: –48601/298,15 = –163,0 J mol⁻¹K⁻¹

$\Delta\sigma = -163,0 - (-957,8)$

$\Delta\sigma = 794,8 \, J \, mol^{-1}K^{-1}$

2-1) Transformation only involving an exchange of heat with the surroundings

Here, we give some examples of such transformations. The calculation of the entropy's changes requires the answer to the question: how is it possible to reversibly raise the temperature of a substance from T_0 up to T?

Let us consider the system as being the substance which will be heated. Evidently, the heat necessary to raise its temperature comes from the surroundings. Let C be the heat capacity of the system which, very often, may be considered as constant and suppose that the substance does not change of phase during the process (see exercise below).

From elementary calorimetry, one knows that the quantity of heat necessary to rise the temperature from T_0 to T of a sample is given by the relation (see Chapter 6):

$Q = C(T - T_0)$

With this in mind, it is *out of the question* to use the following equation to carry out the calculation:

$S \neq C(T - T_0)/T_{ext}$

because of the fact that the transformation would not be reversible since the temperature difference $(T - T_0)$ is too important. A heat exchange between two sources, indeed, can be reversible only if they are at the same temperature (see the previous chapter). The only way is to imagine the transformation under study carried out in multiple successive steps and finally to sum up the successive entropy changes, according to:

$$\Sigma_i \, \Delta S_i = C \, \Sigma_i \, \Delta T_i / T_{ext}$$

It is hence evident that the calculation must be performed according to the integration (see the mathematical appendix II-2):

$$\Delta S_{T0 \to T} = C \int_{T0}^{T} dT/T$$

or

$$\Delta S_{T0 \to T} = C \int_{T0}^{T} d \ln T$$

$$\Delta S_{T0 \to T} = C \ln(T/T_0) \tag{57}$$

For transformations only involving exchanges of heat, the change of entropy is given by Equation (56) if the calorific capacity does not depend on the temperature.

This can be considered as being the case when temperature changes remain weak.

Exercise 2:

4a) Calculate the exchanged entropy with a reservoir at 100°C in order to raise the temperature of 80 g water from 25°C up to 100°C. 4b) What is the change in the entropy of the system? 4c) What is the value of the entropy created? (specific calorific capacity of water 4,18 J g⁻¹ K⁻¹).

Answ:

4a) $\Delta_e S = 4,18 . 75 .80/373,15 = 67,2 \, J \, K^{-1}$

4b) $\Delta S = 4,18 . 80 \ln (373,15/298,15) = 75,0 \, J \, K^{-1}$

4c) $\Delta \sigma = + 7,8 \, J \, K^{-1}$ (natural process)

Exercise 3:

Same process but the reservoir is maintained at 25°C

Answ:

5a) $\Delta_e S = 4,18 . 75 .80/298,15 = 84,1 \, J \, K^{-1}$

5b) $\Delta S = 4,18 . 80 \ln (373,15/298,15) = 75,0 \, J \, K^{-1}$

5c) $\Delta \sigma = -9,1 \, J K^{-1}$ (impossible transformation in these conditions. This is an illustration of Clausius' principle)

Exercise 4:

The fusion heat of water is 334,4 J g⁻¹ at 0°C. Entropy change when 1 g of water is solidifying at 0°C? How the transformation can be reversibly carried out? Surroundings are at 0°C.

Answ:

The transformation is obligatorily reversible since the system (water) and the surroundings are at the same temperature. Therefore, the entropy change is equal to the exchanged one.

$$\Delta S = 334,4/273,15 = + 1,2\ J\,K^{-1}$$

Exercise 5:

Imagine a reversible pathway for the transformation of 10 g water from 25°C to –10°C. Calculate the exchanged entropy, the entropy change and the created one. (Solid water calorific capacity: $C = 2,09\ Jg^{-1}K^{-1}$).

Answ:

During the process, water solidifies. We can imagine 3 steps: a) cooling of liquid water from 25°C down to 0°C; solidification at 0°C; cooling of ice from 0°C to –10°C. Calculations are carried out in the same manner as in the preceding exercises.

- *entropy exchanged:*

  $$\Delta_e S\ (a) = 4,18.\ 10.\ (0 – 25/298,15 = –3,5J\ K^{-1})$$

  $$\Delta_e S\ (b) = –12,2\ J\,K^{-1}$$

  $$\Delta_e S\ (c) = + 2,09.\ 10\ (–10 – 0) = –0,77\ JK^{-1}$$

  total exchanged entropy $= –16,5\ JK^{-1}$

- *entropy change*

  $$\Delta S\ (a) = 4,18.\ 10\ ln(273,15/298,15) = –3,7\ JK^{-1}$$

  $$\Delta S\ (b) = –12,2\ J\,K^{-1}\ (reversible\ transition)$$

  $$\Delta S\ (c) = + 2,09.\ 10\ ln\ (263,15/273,15)\ ) = –0,78\ JK^{-1}$$

  total entropy change $= –16,7\ JK^{-1}$

- *entropy created:*

  $$\Delta\sigma = –0,2\ JK^{-1}$$

Exercise 6:

A glass containing 100 g water at 80°C is left at ambient temperature of 25°C. Water of the glass finishes by taking the latter temperature. Calculate the created entropy during the process.

Answ:

The entropy exchanged between the glass and the ambience $\Delta_e S$ is:

$$\Delta_e S = 4,18.100.(25 – 80)/298,15 = –77,1\ JK^{-1}$$

The entropy change is:

$$\Delta S = 4,18.100\ ln(298,15/353,15) = –70,8\ JK^{-1}$$

The created entropy is:

$$\Delta\sigma = -70,8 + 77,1 = + 6,3 \; JK^{-1}$$

2-2) Transformations involving exchanges of work and heat

In this case, it remains possible to imagine a reversible pathway, but it is necessary to involve a quasi-static process along this pathway. This means that the reasoning implies the aid of the judicious state equations, the plot of which is of great interest.

–   Let us begin by a simple example. Consider n moles of a perfect gas contained in a cylinder shut by a piston. The initial conditions are P_0, V_0, T_0. By a brutal lowering of the piston, the volume of the gas is reduced and one experimentally finds that the temperature of the gas rises. After some time, the temperature of the gas again takes its initial value T_0. The final conditions are now P_1, V_1, T_0. The problem is to imagine a reversible pathway between both states and to infer the entropy change ΔS, thanks to it. Here, it is evident that the transformation is isothermal.

•   From the graphical standpoint, for an isothermal process, the state equation of a perfect gas is a branch of hyperbola P/V:

$$PV = nRT_0 = \text{constant}$$

the term on the right hand being constant. There is no difficulty to locate the initial and final states defined by the coordinates P_0, V_0 and P_1, V_1 at temperature T_0 (see Figure 14). Since the state equation is obeyed all along the pathway, the process is quasi-static, hence reversible.

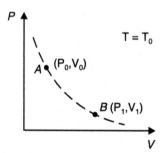

Figure 14. Reversible pathway during the isothermal volume reduction of a perfect gas.

•   For the calculation of ΔS, we follow the reasoning already given in Chapter 8, concerning the determination of some thermodynamic functions accompanying an isothermal expansion. We already know that:

$$dU = 0 \quad \text{(recall: we are in the case of a perfect gas)}$$

and that:

$$dQ = p \, dV \quad \text{(reversible process)}$$

As a result:

$$dS = pdV/T$$

$$\Delta S = \int_{v0}^{v1} nRdV/V$$

$$\Delta S = nR \ln(V_1/V_0)$$

Exercise 7:

Consider an irreversible transformation involving a gas. During it, it is proved experimentally that the exchanged work and heat are null. The same transformation is now reversibly performed. Give the equation permitting the calculation of the entropy change.

Answ:

In both cases, we can write:

$dU = đQ + đW$

$dU = 0$ *(irreversible pathway)*

$dU = TdS - pdV$ *(reversible way)*

Hence:

$TdS - pdV = 0$

$dS = pdV/T$

where P and T are the pressure and the temperature of the system and the surroundings in the reversible experiment.

An interesting remark can be made: *Despite the fact that there is no heat exchange (during the studied process), entropy is created!* This is because the transformation is irreversible.

Exercise 8:

Consider the experiment devoted to the determination of the mechanical equivalent of the calorie, "the paddle-wheel experiment" (see Chapter 4). The fall of the weights provides the mechanical work ∂W permitting the rise of the water temperature. Express the entropy change of water.

Answ:

The most simple means to calculate the entropy change is to consider water as being the system under study. The internal energy change dU is given by the general relation:

$dU = \delta Q + \delta W$ *(irreversible path)*

There is no heat exchange between water and its surroundings, $\delta Q = 0$:

$dU = \delta W$

$dU = dW$

By a reversible pathway,

$dU = TdS - pdV$

There is no change of the volume of the container, dV = 0. As a result:

$$\delta W = T\,dS$$

$$dS = \delta W/T$$

Exercise 9:

Let there be n moles of a fluid starting from an initial state $A(V_0, T_0)$ to the final one $B(V_1, T_1)$. Imagine how one can calculate the ΔS change. Let's give its expression.

Answ:

A perfect gas obeys the data of the problem.

Firstly, it is necessary to conceive a reversible pathway between both states. One consists in following an adiabatic quasi-static pathway up to an intermediary state (point C—Figure 15) and, after, in proceeding to an isothermal reversible expansion from C to B. In the chosen example (Figure 15), $T_1 > T_0$, $V_0 > V_1$.

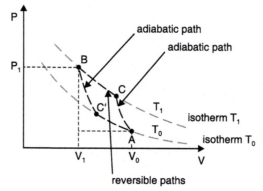

Figure 15. Reversible pathways permitting the calculation of the entropy change when a fluid changes of states is defined by the couples of variables V, T.

The adiabatic first step permits to go from the isothermal at temperature T_0 to that at T_1. According to the study carried out about the reversible adiabatic expansion of a fluid (see Chapter 8), the variables V and T in the final and initial states (in A and C) are linked by the expression:

$$V_C = V_0\,(T_0/T_1)^{1/(\gamma-1)} \quad \text{with} \quad \gamma = C_p/C_v$$

Now, for the isothermal part C → B of the pathway, according to the preceding exercise,

$$\Delta S_{BC} = nR\,ln\,[V_1/V_0(T_1/T_0)^{1/(\gamma-1)}]$$

or

$$\Delta S_{AB} = nR\,ln\,(V_1/V_0 + nCVln\,(T_1/T_0)$$

since, of course,

$$\Delta S_{AC} = 0$$

(there is no transfer of heat on the path A → C).

Remark: There is another reversible pathway between states A and B. It consists in the first step to an isothermal reversible expansion at T_0 up to the point C' and in the second step to an adiabatic reversible path between C' and B. The enthalpy change is the same as before, as it is easily demonstrated from the equation of an adiabatic reversible curve (see Chapter 9).

Exercise 10:

In Joule's experiment, n moles of a perfect gas initially in a container of volume V_A are expended through a stopcock into another container of volume V_B, initially empty. At the end of the experiment, the gas uniformly occupies both containers. The experiment is carried out adiabatically and the experiment shows that the final temperature is the same as in the beginning.

Answ:

The system (gas) does not perform any work and does not receive heat. Hence, the internal energy does not change. However, there is a transformation since the volume (a state variable) of the system has changed. It is irreversible since the expansion of the gas is free. The experiment is an isothermal one. It can be realized reversibly. In this case, the entropy change is given by the relation (see paragraph 2-2):

$$\Delta S = nR \ln (V_A + V_B)/V_A$$

It is interesting to note that there is no exchanged entropy since the system does not receive heat. The entropy change is equal to the one created:

$$\Delta S = \Delta \sigma$$

3) Entropy changes and partial derivatives involving it

Entropy being a function of state, we can express its total differential as being a function of its differential partial coefficients. The reasoning is the same as in the cases of the internal energy and of the enthalpy (see Chapter 5 and mathematical appendix IV-4). Therefore, the entropy may be considered as alternatively being a function of the following couples of state variables p,T; V,T; V,p. These functions are written as:

$$dS = (\partial S/\partial p)_T dp + (\partial S/\partial T)p dT$$

$$dS = (\partial S/\partial V)_T dV + (\partial S/\partial T)_V dT$$

$$dS = (\partial S/\partial V)_p dV + (\partial S/\partial p)_V dp$$

As awaited, the six partial derivatives are not independent. Once the state function relating the variables p, V, T is known, it is possible to find the relations linking these partial derivatives with each other.

The knowledge of these partial derivatives permits to calculate the entropy change accompanying a process by means other than that of finding a reversible pathway. To find out the value of dS it is sufficient to know the partial derivatives of one of the three relations above, and then to integrate. For example:

$$\Delta S = \int(\partial S/\partial p)_T dp + \int (\partial S/\partial T)_p dT$$

4) Expressing the different partial derivatives—Maxwell relations

For the reason which has just been given, it may be interesting to calculate some of these partial derivatives.

We have already found the following relations (see the previous chapter):

$T = (\partial U/\partial S)_V$ and $p = -(\partial U/\partial V)_S$

The fact that U is a state function permits, starting from the latter two relations, to write (see mathematical appendix)

$(\partial T/\partial V)_S = -(\partial p/\partial S)_V$

This relation is based on the use of Schwartz' theorem. Some relations between the partial derivatives are named Maxwell's relations. They are:

$(\partial S/\partial V)_T = (\partial p/\partial T)_V$ $(\partial T/\partial V)_S = -(\partial p/\partial S)_V$

$(\partial S/\partial p)_T = -(\partial V/\partial T)_p$ $(\partial p/\partial T)_S = (\partial S/\partial V)_p$

There exists a mnemonic means to recall these relations. It consists in tidying up the variables by the alphabetic order in a square, line by line. If we consider the first column, we can deduce that $(\partial p/\partial T)_V = (\partial S/\partial V)_T$ and $(\partial p/\partial T)_S = (\partial S/\partial V)_p$. It is analogous if we consider the horizontal lines of the square, but a sign—must be added. For example, according to the first line, we find $(\partial p/\partial S)T = -(\partial T/\partial V)p$.

$$\begin{array}{cc} P & S \\ T & V \end{array}$$

Entropy changes with temperature, implying the two following important relations;

$(\partial S/\partial T)p = C_p/T$ and $(\partial S/\partial T)_V = C_V/T$

We do not demonstrate Maxwell's relations in this book.

Exercise 11:

Let us study a transformation involving 2 moles of a perfect gas. It is non quasi-static and non reversible. The initial state is such that P_1 = 3,5 bars and T_1 = 720 K and the final one by P_2 = 1,3 bars and T_2 = 330 K. Calculate the changes in internal energies and entropy of the gas taken as the system (c_v = 12,5 J K^{-1} mol^{-1}).

Answ:

The internal energy depends only on the temperature. Hence, in the general relation below:

$$dU = (\delta U/\delta T)_V dT + (\delta U/\delta V)_T dT$$

the second term on the right hand side must be neglected and:

$$dU = (\delta U/\delta T)_V dT$$

$(\delta U/\delta T)_V$ is the calorific capacity at constant volume C_V of the system (gas). Hence:

$$dU = C_V dT$$

With $C_V = 2.12,5 = 25$ J K^{-1}

$$\Delta U = 25\ (330 - 720)$$

$$\Delta U = -9750\ J$$

Now, concerning the entropy change, it seems, as a rule, judicious to use the following relation:

$$\Delta S = \int (\partial S/\delta T)_p \, dT + \int (\partial S/\partial p)_T \, dp$$

since $(\partial S/\delta T)_p = C_p/T$ is immediately known. It remains to express the derivative $(\partial S/\delta p)_T$

$$\int (\partial S/\delta T)_p \, dT = 25.1,4 \ln (330/720) = -27,3 \, J \, K^{-1}$$

*(The factor **1,4** takes into account the fact that it is the calorific capacity Cp which must now be handled and not C_v. $\gamma = \mathbf{1,4}$ is the value of the ratio of both capacities).*

According to the mnenomic square:

$$(\partial S/\delta \, p)_T = -(\partial V/\delta \, T)_p$$

Since the gas is perfect:

$$pV = nRT$$

At constant pressure:

$$pdV = nR \, dT$$

$$(\partial V/T)p = (nR/p)$$

$$\int (\partial S/\delta p)_T \, dp = -\int (nR/p) \, dp$$

$$\int (\partial S/\delta p)_T \, dp = -2. \, 8,3. \, \ln(1,3/3,5)$$

$$\int (\partial S/\delta \, p)_T \, dp = -16,4 \, J \, K^{-1}$$

$$\Delta S = -43,7 \, J \, K^{-1}$$

It is interesting to notice how these relations can be obtained. Consider the relation:

$$dU = \partial Q_{rev} - pdV$$

$$dU = TdS - pdV$$

Let us suppose that the volume remains constant, $dV = 0$.

$$dQ_{rev} = TdS$$

The received heat can only raise (or decrease) the temperature of the system. As a result:

$$dQ_{rev} = C_V dT$$

where C_V is the calorific capacity at constant volume of the system. Finally:

$$(\partial S/\partial T)_V = C_V/T$$

The result would be the same if we had considered a transformation at constant pressure. In this case, however, the intermediary variable which must be considered is the enthalpy. This method of calculation may be faster than that consisting in imagining a reversible pathway (Exercise 11).

5) Entropy change accompanying a reversible phase transition

It is possible to maintain two phases at equilibrium at given temperature and pressure. This means that a phase change can be carried out reversibly at constant temperature and pressure. In these conditions,

$\Delta S_{syst} = q$ transition$/T$

(the system being constituted by the substance showing the phase change). In general, transitions are also carried out at constant pressure. No work except the p-V one against the atmosphere is done during the transition. As a result,

q transition $= \Delta H$ transition

$\Delta S_{syst} = \Delta H$ transition$/T$

Chapter 13

Further Considerations on the Meaning of Function Entropy

It is interesting to discuss, even briefly, the significance of the entropy. One excellent reason to do that is the extraordinary, far-reaching significance of this concept.

In this chapter, we focus on its "physical" meaning, that is to say on its practical meaning instead of considering entropy under some mathematical angles as it has been done so far. In the first paragraph, we consider Carnot's cycle, the study of which has aided to define the function entropy in terms of physical variables. In the second paragraph, we relate the fact that it is impossible to fully transform heat into work (whereas the inverse is possible) to the function entropy. Hence, we show that, in some conditions, some heat is unavailable to carry out work and finally that it is a degraded form of energy. Then, we come back to the arguments, coming from experimental physics, which have induced its definition in terms of heat and temperature and which leads to the notions of energies of weak and strong entropy important notions in bioenergetics.

Then, we examine the link between entropy and disorder. In the last part, we begin to consider the concept of entropy with respect to the concept of information theory. This last theory will be widely reconsidered at the end of the book. Finally, we present some values of molecular entropies in order to be familiarized with the order of size of their values. They may permit to better grasp the meaning of the entropy function.

1) Carnot's cycle

A block-diagram of a Carnot's heat-engine is presented in Figure 16. In a cycle carried out by the device, the fluid constituting the system is constituted by 1 mole of an ideal gas. It is contained in a cylinder fitted with a weightless and frictionless piston, thus permitting reversible processes to be performed. The fluid exchanges heat with the two exterior sources at different temperatures. These sources are large reservoirs which remain at the same temperature despite the exchanges of heat. Let T_2 and T_1 be the temperatures of the hot and the cold sources, and q_2 and q_1 the heats exchanged between the system and the sources. From the hotter source at T_2, the system receives the heat q_2 (a positive term) and it gives the heat q_1 to the source at T_1 (a negative quantity). Notice that these directions of the heat changes are the consequence of the second law, more precisely as it has been formulated by Clausius.

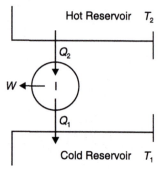

Figure 16. Carnot's cycle.

- Concerning the internal energy balance-sheet, we can say that:
  - $\Delta U = 0$ since the transformation is cyclic,
  - the total change of heat ΔQ is, since there are two sources:

$$\Delta Q = q_1 + q_2$$

  - since there is also exchange of work w and since the process is cyclic, according to the first law:

$$q_1 + q_2 + w = 0 \tag{58}$$

- Concerning the entropy balance-sheet:
  - since the transformation is cyclic, the system comes back to its initial state. Its entropy change is null

$$\Delta S = 0 \tag{59}$$

  - for each exchange of heat:

$$\Delta S_1 = \Delta_e S_1 + \Delta \sigma_1 \tag{60}$$

$$\Delta S_2 = \Delta_e S_2 + \Delta \sigma_2 \tag{61}$$

Since:

$$\Delta S = \Delta S_1 + \Delta S_2 \tag{62}$$

When the transformation is irreversible, the created entropy in a cycle $\Delta \sigma$ is given by:

$$\Delta \sigma = \Delta \sigma_1 + \Delta \sigma_2$$

In the case of a reversible cycle:

$$\Delta \sigma = 0 \tag{63}$$

$$\Delta \sigma_1 = 0 \quad \text{and} \quad \Delta \sigma_2 = 0$$

since $\Delta \sigma_1$ and $\Delta \sigma_2$ can only be positive or null quantities

According to (59), (60), (61), (62),

$$\Delta_e S_1 = -\Delta_e S_2$$

That is to say:

$$\Delta S_1 = -\Delta S_2$$

$$q_{1\,rev}/T_1 + q_{2\,rev}/T_2 = 0 \tag{64}$$

Actually, the relation (63) is the basis of the formal definition of the function entropy (see below):

$$dS = q_{rev}/T$$

Remark: The formalism of relation (63) suggests us to proceed to the analogy: turbine/heat engine, analogy we examine now.

- *In the turbine, the quantity of water entering at the top can be expressed in weight (mg) by the relation:*

  gravitational energy taken in $(mgh_2)/h_2$

  where h_2 is the height of the reservoir. This expression compares favourably with the term taking into account the phenomena developing in a heat-engine:

  thermal energy(heat) taken in/temperature of the reservoir T_2

- *At the height h_1 of the lower point of the turbine, the fluid is expelled with a lower energy, since $h_1 < h_2$. The analogy is all the more judicious as the heat is nothing other than a kinetic energy (see Chapter 1).*

2) Heat is a degraded form of energy

Any quantity of heat cannot be fully transformed into work. Therefore, heat is a degraded form of energy when it is compared to other forms of work. This fact is asserted by considering the transformations of heat into work, when they are carried out:

– in reversible,

– or in irreversible conditions.

To take cognizance of this property, it is judicious to again consider the balance-sheets of energy and entropy in the Carnot's cycle.

2-1) Degradation of the energy in a reversible transformation—Unavailable heat

In order to relate the fact that heat is a degradated form of energy to the entropy, it is sufficient to express w as a function of T_1, T_2 and q_1. According to relation (57):

$$|w_{max}| = + q_{2rev} - |q_{1rev}|$$

and (63)

$$w_{max} = q_{2rev} - q_{2rev}(T_1/T_2)$$

$$w_{max} = q_{2rev}[1 - (T_1/T_2)] \tag{65}$$

This is the relation giving the maximum work, already mentioned in Chapter 10. Recall that the work carried out by the whole system is maximum since the transformation is reversible.

The maximum work performed by the system is equal to the heat it has received from the hot source at T_2 amputated from the quantity $q_{2rev}(T_1/T_2)$ which is obligatorily lower than q_{2rev}.

$$|w| < |q_{2rev}|$$

The part of the heat q_{2rev} (T_1/T_2) is *unavailable* to be transformed into work. It is clear that *through this reasoning, heat appears to be a degradated form energy.*

The unavailable heat occurring in a transformation is related to its entropy change. Now, regarding it during the process occurring at the hot source:

$$q_{2rev}/T_2 = \Delta S_2$$

Injecting this relation into (64), one obtains:

$$w = q_{2rev} - T_1 \, \Delta S_2$$

Given the fact that:

$$\Delta S_2 = -\Delta S_1$$

the following relation is also satisfied:

$$w = q_{2rev} + T_1 \, \Delta S_1 \quad \text{(w and } \Delta S_1 \text{ being negative)}$$

The entropy change, in some sort, quantifies the unavailable energy. It is in relation with the degradation of the heat-energy, even if the process is *reversible*.

2-2) Degradation of heat in an irreversible transformation—Wasted energy

Again, consider the same experiment as above, but now, it is driven in an irreversible manner. Suppose that the system receives heat q_{2irr} at temperature T_2 from the surroundings in an *irreversible* manner, the other heat exchange at T_1 remains *reversible*. The matter here is to compare the irreversible transformation to the previous one. The temperature T_2, T_1, and the heat q_1 are the same as above. The difference is that the heat transfer of q_2 at T_2 is irreversible now. The true heat quantity which is exchanged is $q_{2\,irr}$, with:

$$q_{2irr} < q_{2rev}$$

This is due to the irreversibility of the process. A part of q_{2rev} which would be exchanged is lost, for example by friction. Let us already say that the work $|w'|$ carried out by the system is less than before, since $q_{2irr} < q_{2rev}$.

The entropy change of the surroundings $\Delta S'$ is:

$$\Delta S' = -q_{2irr}/T_2$$

The entropy change ΔS of the system for this exchange is:

$$\Delta S_2 = \Delta_e S_2 + \Delta \sigma_2$$

since the process is irreversible and with $\Delta \sigma_2 > 0$. Actually:

$$\Delta_e S_2 = q_{irr2}/T_2$$

$$\Delta_e S_2 = -\Delta S'$$

$$\Delta S_2 + \Delta S' = \Delta \sigma_2$$

The whole entropy change is:

$$\Delta S = \Delta S_2 + \Delta S_1$$

It is null, since in a complete cycle, reversible or irreversible, the system returns to its original state and, hence, it undergoes no change in its entropy:

$$\Delta S = 0$$

$$\Delta S_2 = -\Delta S_1$$

$$\Delta_e S_2 + \Delta\sigma_2 + \Delta S_1 = 0$$

$$q_{2irr}/T_2 + \Delta\sigma_2 + q_{1rev}/T_1 = 0$$

In the reversible transformation, we found

$$q_{2rev}/T_2 + q_{1rev}/T_1 = 0$$

The work carried out now is:

$$|w'| = q_{2\,irr} - |q_{1rev}|$$

$$|w'| = q_{2irr} - T_2\Delta\sigma_2 - |q_{1rev}|$$

$\Delta\sigma_2$ being obligatorily positive, the result is that:

$$|w'| < |w|$$

We see that there is not only the same unavailable heat as before, but moreover, there is also the supplementary quantity $T_2\Delta\sigma_2$ due to the created entropy which is irremediably wasted.

2-3) Change in entropy of an isolated system and creation of entropy in an irreversible transformation

The preceding considerations permit to establish a relation between these two quantities. We study exactly the same example as in the previous paragraph. To do it, we distinguish the entropy changes at the temperatures T_2 and T_1 (both horizontal lines in Table 6). Moreover, we draw three columns in the same table. In the first one, one considers the entropy changes in the system under study (the heat-engine) at the two temperatures. In the second column, we consider the surroundings of the system, in the same manner. Finally (third column), we regard the isolated system (the "universe") constituted by the system plus its surroundings. Its data are the sum, line by line, of those of the two other columns. All the quantities received by the heat-engine are affected by the positive sign.

Table 6. Change in entropy of an isolated system and creation of entropy in an irreversible process.

system	surroundings	isolated system
$\Delta S_2 = q_{2ir}/T_2 + \Delta\sigma_2$	$\Delta S'_2 = -q_{2ir}/T_2$	$\Delta S_{2isol} = \Delta\sigma_2$
$\Delta S_1 = -q_1/T_1$	$\Delta S'_1 = q_1/T_1$	$\Delta S_{1isol} = 0$

As a result:

$$\Delta S_{isol} = \Delta S_{1isol} + \Delta S_{2isol}$$

$$\Delta S_{isol} = \Delta\sigma_2$$

In an irreversible process, the change in entropy of an isolated system is equal to the created entropy.

In conclusion of this paragraph, we can say that entropy is an index of the capacity for spontaneous change.

2-4) Maximum work performed by a heat engine

Consider a Carnot cycle. The maximum work the heat-engine can carry out is:

$$w_{max} = q_{2rev} - q_{1rev}$$

It is performed in the conditions of reversibility. In these conditions, the overall entropy change is:

$$\Delta S = 0$$

$$q_{2rev}/T_2 = -q_{1rev}/T_1$$

that is to say;

$$|q_{1rev}| = q_{2rev}\, T_1/T_2$$

The maximum work available is:

$$w_{max} = q_{2rev} - q_{2rev}\, T_1/T_2$$

$$w_{max} = q_{2rev}\, (1 - T_1/T_2)$$

The factor $(1 - T_1/T_2)$ which is the fraction of the heat absorbed by the machine which can be transformed into work is its *efficiency*. All reversible heat-engines operating between two given temperatures have the same efficiency. This is Carnot's theorem.

3) On the definition of the entropy in terms of heat and temperature. Energies of "great entropy" and "weak entropy"

Recall that entropy has been defined by Clausius by the relation [see Chapter 11]

$$dS = dq_{rev}/T_{ext}$$

The choice of these two physical quantities came from the consideration of Carnot's cycle (see paragraph 1) which preponderantly has introduced the importance of the ratios q_1/T_1 and q_2/T_2.

It is interesting to notice that when heat is given to the system at high temperature, its entropy increase is lesser than when it is given at colder temperature. In the first case, its energy is of lesser entropy than in the second one. From the standpoint of energetics, an energy of weak entropy is more interesting than one of greater one. This is evident because it is always possible to extract heat from a hotter source than another. Hence, once a hot source has already received some heat, it can, in a second step, still give further heat.

4) Come back on the fact that entropy is a thermodynamic property

The study of the isothermal steps in a Carnot's cycle permits to write:

$$q_2/T_2 + q_1/T_1 = 0$$

or more generally:

$$\Sigma_{cycle}\, q/T = 0$$

This result suggests that S is a state function. Besides, this point has been demonstrated (see Chapter 11). Another demonstration is the following one. Consider the reversible expansion of 1 mole of a perfect gas. We know that in these conditions (see Exercise 11 Chapter 12):

$$dU = đq - pdV$$

$$đq = C_V dT + (RT/V)\, dV$$

The differential đq is inexact. This is confirmed by the consideration of the right-hand side of this equation. It is, indeed, non-integrable because of the presence of the factor T near the differential dV, the direct relation between them being unknown. However, if we divide both sides of the relation by T, we obtain the equation:

$$đq/T = C_V dT/T + (R/V)\, dV$$

It is immediately integrable. It gives the relation:

$$\int đq/T = C_V \ln T + R \ln V + \text{constant}$$

đq/T becomes dq/T

It is clear that the integral only depends on the initial and final states through the values of the variables T and V. The integral is a state function. dq/T is an exact differential even if đq is inexact. (In mathematics, the factor—here $1/T$—which makes the resultant function integrable is named an integration factor).

5) Calculation of entropy changes from thermal data

Such calculations are possible. They are of great theoretical and practical interests. They are not mentioned now because they imply the use of the third law of thermodynamics. They are postponed to Chapter 22.

6) Questions about the meaning of the quantity entropy

6-1) It is possible to obtain one relation in the realm of classical thermodynamics which expresses the function entropy in term of classical variables. It is the entropy of an ideal gas. For the carrying out of its derivation, it is assumed that the transformations the gas undergo are reversible. We have just demonstrated previously that, in these conditions:

$$\int Dq/T = C_V \ln T + R \ln V + \text{constant}$$

or

$$S = C_V \ln T + R \ln V + S_0$$

The integration constant S_0 cannot be obtained from the sole realm of classical thermodynamics.

In any case, this relation, named Sackur and Tetrode's relation, shows that the entropy of a perfect gas depends on its volume and on the temperature in a complex manner.

6-2) Entropy and the atomic theory of matter

The atomic and molecular theories of matter (which classical thermodynamics does not take into account) throw some light on the physical significance of entropy.

6-2-1) Spontaneous processes (such as mixing processes) and entropy

An examination of the various processes spontaneously taking place and which are accompanied with a net increase of entropy shows that they are associated with an increased process of mixing. In most cases, the mixing process is, purely and simply, due to:

– the intermingling of the particles coming from different systems. Due to this phenomenon, there is a spreading of particles over several positions in space, with an increase of the number Ω_1 of their possible arrangements (called complexions) of their location in space;

– the increase of the number Ω_2 of distinguishable micro-states of energy, also called complexions, within a macroscopic system representing the system under study. In statistical thermodynamics, a macro-system is defined by fixed values of some macroscopic variables, such as its energy, volume and the numbers N_i of its different molecules Ω_2 (N_i, E, V). A basic assumption of statistical mechanics is that any of the Ω_2 states (compatible with the values of the variable defining the macrostate) is equiprobable.

Both phenomena of mixing may intervene simultaneously, even sometimes in contradistinction to each other.

The hypothesis, which derives from work of Boltzmann, is that the entropy S is related to its number of complexions Ω by the equation:

$$S = k \ln \Omega \tag{66}$$

k is the Boltzmann's constant.

Let us first say that this relation is demonstrated in the realm of statistical thermodynamics. Secondly, S and Ω are self-consistent. On one hand, they are both functions of the state of the system defined by the variables of the macro-state N_i, U, V. They tend to increase in an irreversible process. Finally, the multiplicative property of the number of complexions Ω is perfectly compatible with the additive properties of entropy. In fact, consider that there are two possibilities of complexions (as above), Ω_1 complexions of the first possibility can be chosen in combination with any of the Ω_2 complexions of the second. The total number of combinations of the system is therefore:

$$\Omega = \Omega_1 \, \Omega_2$$

Taking the logarithm and applying (65):

$$S = k \ln \Omega_1 + k \ln \Omega_2$$

$$S = S_1 + S_2$$

6-2-2) Entropy as a probabilistic quantity

As it has been said above, the relation (65) is demonstrated in the realm of statistical thermodynamics. It is demonstrated within the framework of what is named the canonical macro-state (or ensemble defined by the variables N,V,T). The canonical ensemble is not that corresponding to the conditions of validity of the formula (65) of Boltzmann, which applies to an isolated system.

In the canonical ensemble intervenes the probability P_j that a system (macro-system) is in the state of energy E_j. P_j can be calculated. Then, for the entropy, one obtains the relation:

$$S(N,V,T) = -k \sum_j P_j \ln P_j \qquad \text{(canonical ensemble)} \qquad (67)$$

j being the index of the state. To pass from this canonical ensemble to an isolated system (Boltzmann conditions), it is sufficient, from the standpoint of calculations, to only pick up the systems of the same energy U which are in the initial canonical ensemble. By hypothesis, their number is Ω and $P_j = 1/\Omega$. After replacement, one obtains:

$$S(N,V,E) = k \ln (N,V,E)$$

This reasoning and, overall the relation (66), fully proves the probabilistic nature of the function entropy.

6-2-3) Entropy and disorder

Numerous processes spontaneously taking place are associated with an increased randomness of its distribution, that is to say with an increase of the disorder of the system. For example, the diffusion of one gas into another means that the molecules of both gases become more disordered once mixed than before the process has occurred because then they would be separated. The state of separation consists in the fact that each gas is in separate container which is indeed more ordered than that obtained after intermingling (Cf Maxwell demon Chapter 42). This is the reason why it has been reasonable to postulate a relationship between the entropy of a system and the degree of disorder in a given state.

However, the association entropy/disorder is not perfect for an essential reason which is the fact that the concept of order and disorder is *vague*. It cannot be quantified and hence associated to a numerical value of the entropy. Besides, there exist examples of transformations in which the *order* of the system is increased whereas its entropy also increases!

It is the case, for example, of the crystallisation of a supercooled liquid. If it takes place under adiabatic conditions, the entropy of the resulting crystal becomes greater than that of the supercooled liquid. It is, indeed, difficult to claim that the crystal is more disordered than the initial liquid! The explanation of the paradox lies in an increase of the kinetic energy of the particles during the crystallisation process.

6-2-4) Entropy and information

There exists an entropic theory of information. The association of both concepts— "**lack** of information" + "entropy"—is likely the most pertinent among other ones. This point will be considered again in the Chapter 42.

7) Some molar entropy values—so-called absolute entropy values S_T°

We present some values of molecular entropies. They may permit to better grasp the meaning of the entropy function. There exist in literature numerous values of molar entropies. They are most of the time calculated from thermal data, based on the third principle of thermodynamics (see Chapter 22). We give some values in the Table 7.

Table 7. Absolute entropies $S_T°$ at 298,15 K: J K^{-1} mol^{-1} (according to P.W. Atkins, "Physical Chemistry" 4th edition, general bibliography)

H$_2$	130	C(diamond)	2	C(graphite)	5,6	H$_2$O(l)	69,8	H$_2$O(g)	188,5
CO(g)	197,4	CO$_2$(g)	213,4	CH$_4$(g)	186	C$_2$H$_6$(g)	228	C$_2$H$_4$(g)	220
HCHO(g)	219	glycine(s)	109,1	DL-leucine(s)	206,9				

The adjective absolute be understood with some caution for essentially the following reason. It is not certain at all that all the phenomena which play a part in the entropy value have been taken into account during the calculations, according to the third principle. For example, they do not take into account any change in the nuclear entropies.

Some comments may be done:

– entropy of similar forms of matter (in the same state and at the same temperature) tends to increase with mass as a result of the greater organization of fundamental particles in a large atom compared with many small ones of similar masses;

– molar entropy tends to increase with greater complexity of the molecule, not only on account of a mass effect but also because of more molecular motions. However, it is the converse when there is association of molecules since there is a loss of independent translational motion (of the association) which is not wholly compensated by additional modes of vibration. As a result, entropy decreases;

– entropy increases when substances become mixed or dissolved in one another;

– entropy is the manifestation of molecular motion and, as a consequence, diminishes with temperature.

8) A brief summary of the properties of the entropy and of its implications on the second law

– All real processes are irreversible and when all changes in an isolated system have been taken into account, there is an increase in the entropy of the "Universe";

– the entropy of a circumscribed system, into or out of which heat may flow, may increase or decrease. One more time, the entropy of the system under study must not be confused with that of the isolated system which circumscribes the system under study. The entropy of the latter can only increase or it remains null.

– the entropy change accompanying a transformation is a criterion of its possibility of achievement;

– the second law of thermodynamics points the direction of events in time.

Chapter 14

Free Energy, Free Enthalpy— Helmholtz and Gibbs Energies

Now, we introduce Helmholtz and Gibbs energies, formerly called free energy and free enthalpy. Their utmost importance for our purpose has already been highlighted. Let us just recall that one of the great interests of these two functions is to provide us with a criterion of possibility of spontaneity of a given transformation in certain conditions. A second great interest is the fact that these functions are state functions which are related to equilibrium constants of chemical reactions, here again in some particular conditions. In this chapter, we only consider the first interest. But, before investigating them in some length, it is judicious to briefly define the two functions named free energy and enthalpy versus the external ambience.

1) Monothermal transformation—Free energy and enthalpy related to the surroundings

Transformations are named *monothermal* if the processing system exchanges heat only with one exterior source, the temperature T_{ext} of which being constant. The practical importance of this notion is immense. To take only one example of such a system, let us mention the living organisms. In passing, recall that a process is named *isothermal* if it keeps the same temperature during its course.

1-1) Free energy versus the external ambience

Now, concerning the notion of *free energy* versus the external ambience, let us say that it can be introduced by considering the work ΔW_{rev} received, during a reversible monothermal transformation. ΔW_{rev} received can be considered as a function of the internal energy and entropy changes accompanying the transformation (the external source being at the temperature T_{ext}). According to the first law:

$$\Delta U = \Delta Q + \Delta W$$

and according to the second law:

$$\Delta Q = T_{ext} \, \Delta_e S$$

These relations are valuable if, by hypothesis, the process is reversible:

$$\Delta S = \Delta_e S$$

and

$$\Delta Q = T_{ext} \, \Delta S$$

Finally:

$$\Delta W_{rev} = \Delta U - T_{ext} \Delta S$$

The term ΔW_{rev} represents a change of a state function since it results from a combination of changes in other state functions and of T_{ext}. It is symbolised by A_{ext}.

$$A_{ext} = \Delta U - T_{ext} \Delta S \tag{68}$$

A_{ext} is the *free energy versus the ambience*. The adjective "free" means that it is the part of the internal energy which can be recovered as a work. The term ambience recalls that it depends on the external conditions (T_{ext}).

It can be demonstrated that the work ΔW received by a monothermal system during any process is always greater than the change in the free energy versus the ambience A_{ext}.

$$\Delta W > A_{ext} \tag{69}$$

The demonstration is carried out by taking into account the difference between the entropy changes ΔS and $\Delta_e S$ when the process is reversible in a first place and when the process is not reversible in a second place. For the reversible process:

$$\Delta U = \Delta A_{ext} + T_{ext}\Delta S$$

For an irreversible process:

$$\Delta W = \Delta U - \Delta Q$$

$$\Delta W = \Delta U - T_{ext}\Delta_e S$$

$$\Delta W = \Delta A_{ext} + T_{ext}(\Delta S - \Delta_e S)$$

$$(\Delta S - \Delta_e S) = \Delta \sigma > 0$$

As a result, (68) is satisfied.

1-2) Free enthalpy versus the external ambience

In the work represented by the free energy versus the ambience A_{ext}, two kinds of free energies intervene. One corresponds to the work exchanged with a machine, named the *useful work*, the other to that exchanged with the atmosphere related to the volume changes of the system and to the external pressure p_{ext}.

It is interesting to evaluate the work received by a system, once the one exercised by the external pressure is excluded. We symbolize it as ΔW_R^*. It is directly obtained from A_{ext}. The elementary work dW_p received from the atmosphere is:

$$dW_p = -p_{ext} dV$$

$$dW_R^* = dW_R - dW_p$$

$$dW_R^* = dW_R + p_{ext} dV$$

$$dW_R^* = dU - T_{ext}dS + p_{ext} dV$$

The change of the function:

$$G_{ext} = U - T_{ext}S + p_{ext}V + constant \tag{70}$$

is equal to the work received by the system at the exclusion of that of the exterior pressure. It is called the free enthalpy versus the external ambience.

As before, it is easy to demonstrate that the system receives more useful work when the process is irreversible than when it is reversible for the same identical monothermal process.

1-3) Availability-Exergy

The function $B = [U - T_{ext}S + p_{ext}V + constant]$

is a function of state of the system. U denotes the total energy of the system. B is called the *availability* of the system. Hence:

$$-W_R^* = -(B_2 - B_1)$$

A somewhat similar function to the availability is called the *exergy* of the system. The exergy is defined through the following relation in which the symbol Λ is introduced:

$$\Lambda = U - T_0S + P_0V + constant$$

U denotes the total energy. T_0 and V_0 refer to the system when it has attained equilibrium with the medium.

For a reversible change of the system, from the state 1 to the state 2, the useful obtained work is:

$$w_{u,max} = -\int_1^2 d\Lambda$$

$$w_{u,max} = \Lambda_1 - \Lambda_2$$

or:

$$-W_R^* = -(B_2 - B_1)$$

When the system is in complete equilibrium with the reservoir, its temperature and pressure are therefore T_0 and P_0. It can no longer provide useful energy. It is said to be relaxed. Then $U = U_0$, $S = S_0$ and $V = V_0$. If we choose the above integration constant such as:

$$constant = -(E_0 - T_0S_0 + P_0V_0)$$

the function Λ becomes:

$$\Lambda = (U - U_0) - T_0(S - S_0) + P_0(V - V_0)$$

In these conditions, Λ is the exergy of the system.

The exergy of a thermodynamic system related to a reservoir at defined pressure and temperature is the maximum useful work $w_{u\,max}$ that can be performed by the system without inducing any permanent change in the thermodynamic state of any other system, except the reservoir. According to what has been said previously, it is the maximum mechanical work which may be obtained when a system changes between assigned initial and final states and when the other body which undergoes an overall gain or loss of heat and change of volume is the medium.

(The useful work is that given to the surroundings of the system reduced of the work necessary to the expansion of the system. As a consequence, the chosen reservoir must be sufficiently vast in order for its interaction with the system to only induce infinitesimal changes in its intensive properties).

2) Helmholtz energy

2-1) Generalities

Formerly, this function was named *free energy*. Its symbol is A. It is different from the free energy versus the external ambience A $_{ext}$. The difference between both is that, in the former (Helmholtz energy), the system is constrained to keep the same temperature as that of the surroundings for each infinitesimal transformation, that is to say:

$$T \text{ (system)} = T_{ext}$$

As a result, the free energy versus the ambience:

$$A_{ext} = \Delta U - T_{ext} \, \Delta S$$

becomes the function A:

$$A = U - TS \tag{71}$$

All the quantities involved in this relation are those of the system. It is evident that A is a thermodynamic function as a result of its definition. It exhibits the same properties than A_{ext}, of which it is a particular case. Let us clarify this point.

For the change of the system between states i (initial) and f (final), we can write from (70):

$$A_f - A_i = U_f - U_i - (T_f S_f - T_i S_i) \tag{72}$$

For a closed system:

$$U_f - U_i = q + w$$

and:

$$A_f - A_i = q + w - (T_f S_f - T_i S_i)$$

Now, consider the case in which, on one hand, the heat transferred comes from a reservoir at the constant temperature T, and on the other, the initial and final temperatures T_i and T_f are equal and are also equal to T,

$$T_i = T_f = T$$

$$A_f - A_i = q + w - T (S_f - S_i)$$

$$A_f - A_i = q + w - T \Delta S$$

The transformation may be reversible or irreversible. To take into account both cases, we must consider the two following cases:

$$q \leq T \, \Delta S$$

according to the second law. Therefore:

$$-w \leq - (A_f - A_i)$$

w is the work done on the system. Thus –w is the work done by the system.

The work –w done by a system during a process in which the initial and final temperatures are equal to that of the reservoir is either less than or equal to the Helmholtz energy A change accompanying it. The change in A is therefore a measure of the maximum attainable work under the mentioned conditions. The maximum is given by the relation:

$$-w_{max} = -(A_f - A_i)$$

2-2) Helmholtz energy and the internal energy

Relation (71) may be written:

$$-\Delta U = -\Delta A - T\Delta S$$

Inspection of it shows that the decrease in the internal energy ΔU of the system may be considered as being composed of two parts, the Helmholtz energy decrease $-\Delta A$ and the quantity $-T\Delta S$.

This latter may be considered as a quantity of energy wasted, since we have seen that in a reversible isothermal change, it is equal to the heat exchanged (see the definition of the entropy).

2-3) Helmholtz energy as a criterion of equilibrium and as a potential thermodynamic function

We know that at constant temperature:

$$-dw \leq -dA$$

If no work is performed,

$$dA \leq 0$$

As a result, the Helmholtz energy can only decrease or remain constant. This is the case of systems at constant temperature and volume, such as a system enclosed in a rigid container, held at constant temperature.

When A is minimum,

$$dA = 0$$

the system cannot evolve further. It is at equilibrium. The Helmholtz energy is a criterion of equilibrium, provided, of course, that the conditions in which it is used (constant temperature and volume) are adapted to this function.

The Helmholtz energy is a potential function of thermodynamics. One function is named potential if it is endowed with the following two characteristics:
- its changes represent the work received by a system;
- its value cannot do anything else but to decrease in the conditions in which it is used as a potential function.

Both points have been developed just above.

2-4) Volume and temperature coefficients of the thermodynamic Helmholtz energy function

An easy demonstration shows that the volume and temperature coefficients of Helmholtz energy function are respectively equal to the pressure and entropy with an inverted sign:

$(\partial A/\partial V)_T = -p$ and $(\partial A/\partial T)_V = -S$

The demonstration is the following one:

$A = U - TS$

$dA = dU - TdS - SdT$

taking only account of the expansion work:

$dA = dq - pdV - TdS - SdT$

and with a reversible process:

$dq = TdS$

$dA = -pdV - SdT$

A being a state function (see mathematical appendix II-5):

$dA = (\partial A/\partial V)_T dV + (\partial A/\partial T)_V dT$

The identification of the last two equations leads to the coefficients given above.

3) Gibbs energy function

3-1) Generalities

Formerly, it was named *free enthalpy*. Its symbol is G. It is different from the free energy versus the external world G_{ext}. The difference between both is that, in the former, the system is constrained to keep the same temperature **as** the surroundings for each infinitesimal transformation, that is to say:

$T \text{ (system)} = T_{ext}$ and $p(\text{system}) = p_{ext}$

and also to be at the same pressure as the surroundings. As a result, the Gibbs energy versus exterior G_{ext}:

$G_{ext} = U - T_{ext}S + p_{ext}V$

becomes the function G defined by the relation:

$$G = U - TS + pV \tag{73}$$

Let us clarify its meaning. For a change between initial and final states (i and f), the difference between the Gibbs energies is:

$$G_f - G_i = (U_f - U_i) + (p_f V_f - p_i V_i) - (T_f S_f - T_i f_i) \tag{74}$$

For a closed system:

$U_f - U_i = q + w$

and:

$G_f - G_i = q + w + (p_f V_f - p_i V_i) - (T_f S_f - T_i f_i)$

When

- the only heat transferred to the system is from a reservoir which remains at the constant temperature T,
- the initial and final temperatures of the system T_i and T_f are equal and, moreover, are equal to that of the reservoir T,
- the only body which has undergone a volume change is the surroundings' fluid (atmosphere), this change being carried out at the constant pressure p,
- the initial and final pressures p_i and p_f are equal and are equal to p,

the change in the Gibbs energy is given by the expression:

$$G_f - G_i = q + w + p(V_f - V_i) - T(S_f - S_i)$$

The difference $S_f - S_i$ is the entropy change during the process whether it is reversible or not (entropy is a thermodynamic property). We know that:

$$q \leq T(S_f - S_i)$$

Hence:

$$-w - p(V_f - V_i) \leq -(G_f - G_i)$$

The term $p(V_f - V_i)$ is the work done by the system against its surroundings by displacement at the constant pressure p. Usually, this is not the whole work $-w$ done by the system. Hence, we can introduce a new kind of work $-w'$ such as:

$$-w = -w' + p(V_f - V_i)$$

By handling the latter two relations, we find:

$$-w' \leq -(G_f - G_i) \tag{75}$$

In the given conditions, the work done by the system (not including that of displacement of the surroundings) $-w'$, sometimes called the *useful work*, is either less than or equal to the decrease of the Gibbs function of the system. The change in G is therefore a measure of the maximum attainable useful work under the mentioned conditions. The maximum is given by the relation:

$$-w'_{max} = -(G_f - G_i)$$

By way of examples, let us consider the three following cases, after having setting up $\Delta G = -(G_f - G_i)$:

- $(G_f - G_i)$ positive. The corresponding transformation can occur spontaneously. It is the case of hydrolysis of adenosine triphosphate (ATP—see Chapter 31). The simplified reaction written:

    Adenine-ribose $-P-P-P$ (1 mol L^{-1}) + H_2O →

    Adenine-ribose $-P-P$ (1 mol L^{-1} + HPO_4^{2-} (1 mol L^{-1})

occurs spontaneously in the presence of a suitable catalyst. Its standard Gibbs energy is $\Delta_r G = -29,3$ kJ mol^{-1}. Notice that in this reaction reactants and products are at the concentrations retained for the *standard states (see Chapter 19)*. As a result, the reactional Gibbs energy $\Delta_r G$ is the standard reactional Gibbs energy: $\Delta_r G = \Delta_r G°$

•• Let us now consider the following reaction used in the synthesis of a peptide bond:

benzoyltyrosine (1 mol L^{-1}) + glycinamide (1 mol L^{-1}) →

benzoyltyrosylglycinamide (1 mol L^{-1}) + H_2O

Its standard Gibbs energy is weakly positive $\Delta_r G° = + 1,76\,kJ\,mol\,L^{-1}$. *The peptide synthesis does not occur spontaneously.*

••• Now, consider the reaction:

benzoyltyrosine (0,025 mol L^{-1}) + glycinamide (0,025 mol L^{-1}) →

benzoyltyrosylglycinamide (0,00032 mol L^{-1}) + H_2O

$\Delta_r G = 0$ kJ mol^{-1}. The reaction is at equilibrium. It is interesting to compare this case with the preceding one. We can notice that the difference lies in the concentration values of the species.

3-2) Gibbs energy and enthalpy

Let us consider relation (72) or (73) and remember that enthalpy is defined by:

$H = U + pV$

As a result, the Gibbs function can also be defined by the expression:

$G = H - TS$ $\hspace{4cm}$ (76)

3-3) Gibbs energy as a criterion of equilibrium and as potential thermodynamic function.

For an infinitesimal change at constant temperature and pressure, it is clear from (72) that:

$-dw' \leq -dG$

If, moreover, dw' = 0,

$dG \leq 0$

During a process, the Gibbs energy of a system can only decrease or remain constant. (This is the case of systems at constant temperature and pressure).

Under the conditions required for the judicious use of function G, the criterion of equilibrium of a process is that it has attained its minimum value. Like the Helmholtz energy, the Gibbs function is also a potential function of thermodynamics.

3-4) Pressure and temperature coefficients of the thermodynamic Gibbs energy function

The following demonstration shows that the pressure and temperature coefficients of the Gibbs free energy are respectively equal to the volume and to the entropy affected by the minus sign:

$(\partial G/\partial p)_T = V$ and $(\partial G/\partial T)_p = -S$

Consider the definition:

$G = U + pV - TS$

or

$dG = dU + pdV + Vdp - TdS - SdT$

if only a "pV work" is occurring,

$dU = dq - pdV$

$dG = dq - pdV + pdV + Vdp - TdS - SdT$

If the process is reversible:

$dq = TdS$

$dG = Vdp - SdT$

Remembering that G is a thermodynamic property:

$dG = (\partial G/\partial T)_p dT + (\partial G/\partial P)_T dp$

By identification of the two last relations, one obtains the relations already given.

4) Relationships between Helmholtz and Gibbs energies

According to their definitions, it is evident that:

$G = A + pV$

It is interesting to notice that there are some analogies between the Helmholtz and Gibbs energies. One can remark that A is related to V whereas G is related to p. One can also find that by exchanging A for G and V for p, the equations involving A and V can be converted into analogous ones relating G and p. However, in such an operation, there is a change in a sign. This is due to the fact that an increase of pressure corresponds to a decrease of the pressure.

Let us already mention that the Gibbs energy is more useful for the chemists and biochemists than the Helmholtz energy.

5) Gibbs energy and phase changes

Finally, let us mention that the Gibbs energy function is useful for the study of equilibria between phases.

In brief, Helmholtz and Gibbs energies constitute criteria of possibility of spontaneous evolution of a process and also criteria of the establishment of their equilibrium. If they are less general than that of the entropy evolution of an isolated system because of the conditions involved by the free energy functions, they are by far easier to handle than the former. They, indeed, omit any reference to changes in the surroundings of the studied system, since they are only defined in terms of quantities characterizing the latter.

It is important to insist that the developments given so far apply only in cases of closed systems.

6) Exergonic and endergonic reactions

Reactions which have a negative standard free energy change are said to be exergonic. A reaction which has a positive standard free energy change is not spontaneous and cannot go completion under standard conditions, unless energy is supplied to it. Such a reaction (more generally such a process) is called endergonic. Exergonic reactions are also called "downhill" reactions and endergonic reactions "uphill" ones. We shall see numerous examples of both kinds of reactions in the following chapters.

Chapter 15

Open and Closed Systems–Different Expressions of the Composition of a Solution

So far, we were rather concerned by processes evolving in the realm of pure physics. In fact, these thermodynamic considerations were necessary to introduce chemical thermodynamics which, as it stands, can be considered as being a particular realm for applying the general principles of thermodynamics. Hence, our considerations in thermodynamics are yet to be arrived at a turning point.

Overall, bioenergetics is concerned by chemical reactions carried out in particular conditions which are those of the life. In brief, they are biochemical reactions. They, of course, involve the participation of chemical species which may appear or disappear during the studied transformation. As a result, considering closed systems only, as it has been the case up to now, is not sufficient for the study of bioenergetics. This is the reason why we now begin to tackle open systems.

In the first paragraph of this chapter, we clarify the notions of closed and open systems. In the second, we recall some expressions of the composition of a solution.

1) Closed and open systems

The theory which has been developed so far is only applicable to closed systems. Recall that closed systems are those which can exchange energy (heat and work) with the environment, but the transfer of matter through their boundaries is impossible.

Open systems are those which can exchange both energy and matter with their surroundings. (In passing, notice that systems which would permit exchanges of matter without permitting exchanges of energy are not conceivable. This is, indeed, because some kinds of energy are always associated with matter).

As a result, all the relations such as the following ones (non-exhaustive list):

$dU = dq + dw$

$dS \geq dq/T$

$dU = TdS - pdV$

$dG = -SdT + Vdp$

are no longer applicable to open systems and even to some closed systems which undergo irreversible changes of composition after, for example, a chemical or biochemical reaction. (More details are given in Chapter 20: see the "Gibbs-Duhem relationship").

It is intuitive that an increase (or a decrease) of the amount of a species present in a system may induce a change in its Gibbs function. This is the reason why it is necessary, before studying such systems, to know the principal expressions of their compositions.

2) Different expressions of the composition of a solution

We confine ourselves to the study of the expressions of the composition of solutions for the reason that in cells, biochemical reactions of bioenergetics take place in solution.

The composition of a liquid solution expresses the relative proportions of the solutes and of the solvent in the solution. Among the most usual expressions let us mention:
- the total number of a species i: N_i. It is a large dimensionless number. This is the reason why one rather uses the number of moles,
- the number of moles n_i. The unity is the mole, symbol mol. The number of moles is related to its number of species through the Avogadro number N_A (or L) by the relation:

$$n_i = N_i / N_A$$

- the density number C_i or ρ_i is the number of molecules per unit volume:

$$C_i = N_i / V$$

It is expressed in m^{-3}. Actually, this expression of the composition is mainly used in statistical thermodynamics. ρ_i is then the most often used symbol;
- the molarity, also called amount of concentration (IUPAC), is expressed by the symbol c_i. It is the number of moles related to the volume V of the solution:

$$c_i = n_i / V$$

In SI units, it is expressed in mol m^{-3}. For practical reasons, it is often replaced by the number of moles per dm^3 or moles per liter. A solution 1 mol L^{-1} is often called a molar solution and is often written: solution 1M. The symbol [i] is very often encountered instead of c_i;
- the molality. It is the number of moles of solute i per kilogram of pure solvent. Its symbol is m_i. In the SI system, it is expressed in mol kg^{-1}. Let n_i be the number of moles of solute i dissolved in the mass m_o of pure solvent. The molality m_i is:

$$m_i = n_i / m_o$$

The molality is essentially used in physical chemistry. This unity offers the advantage to be independent of the temperature;
- the molar fraction. it is the ratio of the number of moles of the solute and of the total number of moles in the solution. Its symbol is x. If in a binary solution, n_o is the number of moles of the solvent and n_1 that of the solute, their molar fractions are, respectively:

$$x_0 = n_0 / (n_0 + n_1) \qquad x_1 = n_1 / (n_0 + n_1)$$

Molar fractions are dimensionless quantities. They are very often used in thermodynamics.

Remark: Pathways from molar fractions to the molalities and the molarities.

These pathways are not obvious to establish. However, in some cases, their knowledge may be interesting. We confine ourselves to give the relations between them. Doing that, we show at the same time that in diluted aqueous solutions, the solute molality value of a species differs very little from its molarity and the more diluted the solution is, the truer this assertion.

Let us compare the expressions of the composition in substance A of an aqueous solution.

- One can demonstrate that concerning the relation between the molar concentration and its fraction molar, it is (see appendix I-1):

$$c_A = (1000 \, \rho \, \Sigma n_i / \Sigma n_i M_i) \, x_A$$

This relation is exact. c_A and x_A are, respectively, its molarity and its molar fraction. n_i and M_i are the number of moles and the molar masses of all the species in solution, M_0 being the molar mass of the solvent. ρ is the volumic mass of the solution. We notice that c_A and x_A are not proportional. However, if the solution is sufficiently diluted:

$$\Sigma n_i M_i \approx n_0 M_0$$

and:

$$\Sigma n_i \approx n_0$$

As a result:

$$c_A = (1000 \, \rho / M_0) \, x_A$$

and finally for water at room temperature $\rho \approx 1$:

$$c_A = (1000 / M_0) \, x_A$$

There is now proportionality.

- Now, concerning the relation between the molality and the molar fraction, one obtains:

$$m_A = (\Sigma n_i \, 1000 / n_0 M_0) x_A$$

Again, there is no proportionality. For the same reasons as before, after simplification, one obtains finally:

$$m_A = (1000 / M_0) \, x_A$$

whence:

$$m_A = c_A \, \text{(aqueous solutions, sufficiently diluted, room temperature)}$$

Chapter 16

Escaping Tendency–Gibbs Energy Change Accompanying a Reaction Between Perfect Gases

Biochemical reactions, which are at the heart of bioenergetics, obey the same rules as the chemical ones, although they evolve in somewhat still more restrained conditions than the latter. Hence, it is not surprising that chemical thermodynamics will, therefore, occupy us up to the end of the book.

We begin with the notion of escaping tendency which qualitatively summarizes the chemical and biochemical reactivities. Next, we investigate the Gibbs energy change accompanying a first kind of chemical reactions: that of a reaction taking place between perfect gases. This study involves the definition of the molar Gibbs energy of a substance, especially of a gas.

At first sight, the study of reactions between perfect gases does not seem to be of great interest for us given the fact that biochemical reactions of bioenergetics take place in cells, in particular, in solution. However, in our opinion, such a study is interesting, at least from the educational standpoint. These considerations, indeed, constitute the first step driving towards the concept of chemical potential and of chemical equilibrium... nothing less!

1) The escaping tendency

The expression *escaping tendency* is due to G.N. Lewis. It is the tendency of a substance to leave its thermodynamic state by either a chemical or a physical process (see the following paragraph). Now, we give some examples for which the escaping tendency occurs.

As a first one, we consider the system composed by water and ice. It is judicious to say that the escaping tendency of the chemical substance "water" in both phases is the same at the fusion point. Indeed, at this point the system is at equilibrium. The system does not evolve. There is no effect of escaping tendency at equilibrium. At lower temperature, we can consider that the escaping tendency of liquid water is larger than that of ice, since liquid water disappears by crystallisation. It spontaneously changes its thermodynamic state. The inverse is true for temperatures higher than the fusion point.

As another example, consider the escaping tendency that a substance exhibits when it leaves its thermodynamic state by spontaneously entering into a chemical reaction. Then, its escaping tendency is objected by a modification of its moles number.

Quite evidently, at constant temperature and pressure, the escaping tendency of a substance must be closely related to the decrease of the Gibbs energy of the system, which commands the spontaneous process.

2) The molar Gibbs energy of a substance as a measure of the escaping tendency

Let us again consider the example of the system water-ice at 0°C, under 1 atm. Owing to the fact that the system is at constant pressure and temperature, it is pertinent to it is pertinent to use the Gibbs energies. With the aid of the Gibbs energies of both phases which are composed by a pure substance. The status of thermodynamic potential conferred to the Gibbs function permits to rationalize the evolution of the process.

Consider the transformation:

H_2O (solid, 1 atm) → H_2O (liquid, 1 atm)

and its inverse. Let ΔG be the change in Gibbs energy accompanying it:

$\Delta G = G(liq) - G(s)$

At equilibrium, at the melting point, under the pressure of 1 atm:

$G(liq) = G(s)$

At a temperature higher than that existing at equilibrium, ice disappears. This indicates that:

$G(s) > G(liq)$

and conversely at lower temperature:

$G(liq) > G(s)$

Hence, the molar Gibbs energy may be used to quantify the escaping tendency of a substance, exactly as it is the case of the variables' pressure and temperature. This point has been shown here in the case of a physical process.

In the case of a chemical transformation, several substances in the system obligatorily play a part. It remains to relate their Gibbs energies changes to the thermodynamic parameters of the system.

3) Change of the molar Gibbs energy of a perfect gas with pressure

A first step which must be carried out in order to grasp the relationship between Gibbs energies and some thermodynamic parameters of the system is to consider the simple case of perfect gases.

A perfect gas obeys the state equation (see Chapter 9)

$pV = nRT$

Let us study the infinitesimal isothermal expansion of a pure perfect gas. We know that (see Chapter 14):

$dG = Vdp - SdT$

At constant temperature:

$dG = Vdp$

and from the state equation:

$dG = nRTdp/p$

For a process consisting in a change of pressure from p_A to p_B:

$\Delta G = G_B - G_A$

$\Delta G = nRT \int_{pA}^{pB} dp/p$

$\Delta G = nRT \ln (p_B/p_A)$

The Gibbs energy of a perfect gas at a given temperature depends on its pressure. Notice that since the system is a mixture, the pressures p_A, p_B ....of the gases are called *partial pressures*.

A very important point in the development of the framework of chemical thermodynamics is that the absolute value of the Gibbs energy of a substance is not accessible. Only its changes can be measured. This is a consequence of the very definition of the Gibbs energy in terms of enthalpy and entropy.

Owing to this fact, the Gibbs energy of a gas is usually related to that $G°$ it possesses in a state named "standard state" in which its pressure is $p°$. *The standard state is arbitrarily chosen.* (Notice in passing that the temperature is not an element of definition of a standard state). Therefore, the molar Gibbs energy G of a perfect gas is given by the relation:

$G = G° + RT \ln (p/p°)$ \hfill (77)

Quasi-systematically, the pressure chosen for the standard state is $p° = 1$ atm or 1 bar (see Chapter 19). Thus, its molar Gibbs energy is written:

$G = G° + RT \ln (p/1)$

This is a relation in which 1 stands for 1 atm (in principle now 1 bar). 1 is has a dimension. It is even written as:

$G = G° + RT \ln p$

This last writing is fallacious since, from a pure mathematical standpoint, a logarithm cannot be dimensioned. Under this form, it appears to be the case!

4) Gibbs energy change accompanying a reaction between perfect gases

Let us now consider the following *chemical reaction* going to completion:

$v_M M + v_L L \rightarrow v_N N + v_P P$

v_M ..... v_P are the stoichiometric coefficients. Our goal is to calculate the maximal work which can be done by the system constituted by the four gases at constant temperature and pressure, through a chemical reaction between them. This calculation may be performed by using the Gibbs energy function. In fact, the maximal work available is equal (in absolute values) to the change in the Gibbs energy accompanying the process, which is the chemical reaction.

The reasoning consists in setting up this change equal to the sum of the Gibbs energies of the substances N and P (the sole presence of which defines the final state—the reaction is supposed complete to simplify the reasoning) minus the sum of the Gibbs energies of M and L (constituting the initial state). The reactional Gibbs energy change $\Delta_r G_{syst}$ is given by the relation:

$$\Delta G_{syst} = v_N G_N + v_P G_P - v_M G_M - v_L G_L$$

Since the system is constituted by the reactants and the products of a chemical reaction, we adopt the recommended symbolism:

$$\Delta_r G = v_N G_N + v_P G_P - v_M G_M - v_L G_L \tag{78}$$

where G_M and G_L are the molar Gibbs energies in the initial state and G_N and G_P those of N and P in the final state.

The second step of the reasoning consists in replacing the G_N, G_P, G_M, G_L in relation (77) by their expressions (76).

It is very important to notice, at this point of the reasoning, that relation (76) can be used because the process concerns perfect gases which, in mixtures, exhibit the property that their behavior is the same as that they show when they are alone. This is a recurrent property which is taken into account as soon as perfect gases are under study.

Hence, after replacements, we obtain:

$$\Delta_r G = -\Delta_r G^\circ + RT \ln [p_N^{vN} p_P^{vP}/p_M^{vM} p_L^{vL}] \tag{79}$$

with:

$$\Delta_r G^\circ = (v_N G^\circ_N + v_P G^\circ_P - v_L G^\circ_L - v_M G^\circ_M)$$

after having systematically adopted the value 1 bar for each standard pressure.

At a given temperature, it is evident that $\Delta_r G^\circ$ is a constant, once the choice of the standard states is given.

Now, let us slightly anticipate what is following. Now, we make the hypothesis that the investigated reaction does not go to completion. This means that the equilibrium at a certain extent of the reaction is attained. Then, the reaction does not evolve further. The reasoning remains the same as when there was completion. The formalism also sensibly remains the same except the fact that pressures in relation (78) are those of the different substances present at equilibrium:

$$\Delta_r G = -\Delta_r G^\circ + RT \ln [p_N^{vN} p_P^{vP}/p_M^{vM} p_L^{vL}]_{eq}$$

Since there is equilibrium, the reasoning can be continued further. At equilibrium:

$$\Delta_r G = 0$$

and

$$RT \ln [p_N^{vN} p_P^{vP}/p_M^{vM} p_L^{vL}]_{eq} = \Delta_r G^\circ$$

$$RT \ln [p_N^{vN} p_P^{vP}/p_M^{vM} p_L^{vL}]_{eq} = \text{constant}$$

This is a quantitative relationship between the number of moles of the reactants and products present at equilibrium.

This is the first step towards the notion of equilibrium constant.

Chapter 17

Partial Molar Quantities–Chemical Potential

Once we study the changes in thermodynamic quantities accompanying chemical reactions, the question of the physical interpretation of the measured value may happen. In any case, it is set up as soon as species intervene in solutions as reactants or (and) products. The problem is overcome through the handling of partial molar quantities. We focus ourselves on the chemical potential which is a partial molar quantity. We shall demonstrate later that this notion is a pivotal one in chemical thermodynamics.

1) The need for new variables for systems of variable compositions

Until Chapter 14, we have seen that two variables alone may be sufficient to fix the state of a system. This can be true for bodies of fixed composition. For example, the equation:

$$dU = TdS - pdV \tag{80}$$

called the "fundamental equation for a closed system", shows that the two variables S and V are sufficient in order to describe a closed system (see Chapter 11). This is the case, among other examples, of an homogeneous phase in which there are k different substances, the number of moles $n_1, n_2, n_3 \ldots n_i \ldots n_k$ of which being constant. There is therefore no change in its composition. As a result of this constancy, the internal energy U of the system (the phase) depends only on S and V. However, for variable composition, U depends not only on S and V but also on the n_i, and even on more substance(s) if new ones are formed.

In this case, we admit that the total differential of U can be written:

$$dU = (\partial U/\partial S)_{T,ni} dS + (\partial U/\partial V)_{S,ni} dV + \Sigma_i (\partial U/\partial n_i)_{S,nj,V} dn_i \tag{81}$$

Some authors regard this equation as being a postulate. Since for a constant composition (the $dn_i = 0$), relation (79) is still valid. Hence, we can write:

$$dU = TdS - pdV + \Sigma_i (\partial U/\partial n_i)_{S,nj,V} dn_i$$

Let us anticipate the fact that the partial derivatives $(\partial U/\partial n_i)_{S,nj,V}$ have the special symbol μ_i and bring the name of *chemical potential of substance i*. Hence Equation (80) becomes:

$$dU = TdS - pdV + \Sigma_i \mu_i dn_i \tag{82}$$

An analogous reasoning as that followed above is brought about concerning the total differential of the Gibbs energy when there exists a change of composition in the system or when it is no longer closed. For example, the relation:

$$dG = -SdT + Vdp$$

which entails a mechanical work as the only one developed (see Chapter 13) is not convenient when the matter quantity varies during the course of the transformation. It must be replaced by the equation:

$$dG = -SdT + Vdp + \Sigma_i (\partial G/\partial n_i)_{T,p,nj} \, dn_i$$

Let us still anticipate the fact that the new partial derivatives *also* define the corresponding chemical potentials:

$$(\partial G/\partial n_i)_{T,p,nj} = \mu_i$$

and:

$$dG = -SdT + Vdp + \Sigma_i \mu_i \, dn_i \tag{83}$$

It is interesting, now, to ask the question: why no supplementary partial derivative has been previously introduced in order to take into account the composition change during the chemical reaction between perfect gases? The answer has already be given. It is because in a mixture of perfect gases, a perfect gas exhibits the same behavior as it would be alone. It is also the case when each of the reactants or products constitutes an independent phase.

2) On the necessity to introduce the partial molar quantities when the species are in solution

- In order to set up the problem, let us consider the chemical reaction:

$$Ag(s) + 1/2 \, Cl_2(g) \rightarrow AgCl(s)$$

where (s) and (g) mean solid and gaseous states. Let us focalize on the volume change accompanying the reaction and define the system as being constituted by the chemical substances and by the container. The whole volume V is given by the relation:

$$V = V_{Ag} + V_{Cl2} + V_{AgCl} + V_{(container)}$$

We are interested in the volume change $\partial V/\partial n$ of the system per mole of silver consumed, n being the number of moles of silver. We can write:

$$\partial V/\partial n = \partial V_{Ag}/\partial n + \partial V_{Cl2}/\partial n + \partial V_{AgCl}/\partial n$$

since $V_{(container)}$ is constant. Among the derivatives of the right-hand member, none exhibits any difficulty of interpretation. Each represents the molar volume of the substance, that is to say its molar volume when it is pure. Notice that this is the case because each reactant or product constitutes a pure phase. For each phase, indeed, one can write:

$$V = nv^\bullet$$

where $v^\bullet$ represents the molar volume. It is evident that:

$$\partial V/\partial n = v^\bullet$$

As a result, for the whole system:

$\partial V / \partial n = v^{\bullet}(AgCl) - v^{\bullet}(Ag) - 1/2 v^{\bullet}(Cl_2)$

There is no problem of meaning for that example.

- Now, let us consider the following reaction:

$\frac{1}{2} H_2(g) + AgCl(s) \rightarrow HCl(m) + Ag(s)$

where m is the molality of HCl being in solution. In passing, this reaction is the global reaction of the following well-known electrochemical cell:

$H_2 | HCl(m) | AgCl | Ag$

It may be interesting to know the effect of the pressure on the electromotive force of this cell, that is to say the effect of the pressure on the Gibbs energy change accompanying the reaction cell (see Chapter 27). In order to determine it, we use the general expression of the change in Gibbs energy with pressure at constant temperature (see Chapter 14):

$(\partial G / \partial p)_T = V$

and for the reaction cell:

$(\partial \Delta G / \partial p)_T = \Delta V$

To know the effect of the pressure on the efm of the cell requires to know the volume V of the system and its change as it is indicated by the last two relations:

$V = V_{H2} + V_{AgCl} + V_{HCl\,(solution)} + V_{Ag}$

The volume change per mole of consumed silver $\partial V / \partial n$ is:

$\partial V / \partial n = \partial V_{H2} / \partial n + \partial V_{AgCl} / \partial n + \partial V_{HCl\,(solution)} / \partial n + \partial V_{Ag} / \partial n$

It is clear that the meaning of the derivative $\partial V_{HCl\,(solution)} / \partial n$ remains to be clarified. Here is the problem.

Let us symbolize it by $\overline{v}_{HCl}$.

$\overline{v}_{HCl} = \partial V_{HCl\,(solution)} / \partial n$

As we shall see it in the next paragraph, $\overline{HCl}$ is the partial molar volume of hydrochloric acid at the molality m in the solution. The change $\overline{\Delta V}$ in the volume of the system when one mole of silver has disappeared is given by the relation:

$\overline{\Delta V} = v^{\bullet}(Ag) + \overline{v}_{HCl} - 1/2\, v^{\bullet}(H_2) - v^{\bullet}(AgCl)$

3) Definition of partial molar quantities

According to the previous considerations, it is evident that the relations between the thermodynamic functions X and the variables playing a part in their values must take into account a supplementary kind of variables at least to describe some conditions, that is to say, in the present case, the number of moles of the constituents.

From the mathematical standpoint, the partial molar quantity $\overline{X}_i$ is defined as being its partial derivative with respect to its number of moles n_i, other variables being constant:

$\overline{X}_i = (\partial X / \partial n_i)_{\text{other variables}}$

Its unity is, of course, that of the considered quantity. The introduction of partial molar quantities permits to regard thermodynamic quantities as being function of different variables which command their values, in particular in the case of open systems. For example, the total differential of the Gibbs energy of an open system is written:

$$dG = (\partial G/\partial T)_{p, ni} \, dT + (\partial G/\partial p)_{T,ni} \, dp + (\partial G/\partial n_i)_{T,p,nj} \, dn_i + (\partial G/\partial n_j)_{T,p,ni} \, dn_j + \ldots .$$

or:

$$dG = (\partial G/\partial T)_{p, ni} \, dT + (\partial G/\partial p)_{T,ni} \, dp + \overline{X}_i \, dn_i + \overline{X}_j \, dn_j + \ldots .$$

An important point is the following one. According to what is preceding the "great" functions of thermodynamics, U, G, H, A … can be formally written as:

$U = U(S,V, n_1,n_2 \ldots)$

$G = G(T,P, n_1,n_2\ldots)$

$H = H(S,p,n_1,n_2\ldots)$

$A = A(T,V,n_1,n_2\ldots)$ and so forth.

The variables written with each function are not associated with it randomly. When one set of variables is known (those above facing the function), all the other thermodynamic quantities are accessible. It is not the case with another set. The variables constituting a specific set are named the natural variables of the function.

4) Physical meaning of the partial molar quantities

Let us take the example of the volume of a solution to grasp the physical meaning of a partial molar quantity.

Let us consider a binary solution and the components 1 and 2 be, respectively, the solvent and the solute. (Notice already that, in the following theory, the solvent and the solute play exactly the same part). Their initial numbers of moles are n_1 and n_2 and the initial total volume is V_0. By successively adding some quantities of solute to the solution, its total volume V changes. Let us draw the diagram V as a function of n_2 (Figure 17). The partial molar volume $\overline{V}_2$ is defined by:

$$\overline{V}_2 = (\partial V/\partial n_2)_{n1, \, n'2}$$

It is nothing different from the slope of the curve V/n_2 for the values n_1 and n'_2. The immediate conclusion which may be drawn from this fact is that the partial molecular volume $\overline{V}_2$ may

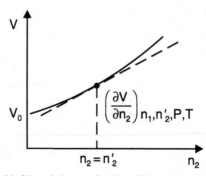

Figure 17. Total volume V of the solution as a function of the number n_2 of moles of solute added.

vary with the instantaneous "composition" of the solution. In rare cases, however, the slope does not change with the composition (see below).

In brief, a partial molar quantity is equal to the increase or decrease of the whole solution when one mole of solute is added to a very large volume of the whole solution in order that the different concentrations do not noticeably change because of the addition.

The same considerations may be addressed to any other quantity.

5) Molar quantities and partial molar quantities

It may happen that the measured thermodynamic quantity is in linear relation with the number of moles of the component. In this case, it is evident that the molar partial quantity is equal to the molar quantity of the pure component. In the example above, in these conditions:

$$\overline{V}_2 = v_2^{\bullet}$$

Remark concerning the use of the term chemical potential: The chemical potential is a molar partial quantity. This term is generally used when a mixture is under consideration. When it is the case of a pure substance under consideration, it is the term molar Gibbs energy which is used.

6) Fundamental equation of the partial molar quantities

Let X be an extensive property of a system constituted by a solution. This can be for example its internal energy. Recall that an extensive property is a property which is a function of the number of moles of each component. Let us suppose that the natural variables (in the case of the Gibbs energy, they are the temperature T and the pressure p) are maintained constant. As a result, the total differential of the function (of the kinds (81) or (82) for example) becomes:

$$dX = \overline{X}_1\, dn_1 + \overline{X}_2\, dn_2 + \ldots.$$

The partial molar quantities $\overline{X}_i$ are intensive quantities since their values are related to a well-defined quantity of water (one mole). Because of this fact, they do not depend on the total quantity of each component but only on the relative composition of each one. As a result, if an identical solution of the same composition is added to a solution containing several components with a given relative composition, the partial molar quantities $\overline{X}_i$ do not change whereas the numbers of moles n_1, n_2…vary. The consequence is that the total differential dX can be immediately integrated and we can write:

$$X = n_1 \overline{X}_1 + n_2 \overline{X}_2 + \ldots. \tag{84}$$

This relation is very important. It is sufficient to consider the case in which an extensive property of a solution is in linear relation with the number of moles of each of the components to be convinced by its interest. In these conditions, we know that partial molar quantities are constant and, moreover, are equal to the molal properties of pure components, that is to say:

$$X = n_1 X_m(1) + n_2 X_m(2) + \ldots. \tag{85}$$

The comparison of Equations (83) and (84) shows that partial molar quantities plays the part of the molar quantities of pure compounds and they can be handled in the same manner.

However, there exists a double difference between both kinds of quantities:

– on the one hand, the partial molar quantities are not constant whereas the molar ones are;
– on the other, the partial molar quantities may be positive or negative. This is inconceivable with the molar ones.

7) Thermodynamic relations between partial molar quantities

The relations between the thermodynamic partial molar quantities are the same as those which exist between the molar ones. For example, the relation:

$$\overline{G} = \overline{H} - T\overline{S}$$

is valid.

8) Experimental determination of partial molar quantities

Partial molar quantities are experimentally accessible:

- either through graphical methods based on the study of the curves extensive quantity/number of moles of the component (or its logarithm);
- or analytically, by starting from the apparent molar quantities.

In some cases, it is the absolute value of the partial molar quantity which is accessible. An example is that of partial molar volumes. In other cases, these absolute values are not. Only their relative values are accessible. For example, it is the case of the partial molar enthalpies and partial molar Gibbs energies. The reason lies simply in the fact that the absolute values of the molar quantities of pure compounds cannot themselves be known. It is the case for example of the internal energy or of the enthalpy.

9) The chemical potential

The chemical potential is by far, for our purpose, the most important partial molar quantity.

9-1) Definitions

- The chemical potential μ_k of a compound k in a given state (temperature T, pressure p, numbers of moles n_i of the other different species making up the system) is expressed, as we have already seen it, by the following mathematical relation:

$$\mu_k = (\partial G / \partial n_k)_{T, p, \, ni} \quad (i \neq k)$$

The quantity G appearing in this relation is the Gibbs energy of the whole solution considered as being the system. Quite evidently, it is the partial molar Gibbs energy $\overline{G_i}$:

$$\overline{G_i} = (\partial G / \partial n_k)_{T, p, \, ni}$$

According to what is mentioned before:

$$\overline{G} = n_1 \overline{G_1} + n_2 \overline{G_2} + \ldots..$$

$$G = n_1 \mu_1 + n_2 \mu_2 + \ldots.$$

Hence, the terms "chemical potential" and "partial molar Gibbs energy" are synonymous. The unity of chemical potential is: $J \, mol^{-1}$.

- Other definitions of the chemical potential are based on the following relations:

$$\mu_k = (\partial U / \partial n_k)_{S, V, ni} \quad \mu_k = (\partial H / \partial n_k)_{S, p, ni} \quad \mu_k = (\partial A / \partial n_k)_{T, V, ni} \quad (i \neq k)$$

All these definitions are strictly equivalent, as it can be demonstrated. Hence, the chemical potential of a substance k turns out to be either a partial molar internal energy, a partial molar enthalpy or a partial molar Helmholtz energy. It is interesting to notice that what is making equivalent these different partial derivatives are their variables maintained constant, which are different from one derivative to another.

9-2) Physical meaning of the chemical potential

The chemical potential of a substance is a quantity which is liable to quantify its tendency to leave its current thermodynamic state by every sort of process, physical, chemical or biochemical one. The chemical potential represents the escaping tendency of a substance, as does the molar Gibbs energy. It is not surprising since the chemical potential is also a molar Gibbs energy, but a partial one. Actually, the chemical potential extends the notion of molar Gibbs energy to complex media.

9-3) An example: the partition of a solute between two immiscible phases

The example given just below is of great importance. It concerns the nature of a *transcellular active transport*.

Let i be the solute being partitioned between two immiscible phases α and β. Suppose that, at the beginning of the process, the whole solute is only present in phase α. Its chemical potential is $\mu_{i\alpha}$ whereas it is null in phase β, $\mu_{i\beta} = 0$. Therefore:

$\mu_{i\alpha} > \mu_{i\beta}$ (initial state of the partition process)

By stirring both phases, a part of the substance spontaneously goes into the phase β. There exists a moment at which the process of partitioning ceases. The concentrations of the solute in both phases do not change further. The partition *equilibrium* is reached. The condition of equilibrium (concerning the partition of the substance) is the equality of the chemical potentials of i in both phases:

$\mu_{i\alpha} = \mu_{i\beta}$ (partition equilibrium)

We notice that the direction of the matter exchange followed that of a decreasing chemical potential. The partition spontaneously occurred because, initially, there existed an inequality of the chemical potentials. The part played by the chemical potential is analogous to that played by an electrical potential difference. Electrons flow between two points of a circuitry because a difference of potential between them exists. To continue analogies, heat transfer and mechanical motion are commanded, respectively, by differences of temperature and pressure.

Likewise, we will see that a spontaneous chemical reaction occurs when a well-defined linear combination of the chemical potentials of reactants and products differs from zero (see Chapter 18).

Hence, we notice for the first time that the notion of chemical potential is in relation with those of equilibrium and evolution of a process.

Remark: Stirring the solutions does not change the position of the equilibrium. In the present case, stirring does not change the concentrations at equilibrium.

9-4) Some properties of the chemical potential

- For a pure compound, the chemical potential is equal to its molar Gibbs energy,
- The chemical potential is an intensive property, as is its molar Gibbs energy,
- It is expressed in J mol^{-1},

- The chemical potential of a perfect gas tends towards $-\infty$ when its pressure tends towards zero. This is a point which is endowed with important practical consequences,
- As all the other partial molar quantities, chemical potentials very often vary with the composition of the system, but this is not obligatory,
- The absolute value of the chemical potential cannot be known since it is a molar Gibbs energy,
- the influence of the temperature on the chemical potential is given by the expression:

$$(\partial\mu_i/\partial T)_{p,nj} = -\overline{S_i} \tag{86}$$

$\overline{S_i}$ is the partial molar entropy of i. The demonstration of this relation is as follows. By definition:

$$(\partial\mu_i/\partial T)_{pnj} = (\partial\,[\partial G/\partial n_i)_{T,p,nj}]/\partial T)_{p,nj}$$

According to Schwartz' theorem (see the mathematical appendix II-6), it is legitimate to write:

$$(\partial\mu_i/\partial T)_{pnj} = (\partial\,[\partial G/\partial T_i)_{p,ni}]/\partial n_i)_{p,T,nj}$$

whence the relation (85), since:

$$(\partial G/\partial T)_p = -S$$

- The influence of the pressure on the chemical potential is given by the expression:

$$(\partial\mu_i/\partial p)_{T,nj} = \overline{V_{mi}}$$

$\overline{V_{mi}}$ is the partial molar volume of i. The demonstration is analogous to the previous one. It results from the relation:

$$(\partial G/\partial p)T = V_m$$

Chapter **18**

Gibbs Energy Change Accompanying a Chemical Reaction–General Equilibrium Condition of a Chemical Reaction

In this chapter, we study the Gibbs energy change accompanying a chemical reaction and we establish the conditions of its equilibrium. The study is carried out by systematically considering the chemical potentials of the reactants and products. The chemical potential, indeed, is the pivotal quantity which commands the evolution of a chemical reaction.

We begin by mentioning the Gibbs energy change accompanying any process.

1) Gibbs energy change in any process

In a completely general case which may refer to a physical, chemical or biochemical process, let us suppose that the system may initially consist of n_1, n_2....moles of constituents 1,2 ...with respective chemical potentials μ_1,μ_2.... The chemical potential being a (partial) *molar* Gibbs energy, the total Gibbs energy of the studied system G_{init} is given by the Equation (86):

$$G_{init} = n_1\mu_1 + n_2\mu_2 + \ldots \ldots \tag{87}$$

If in the final state, the system consists of n'_1, n'_2....moles of substances of chemical potentials μ'_1, μ'_2.....its whole Gibbs energy G_{fin} is:

$$G_{fin} = n'_1\mu'_1 + n'_2\mu'_2 + \ldots \ldots \tag{88}$$

the Gibbs energy change of the system accompanying the process is:

$$\Delta G_{syst} = (n'_1\mu'_1 + n'_2\mu'_2 + \ldots \ldots) - (n_1\mu_1 + n_2\mu_2 + \ldots .) \tag{89}$$

Evidently, the chemical potentials of the substances are different in the final states from those they had in the initial states since the composition of the system has changed owing to the studied process. Moreover, there may exist new products in the system with their own chemical potentials owing to the occurrence of the studied chemical reaction, as some reactants may have completely disappeared for the same reason.

Relation (88) is absolutely general. However, it must not be forgotten that the Gibbs energy decrease (if it decreases during the process) is equal to the maximum useful work which can be done by the system, the pressure and the temperature being identical in the initial and final states.

2) Clapeyron equation—Entropy change during a phase transition

As a first example of the interest that the Gibbs energy function may present, let us study the case of two phases at equilibrium at given pressure and temperature. Its study leads directly to Clapeyron's law and to the entropy change during a phase change.

We are interested in a phase change at constant temperature and pressure, in a closed system. The equilibrium conditions between two phases A and B of the same substance can be obtained with the aid of the Gibbs energy function, since we are in a process at constant pressure and temperature. At equilibrium, any infinitesimal transfer of matter between both phases occurs with a null free energy change:

$$dG_{syst} = 0$$

with:

$$dG_{syst} = G_A dn_A + G_B dn_B$$

G_A and G_B are the molar Gibbs functions of the substance in phases A and B. dn_A and dn_B are the infinitesimal changes in the number of moles in both phases at equilibrium. The whole system (not the phases) being closed:

$$-dn_A = dn_B$$

and:

$$(G_A - G_B)dn_A = 0$$

$$G_A = G_B$$

whatever the conditions are (provided the temperature and pressure are constant). If, now, temperature and pressure are changed in infinitesimal amounts dT and dp while the equilibrium is maintained, the following conditions occur:

$$G_A + dG_A = G_B + dG_B$$

and since:

$$G_A = G_B$$

$$dG_A = dG_B$$

Expressing dG_A and dG_B by their differentials

$$dG_A = V_{mA}dp - S_{mA}d\,T$$

$$dG_B = V_{mB}\,dp - S_{mB}dT$$

where V_{mA}, V_{mB} are the molar volumes of the substance in phases A and B, and S_{mA}, S_{mB} their molar entropies. As a consequence, after rearrangement of these equations, we find:

$(V_{mB} - V_{mA}) \, dp = (S_{mB} - S_{mA}) dT$

$dp/dT = \Delta S_m / \Delta V_m$ (90)

This relation is important. It shows that T and p cannot be varied independently, if in the same time, the equilibrium must be maintained. Once a value of dp or dT is chosen, the value of the other is chosen. Relation (89) expresses Clapeyron's law.

This law permits to immediately establish the entropy change accompanying a reversible phase transition. Hence, we know that it is possible to maintain two phases at equilibrium at given temperature and pressure. Notice that the fact to consider a reversible phase transition at constant temperature implies that the change is also at constant pressure. In general, we are interested in the increase of entropy accompanying the transitions, solid-liquid (fusion), liquid-gas (vaporization) and crystal → crystal. The heats supplied in these conditions are the "latent heats" q transition. No work except the p-V one against the atmosphere is done during these transitions. In these conditions:

$\Delta S_{syst} = $ q transition$/T$

q transition $= \Delta H$ transition

$\Delta S_{syst} = \Delta H$ transition$/T$

Notice that the surroundings gives the quantity of heat q transition to the system. Its entropy change is, hence:

ΔSsurroundings $= -$q transition$/T$

We find:

$\Delta S_{isol} = \Delta S_{syst} + \Delta S$surroundings $= 0$

The process was effectively reversible.

3) Gibbs energy of a chemical system

Let us consider the chemical reaction

$v_A A + v_B B \rightarrow v_M M + v_N N$ (91)

Suppose the numbers of moles of the different species before reaction evolve are n_A, n_B, n_M, n_N. Notice that in the initial mixture, there are not only the reactants A and B but also the final products M and N. This adopted presentation is for the sake of generality of the reasoning. This is not, of course, obligatory. For example, the final products may be already present at the outset. The initial Gibbs energy of the whole system $G_{syst\,i}$ is given by the equation:

$G_{syst\,i} = n_A \mu_A + n_B \mu_B + n_M \mu_M + n_N \mu_N$ (92)

Let n'_A, n'_B, n'_M, n'_N be the numbers of moles of the products when the reaction stops. This can be for two reasons: either when it is complete or when the equilibrium is attained. As in the initial state, some number(s) of moles may be null (complete reaction). The Gibbs energy of the final state $G_{syst\,f}$ is given by the equation:

$G_{syst\,f} = n'_A \mu'_A + n'_B \mu'_B + n'_M \mu'_M + n'_N \mu'_N$ (93)

The Figure 18 summarizes the initial and final states of the chemical reaction.

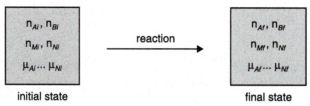

initial state   final state

Figure 18. Definition of the initial and final states of reaction.

The Gibbs energy change $\Delta_r G$ accompanying the reaction is (r for reactional):

$$\Delta_r G = G_{syst\ f} - G_{syst\ i}$$

$$\Delta_r G = (n'_A \mu'_A + n'_B \mu'_B + n'_M \mu'_M + n'_N \mu'_N) - (n_A \mu_A + n_B \mu_B + n_M \mu_M + n_N \mu_N) \tag{94}$$

Relation (93) can be generalized as (the stoichiometric coefficients of the reactants, and not those of the products, are preceded by the minus sign):

$$\Delta_r G = \Sigma_j\, n_j \mu_j \tag{95}$$

If the initial and final pressure and temperature are identical, $\Delta_r G$ is the maximum useful work available from the chemical reaction.

4) Gibbs-Duhem relation

It is interesting to compare relation (94) with the general relation (95) (see Chapter 17 paragraph 1)

$$dG_{syst} = -SdT + Vdp + \Sigma_i\, \mu_i\, dn_i\ (i = 1\ to\ k:\ k\ number\ of\ substances) \tag{96}$$

which at constant temperature and pressure becomes:

$$dG_{syst} = \Sigma_i\, \mu_i\, dn_i \tag{97}$$

In order to do that, let us differentiate relation (94). Here comes:

$$dG_{syst} = \Sigma\, n_j\, d\mu_j + \Sigma\, \mu_j dn_j \tag{98}$$

We notice that, apparently, there exists an inconsistency between Equations (96) and (97). In the former ones, the term $\Sigma\, n_j\, d\mu_j$ is missing. This inconsistency is only apparent since it does not exist. This is because both reactions do not refer to the same conditions. In Equation (97), temperature and pressure are supposed to vary together with the numbers of moles of species. This is not the case of Equation (96).

The consequence is the following one: the chemical potentials of the components of a mixture cannot change independently at constant temperature and pressure. In these conditions, the following relationship, in the case of our chosen example, is satisfied:

$$\Sigma\, n_j\, d\mu_j = 0\ (dT = 0\ and\ dp = 0)$$

It is called the Gibbs-Duhem relation.

5) Actual molar reactional Gibbs function

The changes in the mole numbers of reactants and products during the chemical reaction are linked by the equalities:

$(dn_A/v_A) = (dn_B/v_B) = (dn_M/v_M) = (dn_N/v_N) = d\xi$

ξ is called the extent of the reaction. In these equations, the changes dn_A, dn_B ...are negative because A, B.... disappear during the reaction whereas dn_M, dn_N.....are positive. Taking into account these equalities in (96):

$$dG_{syst} = (-v_A\mu_A - v_B\mu_B + v_M\mu_M + v_N\mu_N)\, d\xi \quad (dT = 0 \text{ and } dp = 0) \tag{99}$$

The entire term in parentheses in (98) is called the *actual molar reaction Gibbs function or molar reaction Gibbs function. With its sign inverted, it is called the affinity of the reaction, the symbol of which is A (de Donder's affinity). The actual molar reaction Gibbs function is the actual Gibbs energy change accompanying the reaction at a given affinity value at an instant of its evolution, that is for an extent ξ for which the instantaneous chemical potentials are μ_i:*

$$-A = -v_A\mu_A - v_B\mu_B + v_M\mu_M + v_N\mu_N$$

The molar reactional Gibbs function varies with respect to the extent of the reaction. From the mathematical viewpoint, it appears, according to the relation (98), as being the partial derivative of the system Gibbs energy with respect to ξ at constant temperature and pressure, for a given ξ:

$$-A = (\partial G_{syst}/\partial \xi)_{T,p}$$

The change dG_{syst} is negative when the process is spontaneous. As a result, at constant pressure and temperature, the molar reactional Gibbs function $(-A)$ must be negative in the case of a spontaneous process:

$(-A) < 0$ (spontaneous process)

that is to say, in the case of our example:

$v_A\mu_A + v_B\mu_B > v_M\mu_M + v_N\mu_N$ $(dp = 0, dT = 0)$

de Donder's affinity is positive for a spontaneous process.

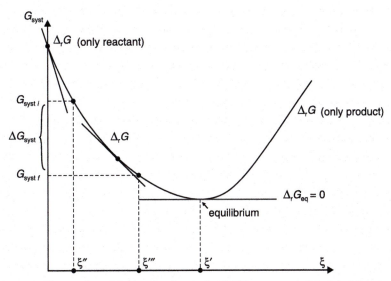

Figure 19. Different values of the actual molar reactional Gibbs energy as a function of its extent ξ.

Their chemical potentials are related to each other through the expression of $-A$. For example, the reaction can be initiated for $\xi = \xi''$ and stopped for $\xi = \xi'''$. The extreme points represent the cases in which only reactants and only products are present in the mixture.

The Gibbs energy change of the system ΔG_{syst} is:

$$\Delta G_{syst} = G_{syst\ fin} - G_{syst\ init}$$

and since the system under consideration is the mixture of the reactants and products of the chemical reaction:

$$\Delta G_{syst} = \Delta_r G$$

The figure shows that $-A$ also changes all along the process. It is sufficient to consider the slopes of the curve G_{syst}/ξ to be convinced. Notice that the slopes are maximum when the sole reactants and products are present in the reaction mixture.

As we have already said, reactions that occur with an increase of Gibbs energy are named *endergonic reactions* whereas reactions that occur with a decrease of Gibbs energy are named *exergonic reactions*.

A question comes unavoidably to mind. What are the conditions of equilibrium which must be satisfied when several chemical reactions can simultaneously evolve? The answer to the question comes from the general criterion: $dG_{syst} = 0$. It is inferred from this general condition that the molar reactional Gibbs functions $-A$ of each reaction must be simultaneously null provided that the different reactions are independent.

Chapter **19**

Activity–Ideal
Solutions–Standard States

The condition of equilibrium of a chemical reaction is of great interest. We shall demonstrate that the actual molar reactional Gibbs function must be null at equilibrium. However, there appears a problem, once the matter is to apply this rule practically. The actual molar reactional Gibbs function, indeed, is a well-definite linear combination of the chemical potentials of the remaining reactants and products at equilibrium. Actually, the notion of chemical potential is essentially abstract. Worst still, this notion may appear to be far from "the chemical reality", that is to say far from the usual parameters describing chemical systems.

Fortunately, G.N. Lewis has introduced two new functions: the activity and the fugacity. Here, we confine ourselves to an elementary introduction of the notion of activity: which firstly requires remembering the definition of ideal solutions. Secondly, it implies to introduce the notions of standard states and of activity coefficients. They permit to quantitatively relate partial pressures or concentrations of reactants and products at equilibrium. Here is the origin of the elaboration of the notion of equilibrium constant, embodied in the so-called "mass action law" of utmost importance.

1) Definitions of an activity

One of the possible definitions of an activity is given through the following relation:

$$\mu = \mu^\circ + RT \ln a \qquad\qquad (100)$$

where μ is the chemical potential of the substance of *activity a* and μ° is its chemical potential in a given state, named its standard state. This relation is absolutely general, even if in some cases it must be completed (see the following paragraphs).

We already notice that the standard chemical potential μ° is the chemical potential of the substance when its activity is equal to unity.

There is another definition of an activity which is based on the notion of *fugacity*. Both definitions are equivalent. Sometimes, especially in biochemistry, an activity is named *an active mass* or *mass unit*.

2) A physico-chemical meaning of an activity

At the outset, we can say that an activity:
– *appears to be a kind of concentration,*
– *may be interpreted as the fraction of the whole concentration of a species. This fraction is the part of the concentration which effectively plays a part in a chemical equilibrium (or even*

in a purely physical process). Quantitatively speaking, it is only this fraction which enters in the equilibrium constant value (see next chapter).

This definition is certainly not perfect, but probably, it has the relevance to clarify the underlying idea of G.N. Lewis when he introduced this notion.

3) Some properties of an activity

– An activity can be defined for every substance, whichever its physical state and whichever the experimental conditions in which it is. However, the interest of this notion is particularly great in the cases of liquid mixtures;

– The mass action law (see the next chapter) is expressed in terms of activities of reactants and products. This is the object of the next chapter to demonstrate this point;

– The activity of a species in a given medium is related to its "concentration" C through the general expression:

$$a = \gamma\, C \qquad\qquad\qquad (101)$$

The factor γ is called its *activity coefficient*. C is the generic symbol of the concentration, whichever its scale is (molality, molarity, molar fraction, etc.). Therefore, the activity of a species and its concentration obey this relation, whatever the concentration scale is. This relation is general. When we gather Equations (99) and (100), we obtain the relation:

$$\mu = \mu^\circ + RT \ln \gamma + RT \ln C \qquad\qquad\qquad (102)$$

This relation throws some light on the meaning of the chemical potential in terms of **the** chemical parameter which is the concentration C of the studied substance;

– an activity *is a virtual quantity*;

– activities are dimensionless quantities and it is the same property for the activity coefficients, whatever the concentration scale is. Hence, the relation (99), although general, is somewhat improper, except when the species concentration is expressed in molar fractions because these latter expressions are also dimensionless;

– the very big difficulty encountered in the handling of activities lies in the fact that relation (100) is not actually a true linear relation. The very origin of this fact is the occurrence of physical interactions between the moles of the species, interactions which vary with its concentration. As a result, the activity coefficient of a species does vary with its "concentration". Actually, the mathematical link between the value of an activity and that of its corresponding concentration seems to be very complex and is very badly known. Only some considerations of statistical thermodynamics throw some light on the problem, but only in some rare cases;

– there exist several kinds of activities which are of different numerical values for the same species in the same thermodynamic state according to

  • the chosen standard state (see paragraphs 4 and 9),
  • the concentration scale to which they are related,
  • eventually, the conditions defining the state of the system.

– the values of the activities of non ionic species are experimentally accessible. This is also the case of a whole electrolyte such as, for example, that of sodium chloride. However, it is impossible to experimentally determine the activity of an ion, but it can be approached by theoretical calculations, notably by those involving the so-called Debye-Hûckel relations. (Although not perfect, they lead to satisfactory results).

4) Standard states and activities

The inconvenience of relation (99) is that it is only a formal definition. So far, in this book, the chemical potential and the activity of a substance are not "anchored" in the chemical reality. This is done by implying a *standard state* related to the corresponding activity. The standard state must be defined in terms of experimental variables.

The principle of the anchorage of an activity is founded on the following reasoning. Consider the definition (99) and more precisely the difference $\mu - \mu°$ which comes from it:

$$\mu - \mu° = RT \ln a$$

Bearing in mind that a chemical potential has the meaning (among other ones) of a Gibbs molar energy and that a difference of a Gibbs energy is experimentally measurable (for example, through the work exchanged during the change), we see that the activity measures the difference in Gibbs energy between the state of the substance in the system under study and its standard state. Relation (99) may be, indeed, written:

$$\mu - \mu° = RT \ln a - RT \ln 1$$

where 1 is the activity in the standard state. As a result, once the physico-chemical properties of the standard state are known, those of the substance in the studied state are also defined, whence the usefulness of the definition in physico-chemical terms of the standard state, that is to say of its chemical anchorage.

The choice of the standard state is purely arbitrary. This is the reason why there exists an infinity of choices for it. However, it turns out that some choices are easier to handle than other ones. Precisely, these choices may change according to some factors such as the physical state of the substance, whether it is pure or in solution or according to its concentration scale. *The result of these considerations is that the notion of activity cannot be dissociated from that of standard state.*

5) Ideal solutions

For our purpose, we are interested in the behavior of solutions, since the reactions involved in bioenergetics occur mainly in aqueous media in cells. This is the reason why it is interesting to briefly study the notion of standard states in solutions. This point impels us to recall some concerning ideal solutions. In fact, standard states in solutions are chosen in relation to the behavior of ideal solutions.

A solution is ideal when the chemical potentials μ_i of all its components is a linear function of the logarithm of its molar fraction x_i, according to:

$$\mu_i = \mu_i^*(T,p) + RT \ln x_i \qquad (103)$$

$\mu_i^*(T,p)$ *is a constant, the value of which depends on the temperature, pressure and identity of the component. It is independent of the composition.* We notice that $\mu_i^*(T,p)$ is the chemical potential of the component i when it is pure ($x_i = 1$). The formalism of this definition looks like that of a pure perfect gas (see Chapter 16):

$$G = G° + RT \ln (p/p°)$$

or most often:

$$G = G° + RT \ln (p/1_{atm})$$

There is still a greater analogy between (102) and another expression of the chemical potential of a gas in a mixture (of gases) (see just below):

$$\mu = \mu_{yi*}(T,p) + RT \ln y_i$$

where y_i is the molar fraction of the component i in the gaseous mixture.

It is interesting to notice that relation (102) is simply an integral solution of the following differential equation:

$$d\mu_i = RT \, d \ln x_i \tag{104}$$

Equation (103) has been that the setting up of which has introduced the notion of activity. It explains the distinction between ideal perfect solutions and ideal sufficiently diluted solutions. The difference between the two kinds of perfect solutions comes from the nature of the integration constant. Some authors, indeed, distinguish:

– the perfect solutions. They are ideal in the whole domain of concentrations. Furthermore, the behavior of each component of the solution is the same. They obey Raoult's law. In its original version, Raoult's law stipulated that in such a liquid solution, the partial vapor-pressure p_i of each component i is proportional to its molar fraction x_i in the solution and to its vapor pressure p_i° when it is pure at the total pressure of the system:

$$p_i = x_i \, p_i^{\circ} \tag{105}$$

It can be demonstrated that Raoult' law is in full compliance with the definition (99).

– the sufficiently diluted solutions. In those solutions, solutes exhibit an ideal behavior only in a limited domain of "concentrations". Experimentally, such behaviors do exist in sufficiently diluted solutions and it is found that:

- the behavior of the solvent tends towards that described by Raoult's law. More precisely, the more diluted the solution is (in solute), the more the solvent tends to have a perfect behavior;

- simultaneously, the solute behavior is not the same as that in a perfect gas. It is experimentally found that in a diluted solution, at constant temperature, the vapor pressure of the solute is proportional to its molar fraction as, at first sight, it is also the case in a perfect solution, *but the proportionality constant is not the same.* These points are expressed by Henry's law. The proportionality constant is called Henry's constant. Henry's law applies to all the diluted solutions, provided they are sufficiently dilute. This is the most frequent case. It is the only one on which we shall focus us.

One can verify that during the linear behavior of the solute, the differential Equation (103) is also satisfied.

In relation to the notion of equilibrium constant, there is another virtual function which has also been introduced. It is the *fugacity*. It has been introduced to study the behavior of imperfect gases. It is a kind of partial pressure. It is endowed with the units of pressure. It is based on the fact that it is admitted that, as a gas, a liquid or a solid may also be endowed with a value of fugacity. There is simple mathematical relations linking the fugacity and the activity of a substance. Besides, it is on these relations that the second definition of an activity is based.

6) Ideal character of a system and interactions between the particles constituting it

The ideal character of a system constituted only by gases is related to the occurrence (or not) of interactions between the particles constituting it. When there is no interaction, the gas or the mixture of gases is called perfect or ideal. In this case, their molar Gibbs energy obeys the relation (76) of Chapter 16:

$$G = G° + RT \ln (p/p°)$$

most often writen:

$$G = G° + RT \ln (p/1_{atm})$$

As we have already said it, the gases behave as if they were sole, their particles being without interaction between each other. In these conditions, the chemical potential being a molar property, it can be written:

$$\mu = \mu° + RT \ln (p/p°)$$

$\mu°$ being the chemical potential of or its molar Gibbs energy when its pressure is p°. We notice the analogy of the latter relation with (76) above. When the behavior of the gas is no longer ideal, there exist interactions between the particles. The molar Gibbs energy or the chemical potential of the gas is given by the relation:

$$\mu = \mu° + RT \ln (f/f°)$$

where f and f° are its fugacities in its state and in its standard state. Hence, the fugacities have been clearly introduced to take into account the interactions. The fugacities differ from the partial pressures but by definition, when the pressure of gas tens to zero so does its fugacity.

The case of ideal solutions is somewhat different from that of gases. Nevertheless, one can still distinguish ideal solutions and non-ideal ones. In the first case, the behaviors of the constituents (solute + solvent, for example) are described by a relation of the type:

$$\mu = \mu° + RT \ln (C/C°)$$

where C and C° are its concentrations in the state under study and in its standard state. When the behavior is non ideal, this relation must be replaced by:

$$\mu = \mu° + RT \ln (a/1)$$

where 1 is, by definition, the value of its activity in the standard state. Again, the more diluted (in the substance) the solution is, the more the value of its activity tends to that of its concentration.

In brief, Lewis has introduced the notions of fugacity and activity in order to treat the non-ideal systems by using a formalism very close to that expressing the chemical potentials of species in ideal systems.

Hence, intermolecular forces operating between the molecules of a pure substance or between the molecules of a mixture command the thermodynamic properties of the system constituted by them.

It is sufficient for our purpose to mention that these interactions are due to different physical forces, and that the greater the concentrations of the solutes in solutions are, the more their behavior differ from the corresponding ideal one.

7) Come back to the activity coefficients

According to the concentration scale, one distinguishes several kinds of activity coefficients of a species i. They are:

$$\gamma_{c,i} = a_{c,i}/c_i \tag{106}$$

$$\gamma_{m,i} = a_{m,i}/m_i \tag{107}$$

$$\gamma_{x,i} = a_{x,i}/x_i$$

The subscripts c, m, x correspond, respectively, to the scales of molarities, molalities and molar fractions. For the solvent, the activity coefficient f_0 is defined by:

$$f_0 = a_0/x_0$$

(f_0 here is not a fugacity!) (Here, we express the activity coefficient of the solvent when its "concentration" is expressed in mole fraction, as it is recommended by IUPAC. It is a quasi-universal convention to express the solvent "concentration" in a mole fraction). We have already said that activities and activity coefficients are dimensionless. Relations (105) and (106) seem in contradistinction with this assertion.

8) Standard states and activity coefficients

By definition, to express an activity requires choosing a standard state. For example, for a solute i, the standard state can be chosen as being the state in which its concentration is c_i° (or its molality m_i° or its mole fraction x_i°), the solution being ideal. (Recall that pressure exerts a very weak influence on the behavior of condensed phases). At concentration c_i° (which is that of the standard state, the chemical potential of i is μ_i° called the standard chemical potential). Hence,

– when the solution is ideal, the chemical potential μ_i at concentration c_i or at molality m_i is given by the expressions:

$$\mu_i = \mu^\circ_{i,c} + RT \ln (c_i/c_i^\circ)$$

or

$$\mu_i = \mu^\circ_{i,m} + RT \ln (m_i/m_i^\circ)$$

– when the solution is non ideal, activities and their corresponding activity coefficients are introduced through the two following relations:

$$\gamma_{c,i} = a_{ci}/(c_i/c_i^\circ)$$

$$\gamma_{m,i} = a_{m,i}/(m_i/m_i^\circ)$$

Activity coefficients are indeed dimensionless. However, standard states which are arbitrary, are chosen usually such as $c_i^\circ = 1$ mol L^{-1} or $m_i^\circ = 1$ mol kg^{-1}. The simplified relations (100), (105), (106) result from these choices.

Therefore, for solutes in real solutions, the chemical potentials are given by:

$$\mu_i = \mu_{i,c}^\circ + RT \ln a_{ci} \text{ or}$$

$$\mu_i = \mu_{i,c}^\circ + RT \ln (c_i/c_i^\circ) + RT \ln \gamma_{c,i} \quad \text{(concentrations scale)}$$

and

$$\mu_i = \mu_{i,m}^\circ + RT \ln a_{mi} \text{ or}$$

$$\mu_i = \mu_{i,m}^\circ + RT \ln (m_i/m_i^\circ) + RT \ln \gamma_{m,i} \quad \text{(molalities scale)}$$

To conclude this paragraph, three points must be emphasized:

a) whatever the chosen scale of "concentration", the chemical potential of the substance i is the same in a given state. This point is obvious. It only possesses one molar Gibbs energy or one partial molar Gibbs energy;

b) for one substance in a given state, there exists several kinds of activities and hence several values, according to its "concentrations" units;

c) once the standard state is chosen in a given system, the chemical potential of the substance in it possesses a constant value (at constant temperature and pressure). This is quite normal since all the parameters in the system are fixed. *This point is of utmost importance for the remaining of our purpose.*

9) Usual conventions for the definitions of the activities

This paragraph concerns the usual conventions adopted for the definition of the activities and, of course, those which prevail to the choice of the standard states, as well.

– For a solute, ion or molecule, the numerical value of its activity is systematically related to its molarity or molality. As a result, in the case of sufficiently dilute solutions (when the behavior tends to be ideal) and since $c_i^\circ = 1$ mol L^{-1} and $m_i^\circ = 1$ mol kg^{-1}, the numerical value of the activity tends towards that of its "concentration":

$a_{ic} \rightarrow c_i$ (numerical value of diluted solution)

$a_{im} \rightarrow m_i$ (numerical value of diluted solution)

Moreover, since in dilute solutions, $m_i \approx c_i$

$a_{ic} \approx a_{im}$

– For the solvent, its activity value is related to its mole fraction. In sufficiently diluted solutions, the value of this quantity tends towards unity because of the expression:

$x_0 = n_0/(n_0 + n_i)$

since $n_i \ll n_0$. As a result:

$a_0 \rightarrow 1$ (diluted solutions)

It is the reason why, when the solvent also participates in the chemical reaction and when the solution is sufficiently diluted, the solvent activity (= 1) is purely and simply omitted in the mass law (see the next chapter);

– For every pure phase (for example a pure liquid or a pure solid), the activity value is taken to be exactly equal to unity. This is why, for example, a pure metal electrode has an activity value of unity;

– For every liquid in a mixture of liquids, its activity value is chosen to be approximately equal to its mole fraction.

10) Osmotic pressure

Here, we somewhat study the notion of osmotic pressure since that of osmotic work will be evoked later when the matter will become the study of the transport of solutes in biological systems under the notion of active transport (see Chapter 40).

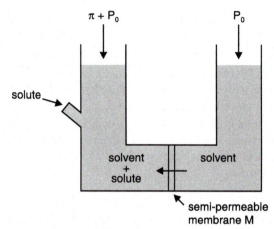

Figure 20. Apparatus to display the occurrence of an osmotic pressure.

It is made up of two compartments separated by a membrane M. At the beginning of the experience, both compartments are filled by the pure liquid 1 which plays the part of the solvent. This liquid can permeate the membrane. The compartment on the left is equipped with an aperture allowing the addition of a solute. The solute cannot pass through the membrane and when it is added it will be confined in the compartment on the left. At the beginning, the solute is not added. The level of the liquid 1 is the same in both compartments because they are under the same pressure P_0. When the solute is added into the left compartment, we notice an enhancement of its level. In order to bring back an identical level of liquid in both compartments, a supplementary pressure π, called osmotic pressure, must be applied on the compartment containing the solute. A thermodynamic reasoning leads, after simplifications are justified when the solution is sufficiently dilute in solute, to the expression:

$$\pi = n_2(RT/V)$$

n_2 is the number of moles of solute and V the total volume of solvent. In principle, the measurement of the osmotic pressure permits the determination of the activity of the solvent.

Notice that in this experience, it is hard to speak of osmotic work. However, we can imagine that it is the mechanical work which is developed to enhance the level of the liquid in compartment 2.

Chapter 20

The Mass Action Law–Equilibrium Constant of a Chemical Reaction

From the general standpoint, this chapter is probably the most important of the branch of the physical chemistry named *chemical* thermodynamics. It mentions the outcome of a series of reasonings, coming from pure "physical thermodynamics" but which are progressively applied to chemistry, as the preceding chapters of this book show. The outcome is the mass action law, the importance of which does not evidently remain to be demonstrated. The mass action law is a result of classical thermodynamics but it has been confirmed, in some conditions, by reasonings of statistical thermodynamics. Beyond the systematic existence of the equilibrium constants commanding chemical reactions which are the mathematical expressions of this law, a very important point concerning the mass action law is the fact that it is expressed in terms of activities.

1) Evolving reactions and equilibrium conditions

According to the meaning of the Gibbs energy function, the equilibrium state is obtained when:

$$dG_{syst} = 0 \quad \text{(equilibrium)}$$

at constant temperature and pressure. Then, the system Gibbs energy G_{syst} must exhibit its minimum value. When the evolving system consists of reactants together with their reaction products, the equilibrium state is obtained for the extent ξ' such as:

$$(\partial G_{syst}/\partial \xi)_{T,p,\,\xi=\xi'} = 0 \quad \text{(equilibrium, dT = 0, dp = 0)}$$

Equation (98) (Chapter 18) shows that therefore:

$$\nu_A \mu_{Aeq} + \nu_B \mu_{Beq} = \nu_M \mu_{Meq} + \nu_N \mu_{Neq}$$

or

$$A = 0 \quad \text{(equilibrium)}$$

The values of the involved chemical potentials are, of course, those at the equilibrium. As a result, for a spontaneous chemical change starting from the sole reactants A and B, the molar reactional Gibbs function—A becomes increasingly less negative when the extent of the reaction increases (Recall that A is de Donder's affinity—Chapter 18). Likewise, the reaction course starting from the sole reaction products is such that the molar reactional Gibbs function is increasingly less positive. Actually, each point of the curve G/ξ curve can represent either the initial or the final instant of the reaction, but not obligatorily the equilibrium. Except for the farthest points, each curve point represents a state where the reactants and products A, B, M, N are all present in the mixture (Figure 19).

2) Obtaining the mass action law

Let us consider the general chemical reaction:

$$v_A A + v_B B + v_C C + \ldots \rightarrow v_M M + v_N N + v_P P + \ldots\ldots \tag{108}$$

We have already (see Chapter 18) defined its actual molar reactional Gibbs energy $\Delta_r G$ and its affinity A related to it:

$$\Delta_r G = (v_M \mu_M + v_N \mu_N + v_P \mu_P + \ldots - v_A \mu_A - v_B \mu_B - v_C \mu_C \ldots)$$

$$A = (+v_A \mu_A + v_B \mu_B + v_C \mu_C \ldots - v_M \mu_M - v_N \mu_N - v_P \mu_P - \ldots)$$

At equilibrium, the actual molar reactional Gibbs energy function (or affinity A) must be null:

$$\Delta_r G_{eq} = 0$$

with:

$$\Delta_r G_{eq} = (v_M \mu_M + v_N \mu_N + v_P \mu_P + \ldots - v_A \mu_A - v_B \mu_B - v_C \mu_C \ldots)_{eq} = 0 \tag{109}$$

(Recall that the subscript eq means that the values of the chemical potentials $\mu_A \ldots \mu_P$ are those at equilibrium. This condition is imperative).

Now, consider the general equation relating the chemical potential of a substance to its activity (see Chapter 19):

$$\mu_i = \mu_i^\circ + RT \ln a_i \tag{110}$$

μ_i° is the standard chemical potential of the species i. It is a constant at given pressure and temperature of the system. Recall also that μ_i and a_i values are related together. They take different values according to the extent of the reaction and the state of the system. The values at equilibrium μ_{ieq} and a_{ieq} are, as we shall see, of special interest.

Now, let us replace the chemical potentials by their expressions (109) in relations (108). We obtain:

$$A_{eq} = (-v_M \mu_M^\circ - v_N \mu_N^\circ - v_P \mu_P^\circ + \ldots + v_A \mu_A^\circ + v_B \mu_B^\circ + v_C \mu_C^\circ + \ldots)$$

$$-RT \ln (a_M^{vM} a_N^{vN} a_P^{vP}/a_A^{vA} a_B^{vB} a_C^{vC})_{eq} = 0 \tag{111}$$

or

$$\Delta_r G_{eq} = (v_M \mu_M^\circ + v_N \mu_N^\circ + v_P \mu_P^\circ + \ldots - v_A \mu_A^\circ - v_B \mu_B^\circ - v_C \mu_C^\circ - \ldots)$$

$$+ RT \ln (a_M^{vM} a_N^{vN} a_P^{vP}/a_A^{vA} a_B^{vB} a_C^{vC})_{eq} = 0 \tag{112}$$

The ratio $(a_M^{vM} a_N^{vN} a_P^{vP}/a_A^{vA} a_B^{vB} a_C^{vC})$ is called the *reaction quotient*. It is symbolized by Q. Q is a ratio in which the activity values may be any one, those of the equilibrium or not. However, at equilibrium, the activity values cannot be anything.

At the chemical equilibrium, indeed, the molar reactional Gibbs energy function and the affinity as well are null owing to the general condition of a chemical equilibrium (110). Thus, one obtains:

$$RT \ln (a_M^{\nu M} a_N^{\nu N} a_P^{\nu P}/a_A^{\nu A} a_B^{\nu B} a_C^{\nu C})_{eq} =$$

$$(\nu_M \mu_M^\circ + \nu_N \mu_N^\circ + \nu_P \mu_P^\circ + \dots - \nu_A \mu_A^\circ - \nu_B \mu_B^\circ - \nu_C \mu_C^\circ - \dots) \qquad (113)$$

The generic subscript eq means that the activities a_i do not have any possible value. They have *only* those at equilibrium.

Indeed, as it has been already said, at constant temperature and pressure, the μ_i° are constants. As a result, after relation (111):

$$RT \ln (a_M^{\nu M} a_N^{\nu N} a_P^{\nu P}/a_A^{\nu A} a_B^{\nu B} a_C^{\nu C})_{eq} = \text{constant } (dp = 0, dT = 0) \qquad (114)$$

and evidently:

$$(a_M^{\nu M} a_N^{\nu N} a_P^{\nu P}/a_A^{\nu A} a_B^{\nu B} a_C^{\nu C})_{eq} = K^\circ \qquad (115)$$

K° is the *standard equilibrium constant* (IUPAC) or the *thermodynamic equilibrium constant*. Equations (112) and (113) express the *mass action law*. It is the quantitative link between the activities (and indirectly the "concentrations") of the reactants and products *at equilibrium*.

We notice that the mass action law is expressed in terms of activities. As a result, the *thermodynamic equilibrium constants are dimensionless*. The law is general. It is satisfied at constant pressure and temperature when the chemical equilibrium is attained. This assertion is true whether it involves one phase or several ones. However, in the latter case, it is true only when the whole closed system is considered and not when one phase is considered solely.

(Remark: in principle, fixing the temperature to a given value is not a factor of fixation of the standard state because every temperature can be retained for the standard state provided it is mentioned. This is not the case of pressure which is fixed once for all).

3) Standard reaction Gibbs energy

Let us consider the first term of the right-hand side of Equation (110)

$$(\nu_M \mu_M^\circ + \nu_N \mu_N^\circ + \nu_P \mu_P^\circ + \dots - \nu_A \mu_A^\circ - \nu_B \mu_B^\circ - \nu_C \mu_C^\circ \dots)$$

It is clear that it has the significance of the *standard molar Gibbs energy* $\Delta_r G^\circ$ accompanying the general reaction (under study) when the reactants and the products are in their standard states. This is immediately proved by setting up all the activities equal to 1 in Equation (110), since activities are equal to unity in the standard states, by definition (see Chapter 19).

$$\Delta_r G^\circ = (\nu_M \mu_M^\circ + \nu_N \mu_N^\circ + \nu_P \mu_P^\circ + \dots - \nu_A \mu_A^\circ - \nu_B \mu_B^\circ - \nu_C \mu_C^\circ \dots) \qquad (116)$$

According to (113) and (114), we can write:

$$\Delta_r G^\circ = -RT \ln K^\circ \qquad (117)$$

With the biochemical standard states (see Chapter 21), Equation (115) must be written:

$$\Delta_r G'^\circ = -RT \ln K''^\circ \qquad (118)$$

The equilibrium constant is not the same as before because the standard states are not the same (see the following paragraph).

4) Consequences of the arbitrary character of the choice of the standard state

A puzzling point concerning the concept of activity lies in the arbitrary character of the choice of the concentration scale to which the chemical activity of a species is related. It is important to mention that any kind of concentration scale can be chosen. Therefore, the following legitimate question comes to mind. Since the thermodynamic equilibrium constant of a chemical reaction results from the mass-action law, since the latter is expressed in activities and since activity values depend on the choice of the scale of concentrations, should they vary and can they not be constant as it is systematically reported in literature? And if it is the case, all the conclusions above, resulting from the consideration of equilibrium constants, become doubtful.

Indeed, according to Equation (114), the standard Gibbs energy $\Delta_r G^\circ$ must change and also the equilibrium constant. This point hardly appears in the literature. The reason of this fact is quite simple. The quasi-whole mondial community of chemists systematically adopts the same standard states. The need to eventually publish several values for the equilibrium constant (each related to different sets of standard states) does not matter.

However, the conclusions resulting from the consideration of equilibrium constants are not doubtful according to the following reasoning. Let us study a reaction for which two sets of standard states have been chosen. The activity values are not the same in both cases. But, at any extent of the reaction, the reaction Gibbs energy (not the standard reaction Gibbs energy) must remain the same, since the Gibbs energy is a state function. *The true invariant is the change in the Gibbs function between two thermodynamic states and not the equilibrium constant. The standard Gibbs energy changes and the thermodynamic equilibrium values are not invariant. There exists a kind of spontaneous compensation between the values of the standard reaction Gibbs energy and those of the activities in order that the Gibbs function change should be a constant, whatever the choice of standard states is. This compensation may be qualified as being subtle.*

5) Formal equilibrium constants—Advantage of the use of activities to express the mass action law

In literature, one finds several other forms of equilibrium constants. They are derived from the thermodynamic equilibrium constant defined above.

The thermodynamic constant must not be confused with any one of the so-called "constants" mentioned now which we symbolise by K. Let us again consider the general relation (107) and the "concentrations" of the reactants and products at equilibrium written in square brackets. Let us also define the new "equilibrium constants" K by the equation:

$$K = [M]^{vM}[N]^{vN}[P]^{vP}/[A]^{vA}[B]^{vB}[C]^{vC} \qquad (119)$$

Relation (117) is a generic one. The term generic means that the brackets embody the different kinds of "concentrations" according to the adopted scale (molarities, molalities, molar fractions and so forth). Let us write now the corresponding thermodynamic equilibrium constant K° by using the general relation $a = \gamma C$ (no matter of the scale of concentrations):

$$K^\circ = [M]^{vM}[N]^{vN}[P]^{vP}/[A]^{vA}[B]^{vB}[C]^{vC} \ \times \ [\gamma_M]^{vM}[\gamma_N]^{vN}[\gamma_P]^{vP}/[\gamma_A]^{vA}[\gamma_B]^{vB}[\gamma_C]^{vC}$$

(The activity coefficients are, of course, different according to the scale of concentrations adopted). The relations between the constants K and the thermodynamic one are:

$$K = K^\circ/\{[\gamma_M]^{vM}[\gamma_N]^{vN}[\gamma_P]^{vP}/[\gamma_A]^{vA}[\gamma_B]^{vB}[\gamma_C]^{vC}\}$$

Since the activity coefficients are not constant as it has already said, constants K are not true equilibrium constants. They are called *formal equilibrium constants*. It is evident that the more diluted the solutions are, the more these formal constants tend towards thermodynamic ones:

$$K \rightarrow K° \quad \text{as} \quad [\,] \rightarrow 0$$

All the formal equilibrium constants exhibit the drawback not to be truly constant on the whole domains of concentrations of the reactants and products or of pressure when the reaction takes place in gaseous phase. The standard thermodynamic equilibrium constant does not exhibit this drawback because of the part played by the activity coefficients and, hence, by the activities. It can be said that the activity coefficients rectify the disturbances brought about to the chemical equilibria when the reactants and products are not sufficiently diluted.

6) Differences of values between activities and concentrations

The goal of this paragraph is to give some figures permitting to appraise the differences which may exist between the numerical values of the activities and the corresponding concentrations, at least in some conditions, bearing in mind that both quantities are linked by the relation:

$$a = \gamma C$$

and that $\gamma \rightarrow 1$ when the concentration tends towards zero.

- Concerning the uncharged species in water, at concentrations less than 0,1 mol L^{-1}, the activity of an uncharged species is within 1% of its concentration. Hence, the activity coefficient of an uncharged molecule can usually be taken to be unity. For "concentrations" in solutions of ionic strength I (see just under) standing in the range 0,5 to 5 mol L^{-1}, the equation:

$$\log \gamma = k\,I$$

is obeyed. The activity coefficients of uncharged species are usually greater than unity.

- Concerning ions, the difference between the activities and the concentration are, by far, more marked. The Debye-Hückel theories permitting to reasonably calculate the activity coefficients of ions in polar solvents (such as water) demonstrate the importance of a quantity named the *ionic strength I* of the solution in this realm. It is defined by the relation:

$$I = \tfrac{1}{2} \Sigma_i \, C_i \, z_i^2$$

where C_i is the "concentration" of every ion in the solution (usually in molarities or molalities), z_i the relative electrical charge of ion i, the sum being expanded over all the ions of the solution. The higher the ionic strength, the higher the difference between the activity and the concentration. We must also notice the influence of the charge of the ions. As examples, the activity coefficients of ions (H^+), citrate^{3-}, PO_4^{3-} for the ionic strength 0,1 mol L^{-1} are, respectively, $\gamma = 0,83 - 0,115$ and 0, 095 (in water at 25°C)!

7) Come back on the reaction quotient and mass action law

We have seen that for the reaction (see paragraph 1):

$$v_A A + v_B B + v_C C + \ldots \rightarrow v_M M + v_N N + v_P P + \ldots\ldots \tag{120}$$

the reaction quotient Q is defined by the expression:

$$Q = a_M^{\,vM} \, a_N^{\,vN} \, a_P^{\,vP} / a_A^{\,vA} \, a_B^{\,vB} \, a_C^{\,vC}$$

It is important to emphasize the fact that Q may have every value depending only on the initial conditions of the reaction and also on its extent, whereas at the equilibrium the activities must absolutely match the value of the equilibrium constant. It is easy to verify that whatever the extent of the reaction:

$$\Delta_r G = (v_M \mu_M{}^\circ + v_N \mu_N{}^\circ + v_P \mu_P{}^\circ + \ldots - v_A \mu_A{}^\circ - v_B \mu_B{}^\circ - v_C \mu_C{}^\circ - \ldots)$$
$$+ RT \ln Q$$

and:

$$\Delta_r G = \Delta_r G^\circ + RT \ln Q \tag{121}$$

We must be careful to distinguish between $\Delta_r G$ which is the actual *Gibbs energy change* and the standard *Gibbs energy change* ΔG° (or $\Delta G'^\circ$). $\Delta_r G$ is sometimes called the Gibbs energy change of the system $\Delta G syst$. Q is the *mass-action* ratio. The great difference between both is that, at a given temperature, $\Delta_r G^\circ$ is a constant (once the standard states for the activities have been chosen) whereas $\Delta_r G$ depends on concentrations (activities of reactants and products).

8) Calculations of Gibbs energy changes accompanying a chemical reaction

The determination of the thermodynamic equilibrium constants permits the calculation of the corresponding standard Gibbs energy changes. This point is postponed to Chapter 22.

9) The Gibbs-Helmholtz equation

As it was shown in Chapter 17, at constant pressure:

$$dG = -S\, dT$$

or

$$d\Delta G = -\Delta S\, dT$$

Taking into account the basic definition of the Gibbs energy at constant temperature and pressure:

$$\Delta G = \Delta H - T\, \Delta S$$

$$\Delta G = \Delta H + T(d\Delta G/dT)$$

This equation divided by T^2 and rearranged gives:

$$(d\Delta G/T) = -\Delta H/T^2 \tag{122}$$

This equation is called the *Gibbs-Helmholtz equation*. It is a relationship giving the temperature dependence of the free energy at constant pressure.

One can immediately deduce the dependence with the temperature of the equilibrium constant which is given by:

$$(d\Delta G^\circ/T) = -R\, d \ln K/dT$$

$$d \ln K/dT = \Delta H^\circ/RT^2 \tag{123}$$

ΔH° is the enthalpy change accompanying the reaction when reactants and products are in their standard states (that is to say in infinite dilute solutions). If ΔH° is independent of temperature, this equation is immediately integrated.

10) Changes of K and ΔG with temperature

One can immediately deduce the dependence of the equilibrium constant which is given by the Gibbs' Helmholtz relation (120) which can be also written:

$$d \ln K^\circ / dT = \Delta_r H^\circ / RT^2$$

$\Delta_r H^\circ$ is the enthalpy change accompanying the reaction when reactants and products are in their standard states (that is to say in infinite dilute solutions). If ΔH° is independent of temperature, this equation is immediately integrated.

$\Delta_r H^\circ$ is the standard reaction enthalpy. It is defined by the relation:

$$\Delta_r H^\circ = (v_M H_M^\circ + v_N H_N^\circ + \ldots) - (v_A H_A^\circ + v_B H_B^\circ + \ldots)$$

or, in general,

$$\Delta_r H^\circ = \Sigma \, nH^\circ \, (\text{final state}) - \Sigma \, nH^\circ \, (\text{initial state})$$

Relation (120) is called the van't Hoff's equation.

Chapter 21

Gibbs Energy Function Changes
Further Comments

At several occasions, we have already mentioned the fact that the Gibbs energy function ΔG plays a pivotal part in the evolving of the biochemical reactions of bioenergetics. In this chapter, we mention some more of its properties. We also give some examples of calculations that have taken this function into account.

1) The Gibbs energy function

- Recall that the Gibbs function change ΔG_{syst} accompanying a chemical reaction should not be mistaken with the molar reaction Gibbs function change at equilibrium $\Delta_r G$ (see Chapter 18, Figure 19). They do not have the same mathematical status. The former change is a difference, the latter is a partial derivative. They no longer have the same physical status. The former is an extensive quantity, the latter is an intensive one.

- Let us mention that the function G is directly related to the isothermal-isobaric partition function (ensemble T, P, N), in statistical thermodynamics.

- If one considers the basic definition of the Gibbs energy,

$$\Delta G = \Delta H - T\,\Delta S$$

one can notice that several origins of spontaneous changes may exist. To study this point, it is judicious to consider the signs of the changes of enthalpy and of entropy which are operating simultaneously during a process. The results are mentioned in Table 8:

Table 8. Enthalpic or entropic origins of ΔG as a function of their signs.

ΔH	ΔS	ΔG
–	+	The reaction is spontaneous (exergonic)
–	–	the reaction is favourized by the enthalpy only. Spontaneous only for temperatures less than $T < \Delta H/\Delta S$
+	+	the reaction is favourized by the entropy only for temperatures such as $T > \Delta H/\Delta S$
+	–	the reaction is always defavourized

Recall that the maximum non-expansion work $-w'$ which can be obtained from a process at constant temperature and pressure is given by the value of ΔG of the process:

$$-w' \leq -(G_f - G_i)$$

2) Coupled reactions

Changes of Gibbs energies are additive. This property has the very important consequence for our purpose that an endergonic reaction may become possible when it is driven by an exergonic reaction. This is often the case for biochemical reactions evolving in bioenergetics. Of course, some conditions must be satisfied.

Let us consider the two following reactions:

$$A + B \rightleftharpoons C + D \quad \Delta G_1 \tag{124}$$

$$D + E \rightleftharpoons F + G \quad \Delta G_2 \tag{125}$$

If $\Delta G_1 \geq 0$, reaction (121) is not spontaneous. However, if simultaneously $\Delta G_1 + \Delta G_2 \leq 0$, both reactions evolve from the left to the right. The net reaction is:

$$A + B + E \rightleftharpoons C + F + G$$

Reaction (1) goes from left to right, the direction for which it is not spontaneous. This is because it is driven by reaction (2) which is more exergonic than (1) is endergonic. Both reactions are *coupled*.

Notice that the coupling is possible not only because of the mentioned values of Gibbs energies but also because there is a common reactant or product in both reactions. In chemistry, the phenomenon is named "equilibrium displacement" (see Chapter 29). Notice also that the coupling may exist between a chemical reaction and a physical process, such as the transfer of one reactant from one phase into another.

There is an interesting mechanical energy to the notion of coupled reactions. Let us consider the Figures 21–23. In Figures 21 and 22, it is evident that masses M_1 and M_2 fall under their weight. When both masses are linked through a pulley (Figure 23), their displacements are coupled. It is clear that if $M_1 > M_2$, the mass M_1 falls spontaneously downwards but, simultaneously, drives M_2 upwards. This is not a spontaneous displacement for M_2. At the borderline, when:

$$M_1 \approx M_2$$

more precisely, when the difference between both masses is infinitesimal, a state of equilibrium is reached (Figure 23);

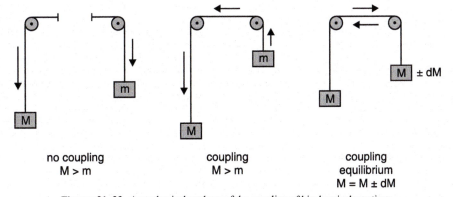

Figures 21–23. A mechanical analogy of the coupling of biochemical reactions.

3) Biological standard states

Biochemists commonly define other standard states which are different from those evoked above. Its characteristics are the following ones:

pH (aqueous solution) = 7; $[H^+] \approx 10^{-7}$ mol L^{-1}; $[H_2O] = 55,5$ mol L^{-1};

$[Mg^{2+}] = 10^{-3}$ mol L^{-1}; T = 298 K; p = 1 bar.

To find the relation between the thermodynamic and biological standard values of the chemical potential of hydrogen ions, we start from the thermodynamic relation:

$$\mu_{H+} = \mu°_{H+} - RT\ln (H^+)$$

where $\mu°_{H+}$ is the standard thermodynamic chemical potential of the (hydrated) proton

$$\mu_{H+} = \mu°_{H+} - RT\ln 10 . pH$$

since (see Chapter 26)

$$pH = -RT \log (H^+)$$

where (H^+) is the activity of the proton.

$\ln 10 = 2,303$.

At pH = 7, the chemical potential of the proton is given by:

$$\mu_{H+} = \mu°_{H+} - RT. 2,303. 7$$

$$\mu_{H+} = \mu°_{H+} - 2,479 . 2,303 . 7$$

$$\mu_{H+} = \mu°_{H+} - 39,96 \text{ kJ mol}^{-1}$$

Let us, now, adopt the biological standard state. The chemical potential of the proton is, now, formally:

$$\mu_{H+} = \mu°_{H+}' + RT\ln (H^+)$$

$\mu°_{H+}'$ is the standard chemical potential of the proton in the biological system. The problem is to set up the relation between $\mu°_{H+}$ and $\mu°_{H+}'$.

Of course, the chemical potential μ_{H+} is the same whatever the writing is (same species in the same solution). By definition, in the standard state, the activity of a species is equal to the unity. Hence, in the biological scale, at pH = 7 (thermodynamic scale), $(H^+) = 1$ (biological scale). As a result:

$$\mu_{H+} = \mu°_{H+}'$$

and, after equalization of both writings:

$$\mu°_{H+} - 39,96 = \mu°_{H+}'$$

At 298,15 K, the two standard states differ by 39,96 kJ.mol^{-1}. An application of this reasoning is given in Chapter 27.

In another convention, when H_2O, H^+, Mg^{2+} are present as reactants or products, their concentrations are not included in the equations defining the formal equilibrium constants. However, their values are taken into account in the calculation of the formal equilibrium constant. In the appendix I-6 such a correction is mentioned.

4) Exercises

Exercise 1:

Calculate the equilibrium constants corresponding to the following standard Gibbs energies $\Delta G'^{\circ}$: 17,09; –11,39; –17,09 J mol^{-1}: T = 298,15 K.

Answ:

   $\Delta G'^{\circ} = -RT\ln K$: $R = 8,315\ J\ mol^{-1}K^{-1}$

   10^{-3}; 10^2; 10^3

Exercise 2:

Calculate the equilibrium constant of the reaction:

   glucose-1-phosphate $\rightleftharpoons$ glucose-6-phosphate

knowing that starting from 20 10^{-3} mole of glucose-1-phosphate alone, one finds, after equilibrium at pH = 7, a result of 19 10^{-3} mole of glucose-6-phosphate + 1 10^{-3} mole of glucose-1-phosphate. (The reaction is catalyzed by the enzyme phosphoglucomutase. The location of the equilibrium is not changed by the presence of the catalyzer).

Answ:

   K = glucose-6-phosphate/glucose-1-phosphate at equilibrium

   K = 19

Exercise 3:

Difference between $\Delta G_{sys}t$ and $\Delta G'^{\circ}$

Let us consider the following transformation:

   fructose-6-phosphate $\rightleftharpoons$ glucose-6-phosphate

1) What is its standard reactional Gibbs energy $\Delta G'^{\circ}$ knowing that K(25°C) = 1,97?
2) What is ΔG_{syst} for the following concentrations: fructose-6-phosphate 1,5 mol l^{-1} and glucose-6- phosphate 0,5 mol l^{-1}?

Answ.

1) $\Delta G'^{\circ} = -RT \ln 1,97$

   $\Delta G'^{\circ} = 1,68\ kJ\ mol^{-1}$

2) $\Delta G_{syst} = \Delta G'^{\circ} + RT \ln(1,5/0,5)$

   $\Delta G_{syst} = 4,4\ kJ\ mol^{-1}$

Chapter 22

Obtention of Standard Reactional Gibbs Energies, Enthalpies and Entropies

The importance of the knowledge of standard reactional Gibbs energies is, among other reasons, justified by the fact that it permits to calculate the equilibrium constant values of chemical reactions. That is to say, they permit to foresee the concentrations of the products and reactants of a chemical or biochemical reaction at equilibrium. Hence, it is interesting to investigate some means of their obtention. The converse is also true. The knowledge of the equilibrium constants permits to obtain the standard reactional Gibbs energies, as we have already seen.

In this chapter, we mention two methods of obtention of values of thermodynamic functions that can be called precise and approximate, at least at first sight. Among the precise ones, we essentially consider the thermal methods which are based on the third law of thermodynamics.

1) Precise methods

1-1) Calculation of the entropy of substances at 25°C. The third law of thermodynamics

The third law permits to calculate the standard change of entropy accompanying a chemical reaction. Calculations involve the values of the molar entropies of the substances which are the reactants and products of the studied reaction. Some values have already been given (see Chapter 13).

Calculations are based on the equation (see Chapter 13):

$(\partial S/\partial T)p = C_p/T$

where S is the molar entropy and C_p the heat capacity at constant pressure of the substance. As a result, molar entropies are given by the relation:

$S(T) = \int_{T1}^{T2} (C_p/T)dT$

The evaluation of integrals imply to know:

- on one hand, data concerning the values of the heat capacities C_p at different temperatures;
- on the other, a numerical value of the entropy at one temperature in order to overcome the problem of the knowledge of the integration constant.

Thermal data permit to develop heat capacities as developments in series as a function of temperatures (see Chapter 8: Kirchoff's rule).

Obtaining the numerical value of one entropy at a given temperature is based on the *third law of thermodynamics*. It stipulates that every perfect crystalline substance exhibits an entropy value which is null at absolute zero: $S(0K) = 0$ J $K^{-1}mol^{-1}$, whence:

$$S(T) = \int_0^T (C_p/T)dT$$

The integration must, of course, take into account the phase changes which may exist in the domain of integration, since they are accompanied by changes in entropy.

1-2) Standard reaction entropy

- The standard reaction entropy $\Delta_r S°$ is defined as being the difference between the sum of molar entropies $S°$ of products and the sum of molar entropy of reactants, all substances being in their standard states at the reactional temperature:

$$\Delta_r S° = \Sigma \, vS°_{(products)} - \Sigma vS°_{(reactants)}$$

Symbols v represent the stoichiometric coefficients of the reactants and products. This definition is analogous to that of the standard reaction enthalpy.

- The standard reaction entropy can be also determined from the fundamental relation:

$$\Delta_r G° = \Delta_r H° - T_r \Delta S°$$

This way of obtention is particularly interesting when a reversible galvanic cell is used to pick up experimental data. The starting equation is (see Chapter 14):

$$(\partial G/\partial T)_p = -S$$

In the present case, for substances participating in the studied chemical reaction in the standard state:

$$(\partial G°/\partial T)_p = -S°$$

and for the standard chemical reaction itself:

$$(\partial \, \Delta G°/\partial T)_p = -\Delta S°$$

If the reaction takes place in a reversible electrochemical cell (see Chapter 27):

$$\Delta S° = nF \, (dE°/dT)$$

where $E°$ is the standard electromotive force, n the number of electrons exchanged in the reaction called the *reaction cell* and F the faraday.

Thus, the sought standard entropy change of the reaction may be determined from the temperature coefficient of the emf (electromotive force) of the cell.

1-3) Standard reaction Gibbs energy

The main methods of determination of standard Gibbs energies are based on:
- the determination of equilibrium constants,
- the measurements of electromotive forces of galvanic cells,

– the measurements of energy intervals in molecules allowing the calculation of molecular partition functions (see statistical thermodynamics),

– the use of the third law of thermodynamics.

In this paragraph, we only confine ourselves to give the principles of the determinations through the equilibrium constants and also through applying the third law. Measurements of electromotive forces are postponed to Chapter 27 devoted to galvanic cells. The determination of energy intervals is deferred to the study of "statistical thermodynamics" which is not carried out in this book.

1-3-1) determination through the equilibrium constants values and *vice versa*

The principle is based on the use of equations (see Chapter 20):

$$\Delta_r G° = -RT \ln K° \tag{126}$$

$$\Delta_r G'° = -RT \ln K'° \tag{127}$$

As an example, let us consider the biochemical reaction (catalyzed with the enzyme *phosphoglucomutase at pH = 7*) (Cf Chapter 34):

glucose 1-phosphate $\rightleftharpoons$ glucose – 6-phosphate

The equilibrium constant $K'°$ at 25°C is:

$K'° =$ glucose 6-phosphate/glucose 1-phosphate

$K'° = 19$

(This value is found by assuming that the activities of the two species are equal to their concentrations). Applying relation (124) gives:

$$\Delta_r G'° = -8,31 \cdot 298,15 \cdot \ln 19$$

$$\Delta_r G'° = -7295 \text{ J mol}^{-1}$$

Let us recall in passing that there are numerous methods of determination of equilibrium constants.

Evidently, the converse experiment (calculating equilibrium constants through standard reaction Gibbs energies) is practised.

1-3-2) determinations through the third law

One may consider that there exist two other ways of obtention of standard reaction Gibbs energies based on the third law. The first one consists in applying the fundamental equation which defines the Gibbs energy ($\Delta G = \Delta H - T\Delta S$). The second consists in using Gibbs energy functions.

• determination through the definition of the Gibbs energy:

The used equation is:

$$\Delta_r G° = \Delta_r H° - T\Delta_r S° \text{ or } \Delta_r S° = (\Delta_r H° - \Delta_r G°)/T$$

Since, according to the Gibbs-Helmholtz equation:

$[\partial(G/T)/\partial T]_p = -H/T^2$

it is easy to obtain:

$d\ln K/dT = \Delta_r H^\circ/RT^2$

This is the van't Hoff equation already encountered.

Two kinds of determinations are involved, that of the reaction enthalpies and that of the reaction entropies.

The term $T\Delta_r S^\circ$ is obtained as it is described in paragraph 2 above, that is to say by applying the third law.

- Concerning the standard reaction enthalpies, we have already mentioned some means to obtain them (see Chapter 8). Here, we mention the use of the *standard heats of formation of species (reactants and products)*, ΔH_f° from their elements *at the temperature T, also called the enthalpy function* $H_T^\circ - H_0^\circ$. As an illustration of the method, let us consider the compound C and its formation reaction by starting from its elements A, B:

A	+	B	$\rightarrow$	C
element		element		resulting species
in		in		in
standard state		standard state		standard state
at temperature T		at temperature T		at temperature T

The formation heats (from the elements) are calculated from the differences of standard enthalpies $H_T^\circ - H_0^\circ$ at temperatures T and 0K. These differences are tabulated (see Table 8)

$C(T) = C(0) - (H_T^\circ - H_0^\circ)_C$

$A(T) = A(0) + (H_0^\circ - H_T^\circ)_A$

$B(T) = B(0) + (H_0^\circ - H_T^\circ)_B$

Let us consider the reaction:

$A(0K) + B(0K) \rightarrow C(0K)$

$\Delta H = \Delta H f_0^\circ$

For the formation of C(T) from its elements:

$\Delta H_T^\circ = \Delta H f_0^\circ + (H_T^\circ - H_0^\circ)_C - (H_0^\circ - H_T^\circ)_A - (H_0^\circ - H_T^\circ)_B$

In the occurrence, ΔH_T° is the standard enthalpy of formation of C at the temperature T and likewise for the other reactants and products of the chemical reaction under study.

Table 9. Enthalpy function $H_T^° - H_0^°$ (after I.M. Klotz and R.M. Rosenberg-chemical thermodynamics—See general bibliography).

	$\Delta Hf_0^°$	$H_T^° - H_0^°$ J mol^{-1} at T (K)			
Substance	kJ mol^{-1}	298,16	400	600	800
$H_2(g)$	0	8459.5	11415.6	17,257.4	23,146.3
$O_2(g)$	0	8671.8	11672.2	17,887.1	24,470.1
C(graphite)	0	1051.5	2100.9	5,008.1	8,701.7
$H_2O(g)$	−238.707	9897.0	13350.9	20,407.6	27,962.5
$CO_2(g)$	−392.789	9355.3	13354.3	22,2476	32,1417
$CH_4(g)$	−66.755	9981.8	13472.1	23,194.8	34,781.8
$C_2H_6(g)$	−69.0411	11938.1	17957	33,5069	53,336.8

1-3-3) determination through the Gibbs energy functions

The Gibbs energy functions are defined at the temperature T by the equation:

$$(G_T^° - H_0^°)/T$$

Their unit is in J mol^{-1}K^{-1}. As in the case of enthalpies (see Table 10), the values of this function for a given substance at a given temperature are tabulated (Table 10). They give the standard Gibbs energy of formation $\Delta G f_T^°$ of one substance by starting from its elements. If we again take the substance C (formed from elements A and B) as an example of a compound participating to the studied chemical reaction, its standard Gibbs energy of formation $\Delta G_T^°$ is given by the equation:

$$\Delta G_T^° = \Delta Hf_0^° + (G_T^° - H_0^°)_C - (G_T^° - H_0^°)_A - (G_T^° - H_0^°)_B$$

This relation simply comes from:

$$\Delta G_T^° = \Delta G_0^° + (G_T^° - G_0^°)_C - (G_T^° - G_0^°)_A - (G_T^° - G_0^°)_G$$

since:

$$G_0^° = H_0^° \quad \text{(third principle of thermodynamics)}$$

$\Delta G_0^°$ is the standard Gibbs energy of formation of substance C at 0 K. Finally, the standard Gibbs energy of formation of substance C is given by the expression:

$$\Delta G f_T^° = [\Delta G_0^° + (G_T^° - G_0^°)_C - (G_T^° - G_0^°)_A - (G_T^° - G_0^°)_G]$$

The same calculation is done for all the products and reactants of the chemical reaction. Of course:

$$\Delta_r G_T^° = \Sigma \Delta G f_T^° \text{ (products)} - \Sigma \Delta G f_T^° \text{ (reactants)}$$

It seems that the last method of obtention of standard reaction Gibbs energies is the best one. The obtention of the Gibbs energy function values avoid the use of empirical equations. Moreover, they are confirmed by calculations of statistical thermodynamics.

Table 10. Gibbs energy functions: $(G_T^\circ - H_0^\circ)/T$ [$G_T^\circ - H_0^\circ$ J mol^{-1}; T K] $(G_T^\circ - H_0^\circ)/T$ at T°K (J mol^{-1} K^{-1}).

Substance	298,16	400	600	800	1000
$H_2(g)$	−102.10	−110.44	−122.07	−130.36	−136.84
$O_2(g)$	−175.81	−184.39	−196.33	−205.00	−211.91
C(graphite)	−1.33	−3.45	−6.17	−8.94	−11.58
$CO_2(g)$	−181.22	−191.56	−205.81	−216.92	−226.18
$H_2O(g)$	−155.38	−165.14	−178.77	−188.64	−196.54
$CH_4(g)$	−152.40	−162.43	−177.19	−188.98	−199.18
$C_2H_6(g)$	−189.23	−201.64	−221.87	−239.47	−255.44
$C_2H_4(g)$	−183.84	−194.83	−211.93	−226.51	−239.47
$C_6H_6(g)$	−221.25	−236.96	−266.27	−294.02	−320.06

In appendix I-8, Gibbs energies of formation of some biochemical compounds are mentioned.

2) Approximate methods

They are empirical methods of correlation which permit to estimate thermodynamic properties permitting, in turn, to calculate standard reaction Gibbs energies and the corresponding equilibrium constants. They also permit to estimate some enthalpies. These methods are based on "extrathermodynamic" relationships.

Several methods are based on the hypothesis that a given thermodynamic property of an organic substance can be resolved into contributions corresponding to groups of atoms constituting a fragment of its molecular squeleton. These groups also exist in other molecules and can be considered as possessing the same value of a thermodynamic quantity whatever the structure of the organic structure is. This is a hypothesis of additivity.

Actually, some thermodynamic quantities which are constitutive functions of molecular structure tend to be additive. Hence, in the physico-chemical literature, there exist numerous *linear quantitative relationships* between a molar property of an organic molecule and the number and the nature of the chemical groups constituting it.

As molar property, it is particularly the case of the Gibbs energy, especially in gaseous phase. The molar values of the property are assumed to be precisely additive functions of independent contributions assignable to part-structures of the molecule. The nature of these part-structures is, of course, subject of arbitrary choice. This is the lowest approximation method. Often, it is not sufficiently adequate. In order to achieve a higher degree of accuracy of the calculated values, further complicated approximations (rules of additivity) may be done. Additivity may be improved by, for example, collating special contributions for each identified group present several times in the same molecule, but not located in the same environment in it. Successively higher approximations improve the accuracy of the calculated values, but there is a cost to increase the number of additivity rules. It is the increase of the number of the parameters permitting to take into account the supplementary rules of additivity. The latter must be evaluated by fitting the calculated values to the experimental data.

Numerous methods of calculation have been proposed. We confine ourselves to only cite the method of Andersen, Beyer and Watson and also the so-called "thermochemical groups method" (see general bibliography "physical chemistry" P.W. Atkins).

The fact that, among other thermodynamic functions, the Gibbs energy function gives the best results with these approximate methods is interesting. This intriguing point may be, perhaps, explained by a "fortunate" mutual compensation between its enthalpic and entropic parts.

All these methods may provide us with reasonable estimates of enthalpies, entropies and Gibbs energies when no adequate information is at our disposal. Actually, it is interesting to have some forecast of the possibility of a reaction. But, in no case, they match the precision of experimental values. That of the latter ones is of the order of size of $\pm$ 1 kJ mol^{-1}. With the approximate methods, variations of the order of 15% are not rare.

In the general bibliography, we present a list of documents in which tables of thermodynamic data are reported. Otherwise, several data are given in this book, overall when they are necessary to buttress some reasonings.

EXERCISES

Exercise 1:

Calculate the molar entropy of chlorine hydride (hydrochloric acid-gas) at 298,15 K. One gives: C_p(solid I) = 16,24 J K^{-1}; C_p(solid II) = 44,03 J K^{-1}; C_p(liquid) = 58,54 J K^{-1}; C_p(gas) = 29,21 J K^{-1}; (It is recalled that hydrochloric gas exhibits two allotropic modifications I and II in the solid state, the phase change temperature of which is 98, 36 K); T_f(fusion variety 2) = 158,91K; T_{eb} = 188,07 K. S (16 K) = 1,25 J mol^{-1}K^{-1}: Enthalpy change (1 → II) = 1188,37 J mol^{-1}; Fusion enthalpy: 1989,68 J mol^{-1}; Vaporisation enthalpy =16134 J mol^{-1}.

Answ:

Owing to the existence of several successive phases in the domain of temperatures 16 K – 292,8 K with the existence of several values of heat capacities and also the occurrence of thermal effects accompanying the phase changes, it is necessary to decompose the process in the following successive transformations:

Step 0: allotrope   I 0 K   →   16 K

Step 1: allotrope I   16 K   →   98,36 K

Step 2: allotrope I   →   allotrope II

Step 3: allotrope II   98,36 K   →   158,91 K

Step 4: allotrope II   →   liquid

Step 5: liquid (158,91 K)   →   liquid (188,07 K)

Step 6: liquid (188,07 K)   →   vapor (188,07 K)

Step 7: vapor (188,07 K)   →   vapor (298,15 K)

The entropy changes for the steps 1,3, 5,7 are calculated with the Equation (A), whereas for steps 2, 4,6 it is Equation (B) which is used (see Chapter 18).

$$S(T) = \int_{T1}^{T2} C_p/TdT \tag{A}$$

$$S(T) = \Delta H(transition)/T \tag{B}$$

After having performing the sum of the changes since 0 K, the standard molar entropy of chlorine hydride is:

$$S(298,15 \text{ K}) = 185,6 \text{ J K}^{-1} \text{ mole}^{-1}$$

Chapter 23

Ligand Binding to Macromolecules

Another aspect of the notion of chemical equilibrium is that concerning the binding of chemical species called *ligands* on *macromolecules*, especially on *proteins*. Such processes are the rule rather than the exception in biological systems. This chapter is of importance for our purpose because of the fact that the functioning of proteins often depends on interactions with other molecules. Thus, for example, ligands bind to a variety of receptors such as enzymes, antibodies, DNA and membrane-bound proteins. Protein binding also plays an important role in pharmacology.

Behind the phenomenon of binding exists all the fundamentals which are the basis of the concept of chemical equilibrium, that is to say, for example, those of Gibbs energy of binding and of binding constants.

Here, we confine ourselves to mentioning the simple theories which permit to justify some simple means of analysis of binding data.

1) Definitions

- A molecule bound *reversibly* by a protein is called a *ligand*. The term reversibly is important because it means that the nature of protein-ligand interactions is transient. This property is critical for life. It permits, indeed, an organism to respond quickly to the changes of the conditions of its functioning. Ligands can be any kind of molecules, small ones such as metabolites or large ones such as another protein, for example.
- The *binding site* of a protein is the place where the ligand binds. The binding site is complementary to the ligand in size, charge, shape and hydrophobic and hydrophilic character. Furthermore, the interaction is specific. A protein may often have several sites.
- An *induced fit* is the structural adaptation that occurs between the protein and the ligand, with a conformational change in the protein. It is a result of the binding. It permits a tighter binding than without the inducing of fit.

2) On the ability of biological macromolecules to interact with various small and large molecules

The first point to highlight is that these interactions are very specific. These interactions are also of very high affinity.

The second point is the following one. For a long-time, the interactions have been envisioned as being the result of the fact that the protein was topologically complementary to the stereochemistry of the substrate. Over the years, the origin of the interactions has evolved. Now, one knows that beyond the stereochemical aspect, the formation of hydrogen bonds, interactions dipole-dipole, and the formation of salts between the ligand and the interacting groups of the binding site also intervene. For example, the phosphate group that may be brought by the structure of a ligand may be able to interact electrostatically with groups instead of rests.

The linking of the ligand on the macromolecule is governed by several points of interactions between them. They define a potential energy surface so-designated to describe the interactions with the ligand.

3) Adsorption, another phenomenon for which theories of binding apply

We have already briefly recalled the part played by the binding in the realm of biochemistry. In physics and chemistry, we encounter other domains in which theories of binding apply. This is the case of adsorption of small molecules or ligands on a surface of a large molecule or of a solid. Mentioning some conditions of adsorption shows the difficulties that the theories of adsorption, and, hence those of binding on proteins, must explain.

Adsorption on a solid or on a protein is realized on portions of surfaces of these substrates, portions called sites.

Some modalities of adsorption are given now. Often,
 − a substrate may possess n classes of sites, each class i having v_i sites with a unique association constant K_i (association constant: see below). In these conditions, all the sites are identical. But they may also not be identical. In this case, the adsorption on a first site may modify that on other of the same class. The association constants are, hence, different:
 − each class may have only one site ($v_i = 1$);
 − the same class of sites may be brought by different parts of the solid or of the protein:
 − there may be multioccupancy of one or several sites;
 − multioccupancy may modify the association constants of the successive ligands of the same site:

and so forth. We shall only study a few of these cases.

4) General equilibrium expression describing the reversible binding of a protein P to a ligand L

At the outset, it must be known that at constant pressure and temperature, the Gibbs energy of the binding reaction decreases during a spontaneous process and cannot do anything else.

Let us suppose the reaction of binding:

$$P + L \rightleftharpoons PL \tag{128}$$

The equilibrium is quantified by the association constant K_a (do not confuse this constant K_a with that of acidic dissociation constant of an acid! See Chapter 26):

$$K_a = [PL]/[P][L_f] \tag{129}$$

In this expression, [PL] is the concentration (mol L^{-1}) of the "aggregate" protein-ligand, [P] the concentration of the remaining protein. This is the concentration in mol L^{-1} of the remaining non-occupied sites. $[L_f]$ is the concentration (mol L^{-1}) of the free ligand. K_a is expressed in (mol $L^{-1})^{-1}$ or M^{-1} where M means "1 molar" and stands for 1 mol L^{-1}. K_a is the constant of association. It is called the standard association constant, defined by:

$$K_a = [PL]_{eq}/[P]_{eq}[L_f]_{eq} \tag{130}$$

in which the concentrations (activities) are those at equilibrium. As the general theory of thermodynamics indicates it, the Gibbs energy $\Delta_r G$ accompanying the association reaction (125) is:

$$\Delta_r G = \Delta_r G° + RT \ln \{[PL]_{eq}/[P]_{eq}[L_f]_{eq}\} \tag{131}$$

where $\Delta_r G$ and $\Delta_r G°$ are the Gibbs energy and the standard Gibbs energy of the binding reaction. It is evident that K_a is the affinity constant of the ligand L for the protein P.

Notice that:

- in this book, association constants are written in terms of concentrations, with brackets, for the sake of simplicity. Actually, they might be defined as usually in activities;
- the binding equilibria are characterized by association constants and by dissociation constants as well (see under), whereas constants defining other types of equilibria, at least in water, are usually dissociation constants.

Of course, a dissociation constant K_D of the "aggregate" PL according to:

$$PL \rightleftharpoons P + L$$

is also defined.

The equilibrium constant K_a is equal to the ratio of the rates constants of the forward k_f and reverse k_r reactions that form the "aggregate" PL (see Chapter 25). Thus:

$$K_a = [PL]/[P][L_f] = k_f/k_r$$

All the theory coming from classical thermodynamics and concerning the chemical equilibrium applies to the binding equilibria. Relations (127) and (128) are examples of this assertion. We can hence write:

$$\Delta G°' = -RT\ln K'$$

and

$$\Delta G°' = \Delta H°' - T \Delta S°'$$

and also:

$$d \ln K/dT = \Delta_r H°/RT^2 \quad \textit{(Van't Hoff relationship—see Chapter 22)}$$

$$\Delta S°' = (\Delta H°' - \Delta G°')/T$$

Concerning these points, it is interesting to mention the sources of thermodynamic changes for the binding of ligands. They include: the change in solvation of the ligand and of the protein—the interactions between the ligand and the binding site (Recall that the corresponding data may concern together the formation of hydrogen bonds, interactions charge-charge, the fixation or loss of protons by the protein and the buffer—the loss of a second buffer owing to the binding of the first—a conformational change of the ligand or of the macromolecule necessary for the fixation—a change in the state of aggregation of ligand or macromolecule or both).

5) The simplest case of binding

In this case, the protein does possess a unique class of sites, but we suppose there are several sites, that is to say v sites and that each site can only contain one molecule of ligand. The "extraction" of the theoretical parameters of binding from experimental data is carried out by a graphical means, the principle of which is founded on the following reasoning.

Let us name $[P_t]$ the total concentration of the protein (of the sites), one can write:

$$[P] = [P_t] - [PL]$$

Otherwise, according to (126):

$K_a [P][L_f] = [PL]$

Substituting the preceding expression of [P] into the latter gives;

$[PL]/[P_t] = K_a[L_f]/(1 + K_a[L_f])$

Let us symbolize the ratio $[PL]/[P_t]$ by r. r is the ratio of ligand bound per mole of total protein. The equation:

$$r = K_a[L_f]/(1 + K_a[L_f]) \tag{132}$$

is nothing else than the Langmuir adsorption isotherm (Figure 24). Another expression is used. It is mathematically equivalent to (129). It is:

$$r = [L_f]/(K_D + [L_f]) \tag{133}$$

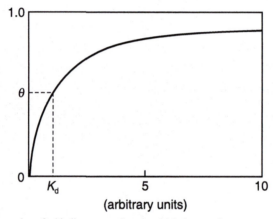

Figure 24. Graphical representation of a binding curve. Case in which the protein possesses a unique class of sites. There are several sites and each site can contain only one molecule of ligand.

The function represented by the expression (129) is a branch of a rectangular hyperbola.

Another expression is used. It is (130).

By way of example, let us cite myoglobin. Recall that myoglobin receives the dioxygen in the muscles and reserves it for further use. The binding of dioxygen is in agreement with the theory developed above, as it is indicated by Figure 25 representing the binding of dioxygen to myoglobin. The experimental data obey the following equations:

$r = [O_2]/([O_2] + K_a)$ and $r = P_{O2}/(P_{O2} + P_{50})$

where P_{O2} is the partial pressure of dioxygen in presence of myoglobin. According to Henry's law (see Chapter 19), there is proportionality between the vapor pressure of a solute and the concentration of the latter in the solution under this partial pressure. The pressure P_{50} is half the pressure P_{O2} for which the binding curve exhibits its horizontal asymptote.

The values of association (or dissociation) constants of binding are located on a large extent. By examples, the dissociation constant of the complex avidine-biotine is $1 \ 10^{-15}$. The complex is very stable. The complex calmoduline/Ca^{2+} is by far less stable ($K_D = 2 \ 10^{-5}$).

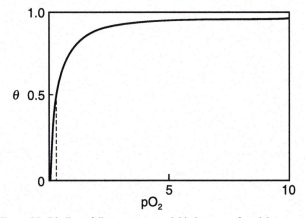

Figure 25. Binding of dioxygen to myoglobin in terms of partial pressure.

6) Achieving experimental data

Several methods are used to determine the amount of ligand bound to a protein. Let us cite equilibrium dialysis, ultrafiltration, electrophoresis, gel filtration, nuclear magnetic resonance, kinetic methods, and radioactive methods.

Treatments of experimental data are often carried out through the study of the *binding isotherms*. A binding isotherm is the diagram: r versus $[L_f]$. The curves $r/[L_f]$ are accessible experimentally.

7) A graphical treatment of the preceding case—Scatchard's plot

Let us again consider the equilibrium (125) and the corresponding mass action law (126). The principle of the graphical Scatchard's plot method is the following one. It is based on the fact that the protein-substrate binding site is saturable. As more ligand is added to a fixed amount of protein, an increasing fraction of protein is occupied by the substrate. It is easy to recognize graphically when the saturation in substrate of protein is obtained, that is to say when $[PL] = [PL_{max}]$. This is done by registering the diagram fixed [PL]/[total substrate added]. The diagram exhibits a hyperbolic form (Figure 26) with a portion nearly horizontal which precisely indicates the saturation. (If it is easy to recognize the saturation, the latter must be marked out, after some parasitic binding corrections are achieved).

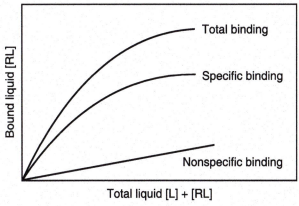

Figure 26. Scatchard's diagram.

Let us name the maximum number of unoccupied sites P_{max}. In these conditions, the mass action law is:

$$K_a = [PL]/[Lf] ([PL_{max}] - [PL])$$

this relation can also be written:

$$[PL]/[L] = Ka ([PL_{max}] - [PL])$$

Notice that the ratio [PL]/[L] is the ratio [ligand bound]/[ligand free]. The experimental diagram [PL]/[total ligand added] permits to obtain all the unknown concentrations. Data coming from the preceding diagram permit to trace the linear plot [Bound substrate]/[free substrate] versus [total ligand added]. The slope gives $-1/Ka$ and the intercept on the x axis [PL max] (see Figure 27).

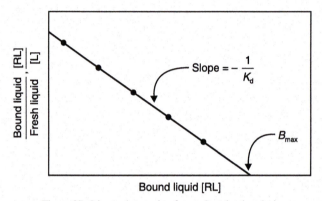

Figure 27. Linear plot coming from a Scatchard analysis.

Equation (129) can be linearized. It can be transformed into:

$$1/r = 1/K_a [L_f] + 1$$

If there are v independent binding sites of the same class (this is the case of the model investigated), the expression of the binding equilibria is:

$$r = v K_a[L_f]/(1 + K_a[L_f])$$

or in an equivalent manner:

$$1/r = (1/vK_a) (1/[L_f]) + 1/v$$

Since, by hypothesis, the sites are identical, their association constants are therefore the same. Another form of this expression is:

$$v/[L_f] = vK_a - rK_a \tag{134}$$

Relation (131) is the basis of the treatment of data according to Scatchard. A Scatchard's plot is obtained by drawing the ratio $v/[L_f]$ versus r (Figure 28).

It is clear that by extrapolating the line $v/[L_f]$ until 0, then $v = r$. The number v of sites is known. Notice that here the data come from an experiment of pharmacology, more specifically, of receptology.

Scatchard plots yield a straight line when only one class of bonding sites exist. Scatchard's technique does not work when there exist several classes of sites.

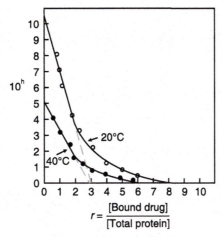

$$r = \frac{[\text{Bound drug}]}{[\text{Total protein}]}$$

Figure 28. Example of a Scatchard's plot.

8) Case in which several classes of sites exist

In this case, the plot $r/[L_f]$ as a function of r is not linear. One way to study it is to seek the fit between the experimental curve and the function:

$$r = v_1 K_1 [L_f]/(1 + K_1 [L_f]) + v_2 K_2 [L_f]/(1 + K_2 [L_f]) + ... v_n K_n [L_f]/(1 + K_n [L_f])$$

As previously, v_n and K_n are the number and the association constant of the site n.

In better cases, the binding diagram may present several successive linear plots, each of them corresponding to a class of sites.

9) Cooperative ligand binding—Hill's equation

Cooperativity may occur between two or several sites or two classes of sites. Cooperativity between two sites means that an event that occurs on one site affects the properties of the second site. In positive cooperative binding, the binding power of all the sites is enhanced when, at least, one site of the molecule is occupied. The binding curve is S-shaped (Figure 29).

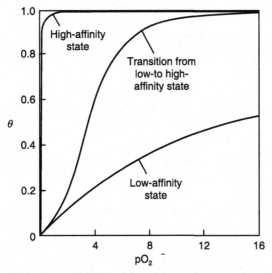

Figure 29. Typical curve of binding when there exists a positive cooperative effect.

We can conceive, indeed, that because of positive cooperativity, the association constant of the ligand with the n^{nd} site is higher than that with the $n-1^{nd}$ one. As a result, the n^{nd} site is associated with all the m molecules of ligand. Finally, when the binding is strongly cooperative, only two kinds of species are of importance. They are P and PL_m. (The phenomenon is analogous to that encountered during the formation of an *ultimate* complex in the chemistry of complexes in solutions).

The equilibrium reaction that is of utmost importance is:

$$P + mL \rightleftharpoons PL_m$$

and the overall equilibrium constant is:

$$K_a = [PL_m]/[L_f]^m [P]$$

The expression for r is:

$$r = [L_f]^m/([L_f]^m + 1/K_a)$$

After rearrangement:

$$r/(1 - r) = [L_f]^m/(1/K_a)$$

The last two relations can be also written:

$$r = [L_f]^m/([L_f]^m + K_D)$$

and

$$r/(1 - r) = [L_f]^m/K_D$$

where K_D is the dissociation constant of the aggregate.

$$\log [r/(1 - r)] = m \log [L_f] - \log K_D \tag{135}$$

where $K_D = [L]^m_{0,5}$.

It is interesting to consider the difference existing between Scatchard's plot and Hill's plot. Recall that Scatchard's plot concerns the case in which there exists a unique class of sites (n = 1), but there exist several (v) sites. The theory of Scatchard's plot is founded on the relation (131) which can also be written:

$$v/(1 - v) = [L_f]/K_a$$

or

$$\log [v/(1 - v)] = \log [L_f] - \log K_a \tag{136}$$

whereas for Hill's plot, it is the relation (132) which is obtained. Hence, these graphical processes constitute a simple means to distinguish both cases.

10) The binding of dioxygen to hemoglobin and myoglobin

The mechanism of transporting dioxygen fom the lungs to other parts of the body has been studied extensively. The main carrier of dioxygen is hemoglobin. It is contained in the red blood cells. Myoglobin receives the dioxygen in the muscles and reserves it for further use.

Figure 30 represents the dioxygen binding isotherms on hemoglobin and on myoglobin.

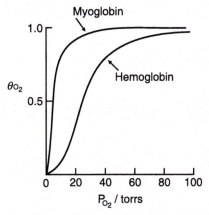

Figure 30. Binding isotherms of hemoglobin and myoglobin with dioxygen.

It is clear that the binding of myoglobin is non-cooperative whereas that of hemoglobin is. Another point to highlight is the fact that the myoglobin curve is everywhere above the hemoglobin curve. From the mathematical standpoint, in order to explain the second fact, it is necessary that the initial slope of the myoglobin curve be larger than that of hemoglobin. From another standpoint, we know that hemoglobin is constituted from four identical subunits which are similar to the unique one of myoglobin. All these facts indicate that myoglobin is constituted by a monomeric polymer having one binding site. Hemoglobin is constituted by four identical polymers of the same kind, each having the same binding site as is the case in the monomer of myoglobin.

The cooperativity of the bindings of hemoglobin facilitates the loading and the unloading of dioxygen. It is clear, according to the cooperative isotherm, that the loading and the unloading can be accomplished within narrow range of concentrations. At the partial pressure in the muscles [about 20 torrs: 1 torr = (101325/760) Pa], the fractional occupation of the sites is about r = 0,2. One can consider that hemoglobin unloads easily for this reason. At the partial pressure of about 100 torr, the fractional occupation takes the value r about 1. Hemoglobin loads easily. It would not be so easy and so complete in both directions with myoglobin alone.

11) Allosterism

The term is used whenever two ligands on two different sites of the same protein can communicate through the medium, that is to say through the protein itself or through the solvent.

Originally, the term "allosteric" was used for some enzymes, so-called regulatory enzymes, where an effector binds to a site other than the active one and thereby changes the properties of the active site. (Regulatory, see Chapter 30). An (allosteric) effector is generally a small metabolite or cofactor which can modulate the activity of regulatory enzymes.

Chapter **24**

Open Systems–Some Rudiments of Non-Equilibrium Thermodynamics*

The thermodynamics principles, recalled so far, only apply to closed systems. However, the living cells are not closed systems. They are open systems. They exchange matter with their surroundings, together with energy and work.

All the principles developed before are devoted to the thermodynamics of the equilibrium, the use of which is not very well adapted in the present case since biological cells are open systems. The latter ones are rather justiciable of a theoretical treatment within the framework of "non-equilibrium thermodynamics". We limit ourselves to recall some results of thermodynamics of non-equilibrium in relation with our purpose. We also limit ourselves to a brief study of the stationary non-equilibrium states. This is the case of living cells.

We can already say that the forecasting of the reactions in these conditions is also based on the values of the entropy changes accompanying the studied processes.

1) Open systems

An open system is a well-defined domain of space through which transfers of matter, heat and work can occur.

In the case of closed systems, when we considered the conservation of energy (the first principle of thermodynamics), we found that it could be taken into account by the expression:

$dE = dQ - pdV$

One property of open systems is that it is impossible that this expression can apply to them. We must pay attention to the fact that an exchange of matter with the surroundings obligatorily involves a simultaneous exchange of heat also. Therefore, the above function Q must be replaced by the function Φ which takes into account both kinds of exchanges (matter and heat):

$dE = d\Phi - pdV$

Φ is the resultant flow of energy due to heat transfer and exchange of matter.

---

* This chapter can be ignored in a first reading.

2) A property of enthalpy

Here, we confine ourselves to the sole consideration of monothermal processes. (Recall that an isothermal process is a process whose course is carried out at a constant and uniform temperature whereas a process is monothermal when, during its course, it exchanges heat with only one reservoir—Chapter 2).

Enthalpy does give rise to a definite application when it is applied to steady-flow processes.

According to the properties of the function enthalpy, for the change of an open system from states 1 and 2, we know that when the pressure is the same:

$$H_2 - H_1 = U_2 - U_1 + PV_2 - PV_1$$

For a closed system:

$$U_2 - U_1 = q + w \quad \text{(first principle)}$$

Therefore:

$$H_2 - H_1 = q + w + P(V_2 - V_1)$$

The last term is the work of displacing the environment of the system at pressure p. If this is the only form of work, the last two terms cancel each other; $w = P(V_2 - V_1)$:

$$H_2 - H_1 = q$$

Hence, in these conditions, when we compare with a closed system, the enthalpy takes the part played by the internal energy.

– Now, let us consider the case of a open system and more precisely that of a steady flow process. In Figure 31, an apparatus C (for example, a turbine, a stopcock) through which there is a steady flow of material, which enters through tube A and leaves it through tube B is represented. Let us consider a fixed quantity δm of the moving material (it is a steady flow system) enclosed at the beginning of the experience between the two virtual pistons a and b.

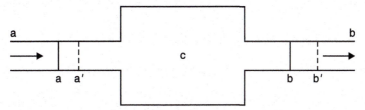

Figure 31. Steady flow process: part played by the enthalpy.

Let the pressures at a and b be p_1 and p_2 and V_1 and V_2 the corresponding volumes per mass unit at these points. (The volume changes per mass unit arise under the same phenomena as those which are at the origin of the notion of partial molar quantities changes—See Chapter 17). We are studying the process when virtual pistons displace themselves, respectively, up to a' and b'. The corresponding works of displacement per mass are in absolute values $|p_1 V_1 \delta m|$ and $|P_2 V_2 \delta m|$. Provided that pressures p_1 and p_2 are constants, the network done on the fluid material being containes in between both virtual pistons is:

$$w = -p_2 V_2 \delta m + p_1 V_1 \delta m + w_u \delta m$$

The term $-p_2V_2\delta m$ is the work done by the sample in displacing the fluid to the right of b and the term $p_1V_1\delta m$ is that done on the sample by the fluid to the right of a. w_u is the useful work done on unit mass of the sample as it passes through C. Let q be the heat absorbed per unit mass of the fluid between a and b, and E_1 and E_2 the total energies per unit mass at a and b. If we suppose

$U \approx H$ (as it is usually the case) we obtain:

$$U_2 - U_1 = q + w$$

with U_2 and U_1 the internal energies of the fluid at the points b and a. Hence, for a closed system:

$$H_2 - H_1 = q + w_u$$

The enthalpy change is directly related to the useful work in a steady-flow process, at least in the conditions given above.

3) The exergy of the system

The exergy of a system is defined by the relation:

$$\Lambda = U - T_0 S + P_0 V + \text{constant}$$

where T_0 and P_0 are the temperature and the pressure of the (unique) reservoir. The term "constant" is an integration constant. Now, suppose that the system (under study) also is in complete equilibrium with the reservoir. One says that the system is completely relaxed. In these conditions:

$$U = U_0; S = S_0; V = V_0$$

Let us set up;

$$\text{constant} = -(U - T_0 S_0 + P_0 V_0)$$

The function Λ becomes:

$$\Lambda = (U - U_0) - T_0(S - S_0) + P_0(V - V_0)$$

Λ is the exergy function (It is also sometimes symbolized by B).

4) Useful maximum work, exergy and free enthalpy versus the ambience

Let us consider a monothermal transformation during which the system exchanges heat with an outer source of temperature T_{ext}. Its energetic balance-sheet is:

$$\Delta U = \Delta Q + \Delta W$$

ΔQ and ΔW are actually the received quantities of heat and work. In particular, ΔW is the total work received by the system. The work ΔW_R received during the course of a reversible monothermal transformation can be expressed in function of the changes in energy and entropy of the system. In the general case:

$$\Delta Q = T_{ext} \Delta S$$

Since the transformation is reversible:

$$\Delta_e S = \Delta S$$

$$\Delta W_R = \Delta U - T\Delta S \quad \text{(reversible transformation)}$$

It can be seen that ΔW_R is a change in a state function. We have already encountered it. It is called the "free enthalpy relative to the ambience", the symbol of which is G_{ext} (see Chapter 14). The Gibbs energy related to the ambience is defined by the function:

$$G_{ext} = U - T_{ext}S + P_{ext}V$$

We have seen that the work ΔW_R^* received by a system, once the external pressure force is excluded, is such as (see Chapter 14):

$$dW_R^* = dU - T_{ext}dS + p_{ext}dV$$

From these considerations, we can notice that the function exergy is linked to the function Gibbs energy related to the ambience.

5) Rate of the exergy decrease and rate of the entropy increase in an irreversible process

One can demonstrate that the rate of decrease of the exergy $-\Lambda_{point}$ in an irreversible process is equal to the rate of creation of the entropy $\Delta\sigma$ multiplied by the temperature T_0 of the reservoir.

$$-\Lambda_{point} = T_0 \Delta\sigma$$

with

$$\Lambda_{point} = -\Delta\Lambda/\Delta t$$

The rate of the decrease of exergy of a system in an irreversible process is equal to the rate of creation of entropy multiplied by the temperature of the reservoir.

6) More on open stationary systems

By definition, in any of the points of their process, the intensive parameters defining open stationary systems (temperature, pressure, concentrations of its components, partial molal energies, etc.) are independent of the time, despite the exchanges which exist between them and the surroundings. Thus, we can in general write:

$$d\zeta/dt = 0 \quad \text{(stationary state)}$$

where ζ denotes any intensive state variable of an arbitrary system. If the system is homogeneous, then the above variables have the same values everywhere. They are invariant with respect to time and position. If we are dealing with a heterogeneous (discontinuous) system, then the intensive variables inside one phase of the system are again constant.

If the amounts of the individual regions of the system, that is for instance the mass of a homogeneous system or the amounts of the phases of a heterogeneous system, are invariant with respect to time, then the extensive quantities of the system no longer depend on time. Let Z be an extensive state function which refers to the total system, we can write:

$$dZ/dt = 0 \quad \text{(stationary state with the masses of all regions constant)} \tag{137}$$

7) Difference between equilibrium and stationary (non equilibrium) states

The difference is particularly noticeable when we consider the total entropy of a system. We have just seen that the stationary state with the mass of all the regions of the system held constant is characterized by (134).

In the case of entropy $Z = S$

$dS/dt = 0$

but according to the second law:

$dS = dS_e + d\sigma$

where dSe and $d\sigma$ are the exchanged and created entropies. As a result:

$dS/dt = dS_e/dt + d\sigma/dt$

For a stationary state, there is continuously produced entropy:

$d\sigma/dt > 0$ whence $dS_e/dt < 0$ (stationary state)

whereas:

$d\sigma/dt = 0$ (equilibrium state)

The difference between equilibrium and stationary states appears clearly. Although the total entropy of the system remains constant, there is a produced entropy during the stationary state whereas the latter is null in the equilibrium state.

No confusion should exist between an equilibrium state and a stationary non-equilibrium state. The equilibrium state is characterized by zero entropy production. This is not the case with a stationary state, in which an entropy production exists.

8) An example of a stationary open system

The Figure 32 provides an example of such a system.

In this example, the constant extensive quantities of the system are its entropy, Helmholtz energy and total energy. A flow of one or several particles i cross over the system (from left to right in this case). Matter and heat also go through the system.

There exist two intermediary parts in the system. On the left, just at the beginning of the crossing over, the temperature and pressure exhibit the values T' and P' which are not the stationary ones T and P. The other intermediary part (located on the right) exhibits the different values T'' and P''.

It is known that a stationary is obtained when a system receives a component from the outside, this component being transformed into several intermediates. A part of these intermediates is returned to the external environment when the concentrations of the latter ones no longer change. Then, the stationary state is attained.

The stationary state may be characterized by the following principle which states that when it is attained, the entropy production has increased but has a minimum value compatible with the conditions defining the system. The concentrations, or more exactly, the chemical composition in the stationary state is a constant. Concentrations are said to be in a dynamic steady state. The rate of formation of a given component is exactly counterbalanced by an equal rate of its removal or breakdown.

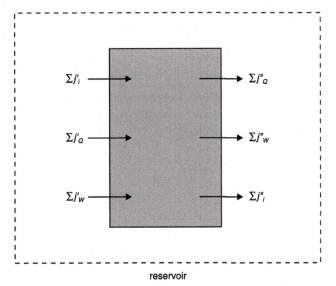

reservoir

Figure 32. Example of an open stationary system—according to P. Chartier, M. Cross and K.S. Spiegler, "Applications de la thermodynamique du non-équilibre", Ed, Hermann, Paris, 1975.

9) Principles of the study of stationary systems

It is important to specify the nomenclature of the parameters used in accordance with the Figure 32. By convention, we point out any current entering in the left by the symbol J' positive and any current going out (on the right) by J" (negative). (A current is a quantity of heat, matter or work entering by second into the system. A current must be distinguished from a flux which is a current per surface unit.) Let us consider one constituent i. If it is introduced by the current J'_i and if it is not chemically transformed in the reactor, the stationary state imposes:

$$J'_i = -J''_i$$

If there is a total chemical reaction, the stationary state imposes:

$$J'_i = \text{some value} \quad \text{whereas} \quad j''_i = 0$$

If it is only partial:

$$J''_i \neq 0 \quad \text{and} \quad J'_i \neq J''_i$$

The signs of the currents of heat are as previously said, but those of work are opposite in order to be in accordance with the signs of Q and w.

It is interesting to proceed to an energetic balance-sheet on the component i for example.

The introduced energy (in second) by the current of matter i is:

$$j'_i = (\overline{E'_i} + p'\overline{V'_i}) = J'_i \overline{H'_i}$$

$\overline{E'_i}$, $\overline{V'_i}$ and $\overline{H'_i}$ are the molar partial energy, volume and enthalpy at the entering of the system (see Chapter 17). The energy associated to the current of matter going outside the system is J''_I $\overline{H''_i}$. But currents of heat j'_{iQ} and j''_{iQ} must also be taken into account. Finally, there also exists the work –J"w which would be recuperated if the current of matter would go through a turbine.

The total balance-sheet is:

$$\Sigma J'_E + \Sigma J''_E = \Sigma j'_i \overline{H'_I} + \Sigma j''_i \overline{H''_i} + \Sigma j'_Q + \Sigma j''_Q - J''_w = 0$$

Of course, the balance-sheet is null because it is a stationary state.

It is also interesting to set up the enthalpic balance-sheet. In the case of a turbine well insulated, $(q = 0)$ where the heat is neither entering nor going out $(\Sigma j'_Q = \Sigma j''_Q = 0)$. In the absence of chemical reaction, the preceding equation gives;

$$j'_w / j_i = \overline{H'_i} - \overline{H''_i}$$

with $J'_i = -J''_i = J_i$

For a system well-insulated $j'_Q = j''_Q = J'' = 0$:

$$\overline{H'_i} = \overline{H''_i}$$

The enthalpy is conserved for the crossing of a fluid through a container which does not produce work as a turbine, whatever reversible or irreversible the process is.

10) Linear thermodynamics of irreversible processes

Applying thermodynamics of irreversible processes consists mainly in the evaluation of the entropy production. The latter can begin by using the Gibbs formula;

$$dS = dE/T + (P/T)dV - \Sigma_\gamma (\mu_\gamma/T) \, dn_\gamma$$

This relation is correct for the equilibrium conditions, as it is well-known. Its use for the non-equilibrium conditions is a postulate which permits to firmly ground thermodynamics of irreversible processes to the classical one. The double use of this formula (in thermodynamics of equilibrium and non equilibrium) means that entropy only depends on the same independent variables, whatever equilibrium or non-equilibrium is. This hypothesis becomes doubtful as soon as the domain of validity of linear phenomenological laws is overpassed.

It can be shown, indeed, that entropy production can be expressed as a sum of the products of generalized forces X_k (or affinities) and of the corresponding rates J_k ("fluxes") of the irreversible processes, according to:

$$d_iS/dt = \Sigma_k J_k X_k > 0 \tag{138}$$

d_iS/dt is the rate of entropy production. The indice k permits to identify the chemical reactions when the studied process results from several chemical reactions. Relations of this kind are empirical laws.

Generally, one can write:

$$J_1 = L_{11} X_1$$

L_{11} is a proportionality constant. There are several cases when two or more processes which can themselves be independent are both taking place. Their interaction results in a new physical or chemical phenomenon. When two such effects are in operation, the previous relation becomes:

$$J_1 = L_{11} X_1 + L_{12} X_2$$

$$J_2 = L_{21} X_1 + L_{22} X_2$$

J_1 is the flow for the first phenomenon, X_1, i.e., force producing it, idem for J_2 and X_2 of the second phenomenon, L_{11} and L_{22} are the proportionality constants for the independent processes and L_{12}, L_{21} are called the phenomenological coefficients. They represent the coupling effect. These relations are called Onsager's relations. Intuitively, it can be set up that $L_{12} = L_{21}$.

The genesis of this relation stems from the observation that the exergy and the entropy are only conserved in the reversible processes. From the same standpoints (exergy and entropy changes), it is proved correct that the property that irreversible processes have in common is that their exergy or entropy is such that, they respectively decrease or increase. Starting from this base, it was logical to define kinds of forces which are at the origin of these changes of exergy and entropy. Of course, since the problem is to treat irreversible processes which evolve in time, the latter parameter must intervene in the theoretical treatment, probably under the form of rates.

Hence, for any irreversible process, a relation of the following general form has been sought:

$$\Delta X_k = S_{kpoint}/j_k$$

where:

$$\Delta X_k \equiv -\Lambda_{kpoint}/T_0 J_k$$

In these relations, J_k is the current transporting k. ΔX_k is the generalized force operating in the studied process. $S_{kpoint} = (d_iS/dt)_k$ is the rate of internal creation of entropy. ΔX_k is the generalized force conjugated to the current J_k. It is defined as being equal to the creation of entropy accompanying the current J_k per second and per current unit. An example is provided by a transfer of heat. A heat current J_k (watts) (a heat quantity circulating in the system per second) flows from a reservoir at temperature T' to another at temperature T" (Figure 33).

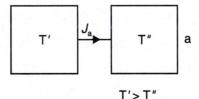

T' > T"

Figure 33. Heat transfer in terms of generalized forces.

The rate of entropy creation S point (watt K^{-1}) is equal to the arithmetic sum of the entropy changes per second in both reservoirs:

$$S_{point\ Q} = J_Q(-1/T' + 1/T'')$$

or with the above symbolism:

$$S_{point\ Q} = J_Q \Delta (1/T)$$

In this example, the generalized force is the entropy creation for one unit of heat current which is: K^{-1}, the inverse of Kelvin degree. Numerous other examples can be taken.

At thermodynamic equilibrium, the following relations which also apply to the irreversible phenomena, are simultaneously satisfied:

$$J_k = 0$$

$$X_k = 0$$

Close to the thermodynamic equilibrium, it is natural to assume that, still, there exist linear relations between the rates and the affinities. Such linear laws are called the phenomenological relations. This is the domain of validity of linear phenomenological laws.

11) Entropy production due to chemical reactions

The following equation which is valid in equilibrium thermodynamics and which is supposed to be valid in non-equilibrium thermodynamics, at least in the so-called "linear range":

$$dS = dE/T + (P/T)dV + \Sigma (\mu_\gamma/T)dn_\gamma$$

can be written:

$$dS = dQ/T + (A/T)d\xi$$

As we have seen (see Chapter 18), A is the affinity of the chemical reaction constituting the process:

$$A = -\Sigma v_\gamma \mu_\gamma$$

The μ_γ are the chemical potentials of the reactants and products and ξ the extent of the reaction. v_γ is the stoichiometric coefficient of the species γ. One demonstrates that the entropy production per unit time is:

$$d_iS/dt = 1/T \; \Sigma A_\rho v_\rho$$

It may happen that a system undergoes two simultaneous reactions such that:

$$A_1 v_1 < 0 \text{ and } A_2 v_2 > 0$$

The reaction 1 is impossible, whereas 2 is possible. The second principle requires that the entropy production resulting from all the simultaneous reactions is positive. Hence, the system can undergo the two reactions simultaneously provided that the sum:

$$A_1 v_1 + A_2 v_2 > 0$$

Both reactions are then "coupled reactions". Thermodynamic coupling allows one of the reactions to progress in a direction contrary to that prescribed by its own affinity. To be effective, this result imposes that some conditions of symmetry, that we do not specify here, are satisfied.

12) General applications in biology

As it has been briefly said, thermodynamics of irreversible processes is essentially concerned with the analysis of entropy production and the study of the relation between rates and affinities. Such a reasoning may be, in the case of the non-equilibrium for example, very fruitful to discover which processes become possible by means of a coupling. Hence, for example, coupled reactions are of great importance in biological processes. A particularly conclusive experimental result states that the total entropy production in biological phenomena is positive

It has been also found that if a stationary state is sufficiently close to an equilibrium state, the production of entropy attains its minimum value for the stationary state compatible with the constraints imposed on the system.

Chapter 25

Some Generalities on the Kinetics of Chemical Reactions

Although this book is not devoted to the kinetics of biochemical reactions playing a part in the bioenergetics, it is interesting for us to recall some elements of chemical kinetics. For example, they are useful for the study of the catalytic effect of enzymes.

1) Some generalities

Let us consider the reaction:

$$v_A A + v_B B + ... \rightarrow ..... v_Y Y + v_Z Z$$

The symbols v_i are the stoichiometric coefficients of the species.

1-1) Total rate of a reaction

The total rate of a reaction is the number of molecules of reactants dn_A, dn_B .... or ..of products dn_Y, dn_Z disappearing or appearing during the time dt. Its value v is related to a species intervening in the reaction. Hence, according to the chosen one, it can be defined by any of the following relations:

$$v_A = -dn_A/dt; \ v_B = -dn_B/dt; \ v_Y = dn_Y/dt; \ v_Z = dn_Z/dt$$

It is negative for the reactants, positive for the products. When the volume V of the system remains constant during the transformation, the rate can be expressed in terms of concentrations since a concentration in the molarity scale is the number of moles related to a volume, as for example: $[A] = n_A/V$. From now on, we shall express the rates in terms of concentrations and the total rate will be given by any of the following relations:

$$v_A = -d[A]/dt; \ v_B = -d[B]/dt; \ v_Y = d[Y]/dt; \ v_Z = d[Z]/dt$$

1-2) Extent of a reaction

According to its definition given above, the total rate of a chemical reaction is different according to the species to which it is related, when the stoichiometric coefficients v_i are not identical. In order to avoid this difficulty, it is judicious to reason in terms of extent of the reaction ξ (see Chapter 8). Recall that the extent of the reaction $d\xi$ is in the present case:

$$d\xi = |dn_A/v_A| : d\xi = |dn_B/v_B| : d\xi = |dn_Y/v_Y| : d\xi = |dn_Z/v_Z|$$

For us in this book, $d\xi$ is expressed in terms of concentrations, that is to say:

$d\xi = d[I]/v_i$

Now, the total rate of reaction v can be defined without any ambiguity by the relation:

$v = d\xi/dt$

1-3) Dependence of the rates of the chemical reactions with the concentrations of the participating species

The experience indicates that v changes with the temperature of the reaction and with the concentrations of the reactants and products. We are now only interested in the effect of the concentrations.

It is an experimental fact that the rate v is very often a function of concentrations [A], [B] ..... Formally, the dependence may be symbolized by the relation:

$v_A = -d[A]/dt = k\ f([A][B] ....)$

where $f([A][B] ....)$ means function of...... For several reactions, the relation is of the form:

$v_A = -d[A]/dt = k\ [A]^\alpha[B]^\beta ...$

k is the rate constant. Its value depends only on the temperature. The sum of the exposants $\alpha + \beta$, etc.... is named the order of the reaction. The values of α and β are coefficients which are purely from experimental origin. When the reaction is, for example, of the type:

$v = k\ [A]$

it is said to be of the first order in [A]. Then, the unit of the rate constant is: $second^{-1}$. When it is of the type:

$v = k\ [A]\ [B]$ or $v = k\ [A]^2$

it is of the second order. The unit of k is then: $L\ mol^{-1}s^{-1}$ (liter per mole per second).

2) Kinetics and equilibria

Let's consider the reversible chemical reaction in solution:

$$A + B \underset{k_{-1}}{\overset{k_1}{\rightleftharpoons}} C + D \tag{139}$$

in which k_1 and k_{-1} are, respectively, the rate constants of the reaction from the left to the right and from the right to the left. The reaction has reached its equilibrium state when x molecules of A and B react in a certain time (say 1 minute) to form C and D whereas the same number x molecules of C and D also react to form A and B. Once the equilibrium is reached, no further *net* reaction occurs. So, concentrations $[A]_{eq}$, $[B]_{eq}$, $[C]_{eq}$, $[D]_{eq}$ do not change with time. This is expressed by the relations:

$-d[A]/dt = 0;\ -d[B]/dt = 0;\ d[C]/dt = 0;\ d[D]/dt = 0$

$[A]_{eq}$, $[B]_{eq}$, $[C]_{eq}$, $[D]_{eq}$ are the concentrations at equilibrium whereas [A], [B], [C], [D] are those at any time. Note that, since A and B are decomposing, the gradients of their concentrations against time are negative.

According to one of the theories governing chemical kinetics—the collision theory-chemical reactions of type (136) are a consequence of molecular collisions between the reactants. The frequency of collisions between A and B is, as a rule, proportional to the product [A] [B]. As a result, the rate of change of concentration [A] due to the occurrence of reaction (136) is given by the relation:

$$-d[A]/dt = k_1 [A] [B]$$

The proportionality factor k_1 is the rate constant. Similarly, the rate of change of the concentration [A] as the result of reaction (136) proceeding from right to left is:

$$d[A]/dt = k_{-1} [C] [D]$$

The net rate of change of [A] is:

$$-d[A]/dt = k_1 [A] [B] - k_{-1} [C] [D]$$

At equilibrium,

$$k_1 [A]_{eq} [B]_{eq} - k_{-1} [C]_{eq} [D]_{eq} = 0$$

or:

$$[C]_{eq} [D]_{eq}/[A]_{eq} [B]_{eq} = k_1/k_{-1}$$

From another standpoint, the term on the left hand side of this relation is the *equilibrium constant* K of reaction (1). This means that:

$$K = k_1/k_{-1} \tag{140}$$

This equation shows the relation between the rate constants and the equilibrium constant for a simple reaction. Both equilibrium and rate constants are only constant at a given temperature.

Remark: As it is in the case of equilibria, activities must be handled instead of concentrations for chemical reactions whose ionic strength is no longer weak.

3) Influence of temperature on the rate of chemical reactions: energetic aspects

When the rate constant of a reaction is determined at different temperatures, it is found that it increases with the temperature. From the quantitative standpoint, a straight line is obtained most often if the logarithm of the rate constant is plotted against the reciprocal of the absolute temperature T (Figure 34). This kind of diagram is named an *Arrhenius' plot*.

- A theory, named theory of collisions, has earlier satisfactorily explained this result. According to it, for two molecules to react with each other, they have to collide. The kinetic theory of gases leads to a value for the number of collisions between two molecules, but the found value is, by far, too large when compared to the values of the rate constants k experimentally found. It has been reasonable to assume that the only reactive molecules are those possessing exceptional amounts of energy. On this assumption, the fraction of molecules possessing energy greater than a certain amount E is, approximately, proportional to the value of the term $\exp[-E/RT]$

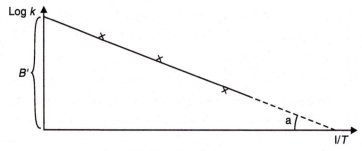

Figure 34. Example of Arrhenius' plot.

according Boltzmann's law. As a result, the rate constant must also be proportional to the same term, that is to say:

k = A exp[–E/RT]

log k = logA – E/2,3RT

(2,3 being the factor permitting to pass from the napieran logarithms to the decimal ones). The angular coefficient (tg α) of the straight line is equal to E/RT and permits to obtain the activation energy. Hence, Arrhenius' plots are, at least in part, justified.

- In the preceding theory, the significance of the constant A has not been clarified. Following Arrhenius' theory, several more or less satisfactory theories expliciting the notion of activation have been developed. They indicated that for the reaction to occur, the molecules must not only possess a sufficient internal energy but must also a definite orientation.

- More recently, the Arrhenius theory has been reinterpreted in terms of the *transition state theory*. It throws light on how bonds are formed or broken in chemical reactions.

In order to begin the explanation, let's study a simple example. Consider the reaction in which chloride ion reacts with methyl bromide in acetone as solvent.

$Cl^- + CH_3Br \rightleftharpoons Br^- + CH_3Cl$

During the reaction, the bond C-Br is broken whereas, simultaneously, the bond C-Cl is formed. There exists an intermediary state called the *transition state* of the reaction in which both ions Cl^- and Br^- are partially bound to the carbon of the methyl rest according to the scheme (see Figure 35):

$Cl^- + CH_3Br \rightleftharpoons [Cl----CH_3----Br]^- \rightleftharpoons ClCH_3 + Br^-$
                    transition state

The transition state differs from an ordinary molecule in, at least, two points:

- there is one direction, named the reaction path, which is the line Cl---C---Br here. Each vibration along this line causes the breaking of the bond C....Br:
- its lifetime is very short, of the order of 10^{-14} s. This value is much shorter than the time interval between two collisions.

Actually, the transition state is a *Gibbs energy barrier* (Figure 36 I and II). Once it has been surmounted, no additional Gibbs energy is necessary for the reaction to reach completion, that is to say to reach its definitive state of equilibrium. The height of the barrier is the

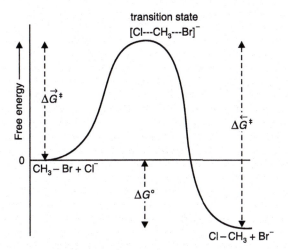

Figure 35. Attainment of the transition state.

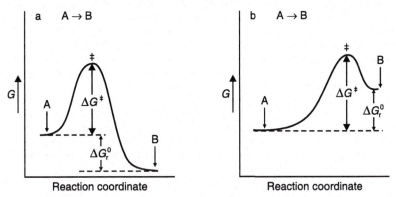

Figure 36. I and II: transition state accessible from the right and from the left—according to Glasstone, Laidler and Eyring "Theory of rate process", Editor Mc Graw Hill, New york, 1941.

excess of Gibbs energy of the transition state over the initial species, whichever is on the left of the transition state (CH_3Br) or on the right (CH_3Cl). The transition state is indeed the same for the two possible directions of the reaction. The excess of Gibbs energy is called the *Gibbs energy of activation*. When the investigated reaction is that going from the left to the right, it is represented by the symbol $\overrightarrow{\Delta G^*}$ and for that going from the right to the left $\overleftarrow{\Delta G^*}$ (Figure 36 I and II).

The Gibbs energies of activation are related to the standard Gibbs energy change for the reaction $\Delta G°$, through the relation:

$$\overrightarrow{\Delta G^*} - \overleftarrow{\Delta G^*} = \Delta G°$$

Owing to the direction of the arrows in this relation, the involved Gibbs energy $\Delta G°$ is that corresponding to the reaction going from the left to the right (and conversely).

According to this theory, the Gibbs energy of activation is proportional to the rate of a reaction. The relation is:

$$k = B \exp[-\Delta G^* \leftarrow \text{or} \rightarrow] \tag{141}$$

The constant B has the same value for all reactions at a given temperature. Its value is given by the equation:

$$B = k_B T/h$$

where k_B is the Boltzmann's constant and h the Planck's constant. For a reversible reaction such as (136), taking into account (138), relation (137) becomes:

$$k_1/k_{-1} = \exp[-(\overrightarrow{\Delta G^*} - \overleftarrow{\Delta G^*})] \tag{142}$$

and according to what is preceding:

$$K = \exp[-\Delta G^\circ]$$

relation already known (see above).

A conclusion of these considerations is that the Gibbs energies of activation govern the rates of the reactions and also the location of the equilibria through relation (139).

Of course, there are other kinds of profiles of activation energies (Figure 37I and II).

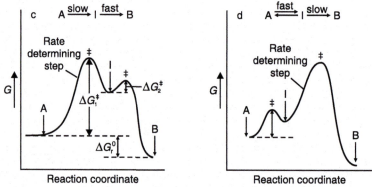

Figure 37. I and II: Other kinds of activation of Gibbs energy profiles—According to N. Isaacs "Physical organic chemistry", 2nd edition, Editor Longman scientific and technical, London 1995.

It is convenient to express the energy change during the course of a reaction in which two geometrical coordinates are important.

Since the first parameters to consider in the transition state theory are the Gibbs energies of activation ΔG^*, these ones (by definition of the Gibbs energy) can be decomposed into an enthalpy of activation ΔH^* and into an entropy of activation ΔS^* (whatever the direction of the reaction is) that is to say;

$$\Delta G^* = \Delta H^* - T\Delta S^*$$

and the relation between a Gibbs energy of activation and the corresponding rate constant k becomes:

$$k = B\exp[-\Delta H^*/RT]\,\exp[\Delta S^*/R]$$

The enthalpy of activation is usually dominated by the breakage and the formation of bonds when the substrate is transformed into the product. The entropy of activation rather takes into account the orientation of the reactants, the changes in flexibility of the conformations during the "induced fit" (see the Chapter 30) and perhaps overall the changes in solvatation effects.

Part II

Some Aspects of Chemical Reactions in Aqueous Solutions

Chapter **26**

Acid-Base Reactions in Aqueous Solutions

Biochemical reactions occurring in bioenergetics obey the same principles as do the chemical ones. In this chapter and in the two following ones, we recall some essential points concerning the principal chemical equilibria occurring in water and encountered during the evolution of the biochemical reactions. We have chosen to essentially develop the acid-base and the redox reactions in water. They are probably the most important equilibria for our purpose. We also mention some other kinds of processes which are also of interest for us, but at a less extent than the preceding ones. As for the choice of water as solvent, it is justified by the fact that a living cell is essentially an aqueous medium.

The goal of this chapter and of the following ones is to facilitate the prediction of the directions of the reactions of bioenergetics, that is to say to facilitate their forecasting. Finally, these studies must justify the directions the reactions actually take.

The contents of these chapters are strongly reminiscent of the physico-chemical theories devoted to the chemistry of aqueous solutions.

In this chapter, we are concerned by acid-base reactions.

1) Definitions of acids and bases and consequences

There are several definitions of acids and bases. We confine ourselves to giving that of Arrhenius' very briefly and, then, to more thoroughly studying the Brönsted-Lowry's theory.

– According to Arrhenius theory, an acid HA is a species that ionizes in water to give one hydrated proton $H^+_{(w)}$ and one anion according to the more or less equilibrated reaction:

$$HA \rightleftharpoons A^-_{(w)} + H^+_{(w)} \qquad (143)$$

A base BOH is a substance that ionizes in water to give one hydroxide anion $OH^-_{(w)}$ and one cation according to:

$$BOH \rightleftharpoons B^+_{(w)} + OH^-_{(w)} \qquad (144)$$

There exist polyacids and polybases. Polyacids give several hydrated protons per molecule, while polybases give several hydroxide anions. The strengths of acids and bases are related to the extent of the ionization processes of reactions (140) and (141).

Arrhenius' theory only applies to aqueous solutions. It permits to correctly predict acid-base reactions (in water) included from the quantitative standpoint.

– According to Brönsted-Lowry's theory, an acid HA is a proton donor:

$$HA \rightleftharpoons A^- + H^+ \tag{145}$$

A base B is a proton acceptor:

$$B + H^+ \rightleftharpoons BH^+ \tag{146}$$

In these schemes, the symbol H^+ does not represent the naked proton. It represents the solvated proton in water. Within the framework of the theory, some authors prefer defining acids and bases after the following reactions (144) and (145). That is to say, the phenomena involve an exchange of protons with water according to:

$$HA + H_2O \rightleftharpoons A^- + H_3O^+ \tag{147}$$

$$B + H_3O^+ \rightleftharpoons BH^+ + H_2O \tag{148}$$

In (144), H_2O (the solvent) also plays the part of a base. In (145), H_3O^+ plays the part of an acid and H_2O that of the solvent. According to this viewpoint, an acid-base reaction may be represented, in general, by the resultant of both Equations (144) and (145):

$$HA + B \rightleftharpoons A^- + BH^+ \tag{149}$$

It appears that the acid-base reaction (146) can be split into the two half acid-base reactions (144) and (145). Thus, an acid-base reaction involves an exchange of protons between two acid-base couples, HA/A^- on one hand and, for example, the couple BH^+/B on the other.

It is interesting to notice that the proton exchange can be done not only directly between the members of the two pairs as indicated by reaction (146) but it can also be exchanged indirectly through the pair H_3O^+/H_2O as indicated by reactions (144) and (145). It is also interesting to notice that half reactions (144) and (145) occur actually. Their evolution can be followed experimentally, and the different formed products identified.

Equations (143) and (144) clearly show that, in the same couple, one member is the acid and the other the base. Both are named *conjugated acid-base*.

Equations (142), (143), (144), (145) also show that the acidic or basic character of a species is independent of its electric charge. For the acidic character, in order to be convinced, it is sufficient to compare the behaviors of HA and BH^+, and for the basic one those of A^- and B. Even a negative species may be an acid. This is the case, for example, of the ion monohydrogenophosphate HPO_4^{2-}:

$$HPO_4^{2-} + H_2O \rightleftharpoons PO_4^{3-} + H_3O^+$$

The assertion is the same on the basic side. A positively charged species may be a base.

Some species can be both acidic and basic. They are called *ampholytes*. The "illuminating example" of this property is water. It gives a proton according to (147):

$$H_2O \rightleftharpoons H^+ + OH^- \tag{150}$$

It accepts a proton according to (148):

$$H_2O + H^+ \rightleftharpoons H_3O^+ \tag{151}$$

Both equilibria (147) and (148) do not represent the same acido-basic couple. Equation (147) defines the pair H_2O/OH^- and (148) the pair H_3O^+/H_2O.

A typical example of ampholyte in the realm of biochemistry is the case of amino-acids (see the end of this chapter).

Some compounds may give several protons. Other ones can accept several protons. They are respectively called polyacids and polybases. The exchange of several protons cannot be achieved once and for all, that is to say fully simultaneously. (This remark anticipates a brief comparison between acid-base and redox processes which is done later see the following chapter).

In aqueous solutions, Arrhenius and Brönsted-Lowry theories can be considered as being equivalent.

2) Quantitative aspects of acid-base reactions

   2-1) Ionic product of water

   Water, even purissime, is slightly ionized. This has been discovered thanks to electrical measurements. Its ionization is the mark of the following equilibrium:

   $$H_2O + H_2O \rightleftharpoons H_3O^+_{(w)} + OH^-_{(w)}$$

   The mass law permits to write:

   $$K = a_{H3O+}\, a_{OH-}/a_{H2O}^2$$

   where K is the equilibrium thermodynamic constant of the reaction above. Electrical measurements give the following concentrations, for pure water at 25°C:

   $$[H_3O^+] = [OH^-] = 10^{-7}\ \text{mol L}^{-1}$$

   Thus, pure water, even "purissime", contains ions but very few. As a consequence, the molar fraction of molecular water can be safely taken to be equal to unity and its activity as well (see Chapter 19). As a result, one can write:

   $$K = a_{H3O+}\, a_{OH-} \tag{152}$$

   The product $a_{H3O+}\, a_{OH}$ is named the *ion-product constant for water or ionic product of water and is symbolized by K_w*:

   $$K_w = a_{H3O+}\, a_{OH-}$$

   The ionic product varies with temperature. Dissociation increases with it:

   at 25°C $K_w = 10^{-14}$

   at 50°C $K_w = 5,6\ 10^{-14}$

   at 100°C $K_w = 6,0\ 10^{-13}$

   In every aqueous solution, which is diluted in ions, the ionic product of water is a constant at a given temperature, no matter what the OH^- and H_3O^+ ions concentrations may be, provided the solution remains diluted. It is said: "the water ion product is satisfied". Solutions for which:

$[H_3O^+] = [OH^-]$ are said neutral,

$[H_3O^+] > [OH^-]$ are said acidic,

$[H_3O^+] < [OH^-]$ are said basic.

2-2) Constant of dissociation acid Ka (pKa)

For one acid, *in dilute aqueous solution*, one defines the acid dissociation constant K_a by:

$$K_a = a_{H+}a_{A-}/a_{HA} \qquad (153)$$

where a_{H+}, a_{A-}, a_{HA} are the activities of the species symbolized in subscript. This definition pertains to equilibrium (142), to equilibrium (144) and to any kind of acids as well. Actually, for the case of an acid HA, the definition could in principle be written:

$$K_a = a_{H+}a_{A-}/a_{HA}\, a_{H2O} \qquad (154)$$

But, one knows that the activity of the solvent is usually taken to be unity because it is related to its molar fraction which is quasi-equal to the unity in diluted solutions. This is because the activity $a_{H2O} = 1$ is omitted in (150);

– for a base (in dilute aqueous solution), one can also define the *basic dissociation constant* K_b by:

$$K_b = a_{BH+}\, a_{OH-}/a_B \qquad (155)$$

which pertains to the equilibrium (143), (145) and to those of other kinds of bases as well. But, actually, the constant K_b is not used because it is simply related to the constant K_a of its conjugated acid. They are related to each other by the expression:

$$K_a K_b = K_w$$

As a result, of course, when the numerical value of K_a is known, so is value of K_b, provided the base and the acid belong to the same conjugated couple.

The higher the value of K_a, the more dissociated the acid and the more strong it is said. Therefore, concomitantly, the weaker is its conjugated base. K_a is a particularly well-suited constant to quantify the acid strength. The more ionized the acid, the higher the numerator and the lower the denominator of the expression of K_a are. Usually, to simplify the writing, the decimal cologarithm of K_a is used:

$$pK_a = -\log_{10} K_a$$

The stronger the acid, the higher its value K_a and the *lower* its pK_a value.

In the case of polyacids, there is one acid dissociation constant per acidic site of the species. The corresponding K_a (pk_a) values are numbered according to the decreasing order of the strengths of the different acidities (or, in an equivalent manner, by increasing the numbering of the pK_a values). For example, phosphoric acid is a triacid, the pK_a values are numbered as follows: $pK_{a1} = 2,10$; $pK_{a2} = 7,20$; $pK_{a3} = 12,35$.

We give pK_a values of some acids in appendice I-8.

3) Notion of pH

In principle, the pH value quantifies the activity of the solvated proton in a solution. This activity can be considered as being the absolute acidity of the solution. Most often, it is an aqueous solution, but the pH is also defined for some other solvents.

The pH of a solution is defined as being the decimal cologarithm of the solvated proton activity $a_{H+\,solv}$ in the given medium:

$$pH = -\log a_{H+\,solv}$$

Let us clarify the assertion that the pH value may be considered as a measure of the "true" acidity of a solution as it is already said but all the more accurately the solution is diluted and is of weak ionic strength.

Considering bioenergetics, it is reasonable, at least to simplify the calculations, to assimilate the activity of the proton to its concentration and to state:

$$pH \approx -\log [H^+_{solv}]$$

where $[H^+_{solv}]$ is the concentration of the solvated proton. The limit values of the scale of pH in water are arbitrarily fixed to 0 and 14 at 25°C. For the value pH = 7, the solution is said to be neutral from the standpoint of the acido-basicity. For the pH value located between 0 and 7, the solution is said to be acidic. For the values located between 7 and 14, the solution is said to be basic. For the values about 0 and 14, the aqueous solution is said to be, respectively, strongly acidic or strongly basic.

If a solution containing both members of an acid-base couple (such as HA and A^-) is not too acidic or too basic and if the activities can be assimilated to the concentrations, Equation (151) leads to Equation (153):

$$pH = pK_a + \log [A^-]/[HA] \tag{156}$$

where K_a is the acid dissociation constant of the couple. Equation (153) is known under the name of *Henderson-Hasselbach* equation. (We notice that to write Equation (153), we have set up $a_H = c_H$ as it is previously explained. a_H is the activity of the solvated proton and c_H its concentration expressed in molarities).

It must be noticed that the pH value represents the absolute acidity of the solution when it is located in a certain domain and when the solution is sufficiently diluted. For example, in water, the domain in which the pH value represents the absolute acidity lies in the range 3–11 and the ionic strength of the solution (the pH of which is measured) must be less than 10^{-2} mol L^{-1}. When it is not the case, the pH value is only indicative. [*] *(The ionic strength I of a solution is defined by the formula:*

$$I = (1/2) \, \Sigma \, m_i z_i^2$$

m_i *is the molality of the ion i and* z_i *its electrical charge. The summation is carried out for all the ionic species of the solution). For the weak ionic strengths, the values of the molalities differ from those of molarities. The ionic strength therefore exhibits the same value, whatever the scale of concentrations (molalities or molarities) on which the activities are based (see Chapter 19).*

---

[*] R.G. Bates in "Determination of pH, Theory and Practice", 1973, p. 28, John Wiley and Sons, Inc Ed, New York.

4) Distribution diagrams and predominance area

Distribution and predominance area diagrams are very useful since their inspection immediately provides information about the fractions of the acidic and of the basic forms of a couple which are present in a given pH value. They are particularly interesting in the case of polyacids.

- In the case of a monoacid HA, it is obvious to see, by considering relation (153) and by assimilating the activities to their corresponding concentrations, that:

$$[A^-]/[HA] = K_a/[H^+]$$

We want to express the fraction of the dissociated acid α_{A^-} defined by:

$$\alpha_{A^-} = [A^-]/C$$

where C is the total (analytical) concentration of the acid:

$$C = [A^-] + [HA]$$

Handling these equations gives the relation:

$$\alpha_{A^-} = K_a/(K_a + [H^+])$$

Of course, the fraction α_{HA} of the non-dissociated acid is given by the expression:

$$\alpha_{HA} = ([H^+])/(K_a + [H^+])$$

Hence, it becomes possible to draw the fractions α_{A^-} and α_{HA} as a function of pH as soon as we know the K_a value. These diagrams are called *distribution diagrams*. In Figure 38 is shown the distribution of the acid form of acetic acid ($pK_a = 4,75$).

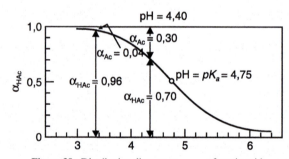

Figure 38. Distribution diagram $\alpha_{CH3COOH}$ of acetic acid.

We immediately see, for example, that at pH = 3,4, acetic acid is still at 96% under the non-ionized form.

We give in Figure 39 the distribution diagrams of the different acido-basic species coming from the successive dissociations of fumaric acid, and in Figure 40 those of orthophosphoric acid.

We symbolize it by H_2A which clearly shows that it is a diacid. The ionization schemes are:

$$H_2A \rightleftharpoons HA^- + H^+ \quad pK_{a1} = 3,05$$

$$HA^- \rightleftharpoons A^{2-} + H^+ \quad pK_{a2} = 4,49$$

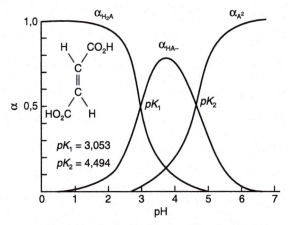

Figure 39. Distribution diagram of fumaric acid.

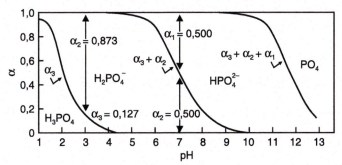

Figure 40. Distribution diagram of orthophosphoric acid.

Such diagrams are of great interest in this case. They permit to immediately see if there are some pH domains in which the different acido-basic species (resulting from the ionization) may exist solely in the solution. In the case of fumaric acid, the species H_2A and A^{2-} can exist solely at pH 0–2 for the former and in the domain 7–14 for the latter. The monoacid (or monobase) HA^- never exists solely. It is always in mixture with forms H_2A and (or) A^{2-}.

– The ionization reactions of orthophosphoric acid H_3PO_4 are:

$$H_3PO_4 \quad \rightleftharpoons \quad H_2PO_4^- \qquad + \quad H^+ \quad pK_{a1} = 2,10$$
dihydrogenophosphate ion

$$H_2PO_4^- \quad \rightleftharpoons \quad H_2PO_4^{2-} \qquad + \quad H+ \quad pK_{a2} = 7,20$$
monohydrogenophosphate ion

$$HPO_4^{2-} \quad \rightleftharpoons \quad PO_4^{3-} \qquad + \quad H+ \quad pK_{a3} = 12,35$$
orthophosphate ion

We notice that contrary to the case of fumaric acid, it is possible to choose domains of pH in which the different species H_3PO_4, $H_2PO_4^-$ and HPO_4^{2-} are the sole species in solution. They are respectively: 1,0–1,5; 5,0–6,0; 10,0–11,0.

- Predominance area

Predominance area provides another means to know if an acid is under its acidic or basic form. According to the Equation (153) above, we know that for pH = pKa, [HA] = [A⁻]. If we draw a line perpendicular to the pH scale to the value pH = pKa, the acidity domain is partitioned in two parts: on the left of the vertical, the form acid is predominant and on the right is the basic form (Figure 41).

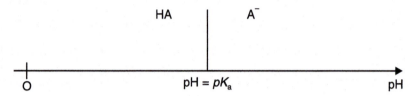

Figure 41. Predominance area of HA and A⁻ in relation with the pH value.

It is important to note the very fast increase (exponential ones) of the ratios [HA]/[A⁻] and [A⁻]/[HA], respectively, on the left and on the right of the vertical line. This fact makes the (approximate) assertion that on the left of the line, it is only the area of the HA form and on the right, that of the A⁻ form, seem very credible.

In brief, there is an approximate rule enabling to immediately know the acidic or basic form percentages of the species. When pH = pK_a, the acid is half under the acidic form and half under the basic form. For values pH = $pK_a - 2$ units, $pk_a - 1$ unit, $pK_a + 1$ unit, $pK_a + 2$ units, the couple is at 99, 90, 10 and 1% under the acidic form.

The concentrations of the acidic or basic forms increase or decrease very quickly once one is far from the value pH = pK_a. This rule is only approximate because it could be expressed in terms of activities and not in terms of concentrations. Nevertheless, it is very useful.

5) Buffer solutions

It is an experimental fact that solutions obtained by dissolving a weak acid and its conjugate base exhibit a very weak pH change when a strong acid or base is added to them, at least in some conditions of concentrations. These solutions are called *buffer solutions*. The fact that the change in the pH value of the solution after addition of an acid or base is very weak is called the *buffer effect*.

The mechanism of the buffer effect can be explained on the basis of two viewpoints.

- The first one may be called the chemical standpoint. Let us consider the buffer HA/A− (or BH+/B) at respective concentrations C_{HA} and C_A. If we reason in terms of the Henderson-Hasselbach equation:

  – before the addition of a strong acid, the pH is given by the relation:

  pH = pK_a + ln [A⁻]/[HA]   (or pH = pK_a + ln [B]/[BH⁺])

  that is to say:

  pH = pK_a + ln C_A/C_{HA}

  where K_a is the acid dissociation constant of the buffer couple;

– after addition of a strong acid at the final concentration C in the solution, we can admit that the following reaction has evolved quasi-totally from the left to the right:

$$A^- + H^+ \rightarrow HA$$

As a result, the concentration [A⁻] decreases from C mol L⁻¹ whereas that of [HA] increases from C mol L⁻¹. The pH value is now given approximately by the relation:

$$pH = pK_a + \ln (C_A - C)/(C_{HA} + C) \tag{157}$$

The change is very weak because it appears, when all calculations are performed, that the C mol L⁻¹ of strong acid added (that is to say the C mol L⁻¹ of hydroxonium ions H⁺ added) has been completely transformed into C mol L⁻¹ of the weak acid HA. An analogous mechanism would prevail for the addition of a strong base.

• The second explanation of the buffer effect is a mathematical one. It lies in the shape of the curve pH/C [Equation (154)]. It exhibits a relative flat domain slightly above and under the pk_a value (Figure 42).

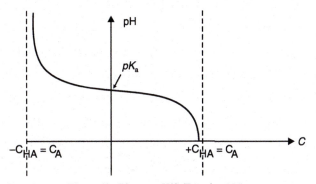

Figure 42. Diagram pH/C (Equation 154).

A measure of the buffer capacity is the amount of strong acid or strong base required to change the pH by a given amount. The larger this quantity is, the better the buffer. The buffer capacity is quantified by the *buffer index β*. In the case of the addition of a strong acid, the buffer index is given by the relation:

$$\beta = -dC_A/dpH$$

where dC_A is the number of moles of a strong acid added to 1 L of the buffer solution and dpH is the corresponding pH change. For addition of dC_B moles of a strong base, β is defined by the relation:

$$\beta = dC_B/dpH$$

The buffer index is conveniently defined in differential terms, since β changes with the pH of the initial solution. A calculation of derivatives (using the chain rule of calculation of derivatives) leads to the following equation permitting the calculation of β, once known as the pH of the solution:

$$\beta = 2{,}303 \ \{K_w/[H^+] + [H^+] + CK_a[H^+]/(K_a + [H^+])^2\}$$

A new calculation of derivatives demonstrates that the buffering power of a couple is maximal for pH = pK_a.

One also defines the buffer range. This is the domain of pH in which the buffering capacity is maintained. On experimental grounds, it is located in the pH interval imposed by the following ratios 1 acid/10 base and 10 acid/1 base, that is to say:

pKa – 1 < pH < pKa + 1

This is the buffer range.

6) Acid-base equilibrium constants

In the polyacid case, there are actually two sorts of equilibrium constants of dissociation acid:
– the macroscopic constants,
– the microscopic ones.

Both are identical in the case of monoacids.

Let us consider the simplest case in this matter, that of the diacid H-A-H. It exhibits two acid-base sites. Its ionization can follow the two ways shown in Figure 43.

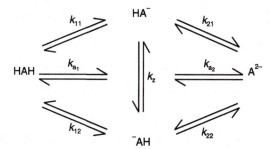

Figure 43. Definitions and symbolism of microscopic constants. The first number of the subscript indicates the order of the ionization, the second number the way.

The microscopic dissociation acid constants are defined by the following relationships (mixing activities and concentrations):

$k_{11} = [HA^-][H^+]/[H\text{-}A\text{-}H]$ $k_{21} = [A2^-][H^+]/[HA^-]$

$k_{12} = [^-AH][H^+]/[H\text{-}A\text{-}H]$ $k_{22} = [A2^-][H^+]/[^-AH]$

The equilibrium constants, which are determined experimentally, are the macroscopic ones. They *quantify* together the two ionization ways (see the Figure 43). They are *overall* acid-dissociation equilibrium constants. They are defined as follows:

$K_{a1} = [H^+] \{[^-AH] + [HA^-]\}/[H_2A]$

$K_{a2} = [H^+][A^{2-}]/\{[^-AH] + [HA^-]\}$

The comparison of the expressions of macroscopic and microscopic constants leads to the following relationships that link them:

$$K_{a1} = k_{11} + k_{12} \tag{158}$$

$$1/K_{a2} = 1/k_{21} + 1/k_{22} \tag{159}$$

$$K_{a1} \, K_{a2} = k_{11} \, k_{21} = k_{12} \, k_{22}$$

and:

$$[HA^-]/[^-AH] = k_{11}/k_{12} \quad \text{or} \quad k_{22}/k_{21} = k_z$$

with:

$$k_{11}/k_{12} = k_{22}/k_{21} = k_z$$

The last two equations are not independent from each other in the mathematical sense. As for the four last equations, they form a mathematical system of three independent relations for four unknowns, the four microscopic constants k_{11}, k_{12}, k_{21}, k_{22}, whereas the macroscopic ones K_{a1} and K_{a2} are experimentally accessible. Hence, microscopic constants cannot be determined without ambiguity. Additionally, the framework of classical thermodynamics does not include the notion of microconstants. However, their values may be approached reasonably with the aid of extrathermodynamic hypothesis. Often, such hypothesis are founded on structural analogies. Another point arising from the preceding reasoning is that the ratio k_z of the concentrations of both intermediary monoacids is (perhaps surprisingly at first sight) independent of the pH value. Finally, an important result is that, in the case of a diacid, the macroscopic measured acid dissociation constants are always combinations of two microscopic ones.

As a class of compounds, of utmost interest for our purpose, for which the preceding reasoning is particularly important to adopt, is that of amino-acids. We shall reason with glycin (other name glycocolle) for the sake of economy of writing, since it has the simplest molecular structure:

$$NH_2 - CH_2 - COOH$$

It is a "classical" amino-acid since it is a 2-aminocarboxylic acid. In a medium sufficiently acidic, the basic rest amino $-NH_2$ is protonated giving the conjugated corresponding rest acidic $-NH_3^+$. Thus, with such a pH value, the obtained species is the diacid:

$$NH_3^+ - CH_2 - COOH$$

which, henceforth, we symbolize by A^+. This diacid dissociates according to the two microscopic ways (Figure 44):

$$NH_3^+ - CH_2 - COOH \rightleftharpoons NH_2 - CH_2 - COOH \ (A^\circ) + H^+$$

$$NH_3^+ - CH_2 - COOH \rightleftharpoons NH_3^+ - CH_2 - COO^- \ (A^\pm) + H^+$$

Let us represent the dibasic form $NH_2 - CH_2 - COO^-$ by A^-. It appears that in solution, the amino-acid, usually represented by A° (NH_2-CH_2-COOH), stays in aqueous solution, under the mixture of A° and $A^\pm$ (NH_3^+-CH_2-COO$^-$) in a constant ratio whatever is the pH value (Figure 44).

The macroscopic constants qualify the two following equilibria:

$$A^+ \rightleftharpoons \{A^\circ + A^\pm\} + H^+ \ (pK_{a1} = 2{,}35)$$

$$\{A^\circ + A^\pm\} \rightleftharpoons A^- + H^+ \ (pK_{a2} = 9{,}82)$$

The macroscopic constant $pK_{a2} = 9{,}82$ is of the same order as the pk_a values of the protoned aliphatic amines ($pK_a \approx 9{,}5$). It results from the preceding equations that:

$$k_{22} = K_{a2}$$

The chemical meaning of this result is that the amino-acid is quasi-completely under the zwitterionic form $A^\pm$ in aqueous solution.

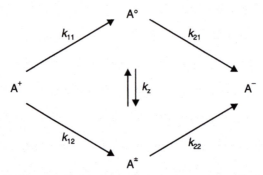

Figure 44. Macroscopic and microscopic ionization constants of amino-acids.

The problem of microscopic constants also occurs in the case of several acidities, but in a more complicated manner because the number of microscopic constants increases markedly faster than that of the number of acidities.

7)　Prevision of acid-base reactions in aqueous solutions

The matter of predicting reactions is to foresee if they are possible in a given direction and also, if it is possible, to know their quantitative character. Such a forecasting is not necessarily an easy task. It involves a thorough examination of the experimental conditions of the reaction. Especially, the influence of other chemical reactions coupled with that under study must be examined.

Let us consider the following possible acid-base reaction:

$$\text{acid}_1 + \text{base}_2 \rightleftharpoons \text{base}_1 + \text{acid}_2 \tag{160}$$

It involves the two acid-base pairs $\text{acid}_1/\text{base}_1$ and $\text{acid}_2/\text{base}_2$. Let $K°$ be its thermodynamic equilibrium constant. Two questions can be asked:

－ the first involves the direction of the spontaneous reaction. Does the reaction evolve spontaneously from the left to the right, or is it the reverse direction?

－ the second is that of the reaction extent.

From the qualitative viewpoint, the reaction evolves spontaneously from left to right when the equilibrium constant $K°$ is higher than unity. (When it is lower than unity, it *also* evolves to the right but in a very minute manner in such a way that the mass action law remains obeyed.)

From the quantitative viewpoint, the knowledge of the equilibrium constant $K°$ provides a first information. $K°$ can simply be calculated from pK_a values of both couples 1 and 2. The expression of $K°$ is indeed (in terms of activities):

$$K° = a_{\text{base1}} \, a_{\text{acid2}}/a_{\text{acid1}} \, a_{\text{base2}} \tag{161}$$

It is sufficient to multiply the numerator and the denominator of (158) by the activity of the proton in the solution to see that:

$$K° = K_{a1}/K_{a2}$$

or:

$$\log K° = pK_{a2} - pK_{a1}$$

Once and for all, numerous pK_a values are tabulated. We see that reaction (157) evolving from left to right is all the more quantitative when the pK_{a2} value is high and the pK_{a1} value is low.

An important point to realize is that the reaction extent does not only depend on the equilibrium constant, but also on the initial concentrations of the species (reactants and products) participating in the reaction. Calculations of the different concentrations at equilibrium can be made by using the following basic equations which express the notions of equilibrium, of the conservation of the matter and the stoichiometry of the studied reaction. These reactions are always satisfied.

Let us consider the reaction:

$$\text{acid}_1 + \text{base}_2 \rightleftharpoons \text{base}_1 + \text{acid}_2 \tag{162}$$

and assimilate the activities to the concentrations. The necessarily satisfied equations are:

$$K_{a1} = [\text{base}_{1\,eq}][H^+_{eq}]/[\text{acid}_{1eq}] \text{ and } K_{a2} = [\text{base}_{2eq}][H^+_{eq}]/[\text{acid}_{2eq}] \tag{163}$$

$$[\text{base}_{1eq}] + [\text{acid}_{1eq}] = C_1 \tag{164}$$

$$[\text{base}_{2eq}] + [\text{acid}_{2eq}] = C_2 \tag{165}$$

$$[\text{base}_{1eq}] = [\text{acid}_{2eq}] \tag{166}$$

Notice that the concentrations involved in these equations are those at equilibrium. In these kinds of problems, there are always the same number of unknowns as equations: in the present case, 5 unknowns (the 5 concentrations) for 5 equations. The system of equations 159–163 is mathematically soluble.

The case of the occurrence of several simultaneous equilibria has already been tackled with the notions of microscopic and macroscopic constants. Such a case may be horribly complicated in biochemistry. This is the case, for example, of ribonuclease. This protein contains 36 amino-acids possessing side-chains containing either an acidic carboxylic or a basic amino rest! However, by studying the acid-base titration curves of such compounds, it is possible to determine the number of acidic or basic (and even quasi-neutral) rests since they appear on the titration curve in statistically well known domains of pH.

It is also interesting to consider the *kinetic aspects of the acid-base reactions in water*. Thermodynamics, indeed, permits to say if a given reaction in given conditions is possible or not. The answer is without any appeal. But, when the reaction is possible, thermodynamics does not say if the reaction is fast or low. The answer can only come from the realm of kinetics. However, concerning the reactions of acid-base in water, there is no problem. They are among the *fastest reactions* in solutions. They can be considered as immediate. There are very few exceptions to this rule. They concern some kinds of unusual organic acids.

Chapter **27**

Redox Reactions–Redox Couples–Brief Description of an Electrochemical Cell

Redox reactions are numerous in biochemistry. Among them, perhaps the most known are those involving cytochromes. The definition of couples redox and the measurement of their standard potentials permit to class them according to their oxidative and reductive power. In turn, this ranking permits to predict the direction of redox reactions and even to calculate their equilibrium constant values. Electrochemical measurements, which permit the determination of standard potentials, may also permit, in some cases, to obtain the standard thermodynamic functions accompanying chemical and biochemical reactions.

1) Redox equilibria

A redox reaction results from the exchange of electrons between two redox couples or pairs. A redox couple is defined by the following half redox reaction:

Oxidant + n electrons $\rightleftharpoons$ reductant (167)

For example:

$Fe^{3+} + 1e- \rightleftharpoons Fe^{2+}$

Fe^{3+} is the oxidised form of the couple Fe^{3+}/Fe^{2+} and Fe^{2+} is its reduced form. Ferric ions Fe^{3+} are the oxidant and ferrous ions the reductant. A species is said as oxidised when it has lost electron(s) and as reduced when it has gained electron(s). An oxidation corresponds to a loss of electrons by the oxidised species, and a reduction to a gain of electrons by the reduced species.

In order to equilibrate redox reactions, one defines *oxidation numbers*. They characterize the oxidation state of one element. They are symbolized by a Roman number which may be positive, negative or null. They are located as superscripts to the right of the chemical symbol. For example, the element manganese in the permanganate ion has for oxidation number + VII. The rules permitting to assign an oxidation number to an element are somewhat arbitrary. They are not devoid of any ambiguity (for further details, see the following paragraph).

Half redox reactions are never "seen". They never evolve alone. They are only "seen" indirectly. Actually, they are always coupled to another half redox reaction (which, itself, cannot be "seen" solely). The coupling of both half-reactions can occur in a homogeneous phase (that is to say in solution). In this case, it is a chemical coupling. It can also occur in a heterogeneous medium such as in an electrochemical cell. The coupling is then said to be electrochemical.

For example, let us consider the reaction of ions Cu^{2+} and Zn^{2+}. It is (s: solid; w: in water chosen as solvent):

$$Zn_{(s)} + Cu^{2+}_{(w)} \rightleftharpoons Zn^{2+}_{(w)} + Cu_{(s)} \tag{168}$$

Reaction (165), the only one "seen", results from the coupling of the following two half redox reactions occurring simultaneously:

$$Zn^{2+}_{(w)} + 2e^- \rightleftharpoons Zn_{(s)} \tag{169}$$

and:

$$Cu^{2+}_{(w)} + 2e^- \rightleftharpoons Cu_{(s)} \tag{170}$$

Of course, redox reactions may be more complicated than (165). For the sake of generality, a better formalism is:

$$aOx_1 + bRed_2 \rightleftharpoons aRed_1 + bOx_2 \tag{171}$$

The different stoichiometric coefficients a and b result from the difference of the numbers electrons exchanged (virtually) in each redox half-reaction $Ox_1 \rightarrow Red_1$ and $Ox_2 \rightarrow Red_2$.

In a first approximation, the "oxidative (or reductive)" force of a redox pair is characterized by the value of its standard potential $E°$. The standard potential is a kind of equilibrium constant of the half reaction (164). $E°$ is expressed in volts.

2) Oxidation numbers—A discussion

Oxidation numbers (o.n.) characterize the oxidation state of one element within a chemical species. They can be specified by a Roman number facing the element or, alternatively, they can be located to the right and on the same line as the complete name of the species.

In most cases, the element of the species that is oxidized or reduced is not clearly defined. Even attributing an o.n. to an element in an organic molecule may offer serious difficulties.

To overcome them, some arbitrary conventions and definitions have been devised.

According to the IUPAC, both electrons shared by the two atoms (forming the bond between them) must be assigned as belonging to the more electronegative one of both. If the two atoms sharing them are identical, the number of electrons must be divided equally. The formal charge remaining on one atom, once the assignment is made, is its oxidation number. Another convention which extends and completes the preceding one is very useful. On one end, it stipulates that in a compound containing hydrogen, oxygen nitrogen and carbon atoms, one assignates the values +I, –II, –III as oxidation numbers, respectively, for hydrogen, oxygen and nitrogen atoms on one hand and, on the other, the sum of all the o.n. and of the electrical charge of a neutral molecule or of an ion is null. However, these three atoms may have different values for their o.n. than those given, in some unusual compounds.

The following question may be asked: what is the utility of oxidation numbers?

A first positive interest is that o.n. extend the oxido-reduction concept to covalent derivatives. A second is that it facilitates the equilibration of redox reactions. A third interest is that it facilitates the description of the properties of an element by providing a logical presentation of them. The major drawback is the following one. It is the possible existence of several sets of values for the same element in the same molecule.

As an example of the determination of an o.n., let us mention the case of the element manganese in the ion permanganate MnO_4^-. Attributing the value –II to the oxygen and the unit negative value for the whole charge of the species, we immediately find the value +VII for the manganese. This does not mean at all that the ion Mn^{7+} exists! Indeed, it does not exist.

We shall encounter the concept of o.n. in several places of the book, as for example, during the discussion of the Emden-Meyerhof Chain (see Chapter 34).

3) Definition of the global reaction of an electrochemical cell

Redox reactions can take place in a homogenous phase (as it is already said in a solvent) or in a heterogeneous medium, on the surface of electrodes, that is to say in an electrochemical cell. The functioning of electrochemical cells is based on two mutually coupled redox reactions occurring simultaneously but on two different electrodes. The two mutually coupled redox reactions are the same as the half redox reactions mentioned above, reacting together in a homogenous medium. In the electrochemical cell, they occur separately at the surface of two electrodes.

Electrochemical cells are devices which may permit to study the thermodynamics of redox reactions, at least in some cases. Let us consider reaction (168). Its molar reaction is:

$$\Delta_r G = -a\mu Ox_1 - b\mu Red_2 + a\mu Red_1 + b\mu Ox_2 \qquad (172)$$

As stated previously (see Chapter 18), the values of these terms change with the extent of the reaction ξ. For example, in the case of reaction (168), applying relation (169) (see Chapter 18) gives:

$$\Delta_r G = \Delta_r G° + RT \ln \{[a_{Red1}{}^a\, a_{Ox2}{}^b]/[a_{Ox1}{}^a\, a_{Red2}{}^b]\} \qquad (173)$$

In this relation, terms a_{Red1}, a_{Ox2} and so forth are the activities of the species indicated in subscript. (Do not confuse them with the stoichiometric coefficients).

We shall see that global redox reactions of the kind (165) or (168) may be considered as being a global redox reaction evolving in a homogenous medium. This is the reason why it is named "cell reaction". Actually, this reaction does not exist as being only one reaction since it is the result of two separate reactions occurring simultaneously on each electrode.

4) Description of an electrochemical cell—The galvanic and electrolytic cells

* Galvanic cell

Let us consider the electrochemical cell represented in Figure 45. It is named Daniell's cell. It contains two compartments. One consists of a zinc strip dipping into a zinc sulfate solution and the other of a copper strip dipping into a copper sulfate solution. The two metallic conductors are called the *electrodes*. Both compartments are linked by a conducting bridge. It precludes the mixing of the two electrolyte solutions, but its permits the current to pass from one compartment to the other. Finally, both electrodes are in mutual electric contact through a metallic thread, for example a platinum one. One galvanometer and possibly an electrical motor are inserted in the circuit. A millivoltmeter is connected in parallel between the two platinum threads.

When the circuitry is closed, a spontaneous current passes through it until equilibrium potential has been attained. Then, no current passes further.

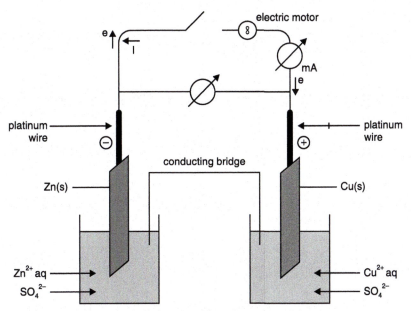

Figure 45. Daniell's electrochemical cell.

Actually, two kinds of electrical current exist in the cell. In the external circuitry, the current is purely and simply the displacement of the electrons. It is the metallic current. In the electrolytic solutions, the current is due to the displacement of the ions. It is named the *ionic current*. It also exists in the bridge.

At this point of the description, the following question arises: what happens at the interface of both kinds of current, that is to say on the surfaces of the electrodes? The answer is the following one: according to Kirchoff's law, the current continuity must exist. It can be realized only if the two following reactions take place simultaneously and separately at the surface of the electrodes. In the case, for example, of the redox reaction (165) studied, this means that:

$$Zn_{(s)} \rightleftharpoons Zn^{2+}_{(w)} + 2e^-_{(metal)} \tag{174}$$

$$Cu^{2+}_{(w)} + 2e^-_{(metal)} \rightleftharpoons Cu_{(s)} \tag{175}$$

The formed zinc ions at the surface of the electrode go into the solution to give the hydrated ones $Zn^{2+}_{(w)}$. Thus, they contribute to the ionic current. The electrons liberated simultaneously at the same electrode are going into the electric conductor. They go to the copper strip. They constitute the electronic current. At the surface of the copper electrode, the cupric ions $Cu^{2+}_{(w)}$ capture the electrons coming from the metallic conductor. Displacements of ions Cu^{2+}, Zn^{2+} and SO_4^{2-} also contribute to the ionic current. As a consequence of these phenomena, the current continuity is ensured. Reactions (171) and (172) are called *electrochemical reactions* because they take place at the two interfaces. The chemical reaction, which formally corresponds to the sum of the two preceding electrochemical reactions, is called the *global cell reaction*.

When the cell reaction is equivalent to a spontaneous chemical reaction occurring in the same conditions of composition, temperature and pressure as in the cell, the latter is called a *galvanic cell*. It is an energy-producing device. In Daniell's cell, electrons spontaneously circulate from the zinc electrode to that of copper, when the circuitry is closed. A spontaneous current passes through it until equilibrium has been attained. This indicates that, spontaneously, the copper strip is less negatively (or more positively) charged than the zinc one.

Daniell's galvanic cell, thanks to the current it generates, permits to recover energy of chemical origin in the occurrence of the chemical energy contained in the electrodes. A galvanic cell is also named an *energy producer device*.

* An electrolytic cell

Let us consider an electrochemical system analogous to the galvanic Daniell's cell but differing from the latter by the presence of a power supply instead of the electrical motor. It permits to apply a potential difference sufficient to make the electrons go in a direction opposite to that followed in Daniell's galvanic cell in the external circuitry. In these conditions, the promoted reaction is:

$Zn^{2+} + 2e^- \rightleftharpoons Zn$

at the surface of the zinc wire, and

$Cu \rightleftharpoons Cu^{2+} + 2e^-$

at the surface of the copper wire. The reaction cell is:

$$Zn^{2+} + Cu \rightleftharpoons Zn + Cu^{2+} \qquad (176)$$

It is just the opposite of that occurring in Daniell's galvanic cell. This reaction cannot be achieved spontaneously in a pure chemical manner without receiving energy (heat for example) from the surroundings. If it were the case, the success of obtaining reaction (173) would be miraculous!

Such cells are called *electrolytic cells* because they permit to obtain chemical substances which are not spontaneously accessible. They are also named "*substance—producer devices*".

5) Some other definitions found in electrochemistry

By definition, the *cathode* is the electrode where the electrochemical reduction reaction occurs. The *anode* is where the electrochemical oxidation occurs. The fact that a cell may behave either in a galvanic mode or in an electrolytic mode does not modify these definitions which are quite general. In Daniell's galvanic cell, the cathode is the copper wire and the anode, the zinc wire. In the corresponding electrolytic cell, it is the reverse. The cathode is not necessarily the electrode toward which cations go and the anode that toward which anions go. This may happen, but it is not always true. Actually, the cathodic or anodic behavior of an electrode is disconnected from its charge.

An electrochemical cell is said to be *reversible* if the direction of the reaction cell is inverted when the electron flow is inverted. It is *irreversible* when a new reaction cell appears.

When a power supply generates a potential difference which exactly counterbalances that existing between the electrodes, no current flows. The system is said to be *at equilibrium*.

The potential difference E determined at equilibrium (the "zero-current potential cell") E° is called the *electromotive force* of the cell.

6) Electromotive force of a galvanic cell—Cell potential difference

It is an experimental fact that global reactions (168) performed by purely chemical means lead to the same final states as the same reactions performed by electrochemical means (through the corresponding electrochemical reactions) provided, of course, that the initial and final states are the same in both experiments and provided that the electrochemical cell has not furnished work since the chemical reaction, the behavior of which is compared to that of the electrochemical process, does not furnish work in the experience. This result is general. A galvanic cell discharge is equivalent to a chemical process provided the initial and final thermodynamic states are the same.

7) Nernst's equation

Now, we consider a very important law in electrochemistry, the *Nernst's law*. It is important for our purpose since it leads to the concept of standard potentials of electrodes and likewise to the notion of standard Gibbs energy decline accompanying chemical and biochemical reactions.

Nernst's equation results from the equality of work supplied by the electrochemical system *under conditions of reversibility* with the standard Gibbs energy decrease of the corresponding chemical reaction. (Notice that the conditions of reversibility were not prevailing in the comparison experience mentioned just above).

To again take the above example, the work performed under the reversibility in the cell is that of transport of the $Cu^{2+}{}_{(w)}$ and $Zn^{2+}{}_{(w)}$ in both compartments against the electrical field since the copper electrode is positively charged. The charge q brought by dn mol L^{-1} of the $Cu^{2+}{}_{(w)}$ and $Zn^{2+}{}_{(w)}$ (both ions of valence 2) crossing the cell during a very brief time interval dt from the left to the right is:

dq = 2F dn

Since the interval dt is very brief, the potential difference between both electrodes can be considered as being constant during this period. If its value is E, the work dw' done by the system for the displacement of positive ions is in absolute value:

|dw'| = |Edq|

that is to say:

|dw'| = |2FE dn|

This equality results from the law of electrostatics. Since the work is carried out by the system, one can write according to the usual conventions of thermodynamics:

|dw'| = –2FE dn

dG_{syst} = –2FE dn

The Gibbs energy change accompanying the reaction at every stage of the process is:

$dG_{syst} = -(-\mu_{Zn} - \mu_{Cu2+} + \mu_{Zn2+} + \mu_{Cu})\, d\xi$

By comparison with the preceding relation, we find:

$$-\mu_{Zn} - \mu_{Cu2+} + \mu_{Zn2+} + \mu_{Cu} = -2FE \qquad (177)$$

since:

$d\xi$ = dn   (since $v_{Cu2+} = v_{Zn2+}$).

and E is the electromotive force of the cell.

The left-hand of relation (174) is the molar reaction Gibbs function change of the chemical reaction equivalent to the reaction cell. This reasoning can be generalized. For example, for reaction (168) performed through an electrochemical cell, we can write:

$$\Delta_r G = -nFE \tag{178}$$

$$(-a\mu Ox_1 - b\mu Red_2 + a\mu Red_1 + b\mu Ox_2) = -nFE \tag{179}$$

where $n = ab$ is the number of electrons exchanged by the two pairs. Relations (175) and (176) constitute the Nernst's law.

Nernst' law is of enormous interest in physical and analytical chemistries. It permits to predict the direction and the quantitative character of redox reaction.

– The molar reaction Gibbs function possesses an instantaneous value. It depends on the reaction extent. As a result, the value of E found in Nernst's law is also an instantaneous one.

The electromotive force mentioned in Nernst's law are measured at null current. This is the condition of reversibility. They are the "zero cell potentials". Actually, without any particular precaution to maintain the reversibility, an electrical current passes in an electrochemical process. For example, it can drive an electrical motor. As a result, there is an electrical energy recovered from the Gibbs energy, initially contained in the chemical system. Due to the current's occurrence, there is thus a release of heat due to the joule effect in the circuitry and, hence, an entropy creation. The process is irreversible. This is why measurements are carried out with very weak currents with the use of an opposition montage and by avoiding any other source of irreversibility.

8) Standard reaction entropy change from the temperature coefficient of the emf. of a reversible cell-Determination of the enthalpy change

The last considerations justify the use of the following relation for the determination of the standard reaction entropy change from the temperature coefficient of the emf. of a reversible cell (see Chapter 22):

$$\Delta S° = -d (\Delta G°/dT)$$

$$\Delta S° = nF (dE°/dT)$$

Furthermore, there are other possibilities offered by this relation and even by those related to it.

• the first one is to determine the molar entropy of one reactant or product of the chemical reaction under study. This is only possible if the standard molar entropies of other products and reactants are known. In these conditions, measurements of the standard reaction Gibbs energies, that is to say their corresponding emf, permit to obtain the standard molar reaction entropy unknown through the relation (see Chapter 22):

$$\Delta_r S° = \Sigma \, vS°_{(products)} - \Sigma vS°_{(reactants)}$$

because those of other products or reactants are known.

• the second possibility is to obtain the reaction enthalpy.

9) Electrode potentials

The values of electrode potentials permit to easily predict redox reactions.

In the standard conditions, reaction (170) becomes:

$$\Delta rG° = -nFE°$$

Equation (170) may be written equivalently:

$$E = E° – (RT/nF) \ln [(a_{Red1}{}^a/a_{Ox1}{}^a)] + (RT/nF) \ln [(a_{Red2}{}^b/a_{Ox2}{}^b)] \tag{180}$$

It is possible to set the standard potential E°, which is a constant, equal to a difference of two constants, temporarily called $E_1°$ and $E_2°$, that is:

$$E° = E_1° – E_2°$$

Next, regarding (177) and after having replaced E° by this difference, we see that two submembers appear on its right-hand side. They are written in brackets in the following relation:

$$E = \{E_1° – (RT/nF) \ln [(a_{Red1}{}^a/a_{Ox1}{}^a)]\} – \{E_2° – (RT/nF) \ln [(a_{Red2}{}^b/a_{Ox2}{}^b)]\} \tag{181}$$

Since the measured cell potential difference is actually the potential difference between two electrodes, it immediately comes to mind to assimilate each of the preceding terms in brackets to the potential of each of the electrodes. They are called *electrode potentials* E_1 and E_2. $E_1°$ and $E_2°$ exhibit characteristic values of both couples Ox_1/Red_1 and Ox_2/Red_2. They are called *standard potentials of* both couples and are symbolized $E°(Ox_1/Red_1)$ and $E°(Ox_2/red_2)$.

The electrode potentials E_1, E_2 are measurements of the oxidizing strength of the couples 1,2.... in the conditions of the experience.

Assigning numerical values to $E_1°$ and $E_2°$ has been a problem since the experimental determination of absolute electrode potentials is (probably) definitively impossible. However, it has been solved by assigning *relative* values to them. This strategy is based on the fact that if absolute electrode potentials are not measurable, their differences can be. Thus, an electrode potential standard value has been conventionally chosen for the couple $H^+_w/H_2(g)$, which constitutes the hydrogen electrode (w: water). Its standard electrode has been set definitively to the value 0,0000 V at every temperature:

$$E° (H^+_w/H_{2(g)}) = 0,0000 \text{ V} \quad \text{(every temperature)}$$

The standard conditions for both members of the couple are $P_{H2} = 1$ bar and $a_{(H+w)} = 1$. These values are those of the so-called *normal hydrogen electrode* (NHE).

The electromotive force of a cell consisting of the couple under the study and by the couple $H^+_w/H_2(g)$ in these conditions is by definition the standard potential of the first one (Figure 46).

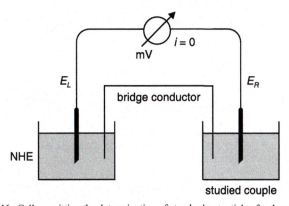

Figure 46. Cell permitting the determination of standard potentials of redox couples.

Standard potential electrodes have been established according to this principle.

It is important to notice that the cells which permit such determinations must be built so that the hydrogen electrode is on the left of that under study. The accepted value E°(Ox/Red) is (R: right; L: left):

$$E°(Ox/Red) = E_R - E_L$$

10) Some standard electrode potentials

In Table 11, we give some reduction electrode potentials E°. In Table 12, we give some reduction standard potential values E° of some redox couples at 298 K. Table 13 mentions the values for some organic couples but with the biochemistry conventions (see Chapter 21).

Table 11. Some reduction electrode potentials values at 298 K.

Organic redox couples	E'°(V)
o-quinone $+ 2H^+ + 2e^- \rightleftharpoons$ pyrocatechol	0,43
adrenochrome $+ 2H^+ + 2e^- \rightleftharpoons$ adrenaline	0,38
oxidized cytochrome a+e⁻ $\rightleftharpoons$ reduced cytochrome a *	0,29
oxidized cytochrome c+e⁻ $\rightleftharpoons$ reduced cytochrome c	0,26
oxidized cytochrome b+e⁻ $\rightleftharpoons$ reduced cytochrome b	−0,04
met Hb (Fe^{III}) + e⁻ $\rightleftharpoons$ Hb (Fe^{II}) (hemoglobine) **	0,15
fumarate + 2H⁺ + 2e⁻ $\rightleftharpoons$ succinate	0,00
oxaloacetate + 2H⁺ + 2e⁻ $\rightleftharpoons$ malate	−0,17
pyruvate + 2H⁺ + 2e⁻ $\rightleftharpoons$ lactate	−0,18
acetaldehyde + 2H⁺ + 2e⁻ $\rightleftharpoons$ ethanol	−0,20
FAD + 2H⁺ + 2e⁻ $\rightleftharpoons$ FAD H_2	−0,22
NAD + H⁺ + 2e⁻ $\rightleftharpoons$ NADH, H	−0,32
cysteine + 2H⁺ + 2e⁻ $\rightleftharpoons$ Cystine	−0,39
HCO_3^- + 2H⁺ + 2e⁻ $\rightleftharpoons$ $HCOO^-$ + H_2O (bicarbonate / formiate)	−0,41

* Heteroproteins in a ferroporphyrinic prosthetic group. Catalyze the oxidation of many substrates in the cell metabolism.

**Porphyrinic erythrocytic chromoproteins transporting oxygen along with one part carbon dioxide, contributing to the buffering capacity of the blood.

Table 12. Some reduction standard potential values E° at 298 K.

Redox semi-reaction	E°(V)
$F_{2(g)} + 2e^- \rightleftharpoons 2F^-$	2,87
$S_2O_8^{2-} + 2e^- \rightleftharpoons 2SO_4^{2-}$	2,01
$O_{3(g)} + 2H^+ + 2e^- \rightleftharpoons O_{2(g)} + H_2O$	2,075
$H_2O_2 + 2H^+ + 2e^- \rightleftharpoons 2H_2O$	1,77
$HClO + H^+ + e^- \rightleftharpoons \frac{1}{2}Cl_{2(g)} + H_2O$	1,63
$H_5IO_6 + H^+ + 2e^- \rightleftharpoons IO_3^- + 3H_2O$	1,60
$BrO_3^- + 6H^+ + 5e^- \rightleftharpoons \frac{1}{2}Br_2(l) + 3H_2O$	1,52
$BrO_3^- + 6H^+ + 6e^- \rightleftharpoons Br^- + 3H_2O$	1,44
$MnO_4^- + 8H^+ + 5e^- \rightleftharpoons Mn^{2+} + 4H_2O$	1,52
$Cl_{2(g)} + 2e^- \rightleftharpoons 2Cl^-$	1,36
$Cr_2O_7^{2-} + 14H^+ + 6e^- \rightleftharpoons 2Cr^{3+} + 7H_2O$	1,33
$O_{2(g)} + 4H^+ + 4e^- \rightleftharpoons 2H_2O$	1,23
$IO_3^- + 6H^+ + 5e^- \rightleftharpoons \frac{1}{2}I_{2(s)} + 3H_2O$	1,20
$IO_3^- + 6H^+ + 5e^- \rightleftharpoons \frac{1}{2}I_2 + 3H_2O$	1,18
$Br_2 + 2e^- \rightleftharpoons 2Br^-$	1,09
$Br_2(l) + 2e^- \rightleftharpoons 2Br^-$	1,07
$ICl_2^- + e^- \rightleftharpoons \frac{1}{2}I_{2(s)} + 2Cl^-$	1,06
$AuCl_4^- + 3e^- \rightleftharpoons Au_{(s)} + 4Cl^-$	1,00
$HNO_2 + H^+ + e^- \rightleftharpoons NO_{(g)} + H_2O$	1,00
$2Hg^{2+} + 2e^- \rightleftharpoons Hg_2^{2+}$	0,92
$Cu^{2+} + I^- + e^- \rightleftharpoons CuI_{(s)}$	0,86
$Hg_2^{2+} + 2e^- \rightleftharpoons 2Hg(l)$	0,79
$Fe^{3+} + e^- \rightleftharpoons Fe^{2+}$	0,77
$PtCl_4^{2-} + 2e^- \rightleftharpoons Pt_{(s)} + 4Cl^-$	0,73
$I_2 + 2e^- \rightleftharpoons 2I^-$	0,62
$H_3AsO_4 + 2H^+ + 2e^- \rightleftharpoons H_3AsO_3 + H_2O$	0,56
$I_3^- + 2e^- \rightleftharpoons 3I^-$	0,54
$I_{2(s)} + 2e^- \rightleftharpoons 2I^-$	0,54
$Fe(CN)_6^{3-} + 1e^- \rightleftharpoons Fe(CN)_6^{4-}$	0,36
$UO_2^{2+} + 4H^+ + 2e^- \rightleftharpoons U^{4+} + 2H_2O$	0,33
$Hg_2Cl_{2(s)} + 2e^- \rightleftharpoons 2Hg(l) + 2Cl^-$	0,27
$AgCl_{(s)} + e^- \rightleftharpoons Ag_{(s)} + Cl^-$	0,15
$Cu^{2+} + e^- \rightleftharpoons Cu^+$	0,15
$Sn^{4+} + 2e^- \rightleftharpoons Sn^{2+}$	0,15
$S_4O_6^{2-} + 2e^- \rightleftharpoons 2S_2O_3^{2-}$	0,08
$2H^+ + 2e^- \rightleftharpoons H_{2(g)}$	0,00
$V^{3+} + e^- \rightleftharpoons V^{2+}$	– 0,26
$Cr^{3+} + e^- \rightleftharpoons Cr^{2+}$	– 0,41
$U^{4+} + e^- \rightleftharpoons U^{3+}$	– 0,61

Table 13. Reduction potential values of some organic couples (biochemical conventions pH = 7, T = 37°C).

Reaction to the electrode	E°(V)	Reaction to the electrode	E°(V)
$Li^+ + e^- \rightleftarrows Li_{(s)}$	$-3,05$	$Sn^{2+} + 2e^- \rightleftarrows Sn_{(s)}$	$-0,15$
$K^+ + e^- \rightleftarrows K_{(s)}$	$-2,93$	$Pb^{2+} + 2e^- \rightleftarrows Pb_{(s)}$	$-0,13$
$Ca^{2+} + 2e^- \rightleftarrows Ca_{(s)}$	$-2,87$	$2H^+ + 2e^- \rightleftarrows H_{2(g)}$	$0,00$
$Na^+ + e^- \rightleftarrows Na_{(s)}$	$-2,71$	$Cu^{2+} + 2e^- \rightleftarrows Cu_{(s)}$	$0,34$
$Mg^{2+} + 2e^- \rightleftarrows Mg_{(s)}$	$-2,37$	$Hg^{2+} + 2e^- \rightleftarrows Hg(l)$	$0,79$
$Mn^{2+} + 2e^- \rightleftarrows Mn_{(s)}$	$-1,18$	$Ag^+ + e^- \rightleftarrows Ag_{(s)}$	$0,80$
$Zn^{2+} + 2e^- \rightleftarrows Zn_{(s)}$	$-0,76$		
$Fe^{2+} + 2e^- \rightleftarrows Fe_{(s)}$	$-0,44$		

In appendix I-9 are given some other values of standard reduction potentials of some biologically important half-reactions.

These potential values are those of reduction potentials. The values are those of zero-current cell potentials in which the hydrogen electrode is located on the left and that under study on the right (Figure 46). All the species that participate in the half-reduction equilibria are in their standard state. Their activity is equal to unity. The hydrogen electrode necessarily plays the part of the anode and the studied electrode that of the cathode. Hence, the studied system suffers the electrodic reaction:

$$Ox + ne- \rightarrow Red$$

hence the name "standard reduction potentials". This point is very important especially for the calculation of the Gibbs energies of the half-redox reactions. (Actually, let us recall that summing the Gibbs energies of both half redox reactions in the right direction permits to determine the accurate Gibbs energy of the whole reaction. For example, if we are interested by the standard Gibbs energy of reaction (165), we must add those of half reactions (166) and (167) and write these reactions taken in the judicious directions. That is to say, the values $E°_{(Zn/Zn2+)} = + 0,76V$ and $E°(Cu^{2+}/Cu) = + 0,34V$ must be taken. Gibbs energies of half redox are, then, calculated through the relation $\Delta G° = -nFE°$.

11) Prevision of redox reactions

From the qualitative standpoint, the simplest way to predict the direction of a redox reaction is to compare the standard potentials of the two couples which may react together in the investigated reaction. The rule is that the oxidized form of the couple that has the highest standard potential spontaneously react with the reduced form of the couple that has the lowest standard potential. As an example, let us suppose that the couples Zn^{2+}/Zn (solid) ($E° = -0,77V$) and Cu^{2+}/Cu (solid ($E° = +0,34V$) are placed face to face, then, according to this rule, we can predict that the spontaneous reaction is:

$$Zn(s) + Cu^{2+} \rightarrow Zn^{2+} + Cu(s)$$

We already know that this is true. This reaction is, indeed, that of a galvanic electrochemical cell. *But this is a crude rule.* Its prediction, which may or may not be good, is, however, not wholly justified. Let us consider the Equation (171) which gives the emf E of the cell (embodying the reaction under study) and recall that E has the deep meaning of the Gibbs energy of the studied reaction, that is to say the tendency of the reaction to react in the indicated reaction. This equation shows that the above rule does not take into account the logarithmic terms. For example, it is quite possible (and sometimes it happens) that the difference between the standard electrode potentials $E_1° - E_2°$ predict the reaction to evolve in one direction, whereas the difference between the electrode potentials $E_1 - E_2$ predict the inverse direction. In this case, it is the last direction which must be taken into account.

From the quantitative standpoint, as for the acid-base reactions, the quantitative character of the reaction depends on the equilibrium constant K°. It is related to the standard efm of the cell E° through the Nernst relation:

$$RT \ln K° = -nFE° \tag{182}$$

But, here also, the sole value of the equilibrium constant does not suffice for an accurate prediction of the quantitative character of the reaction. The values of the concentrations (activities) of the reactants, and eventually of the products of the reaction, must be taken into account.

A first point to notice is that, here, we uniquely study the thermodynamic aspects of the prevision of redox reactions. Contrary to the reactions acid-base, the kinetics of redox reactions are variable in aqueous solutions and can play a part. For example, they may be very sluggish.

The second point is that determining the quantitative character necessitates to evaluate the concentrations of the different species in the initial and final states. The calculation of these concentrations implies to handle the different mathematical relations which govern the equilibria and that are obligatorily satisfied. For example, let us study the equilibrium:

$$Red_1 + Ox_2 \rightleftharpoons Ox_1 + Red_2 \tag{182'}$$

Let us consider the calculation of the equilibrium constant of a reaction of biochemical importance, that of the reduction of acetaldehyde by NADH at pH = 7. The products are NAD⁺ and ethanol (notice that the standard potentials are the biological ones —see Chapter 21). (The molecular structures of these reactants and products are given during the course of this book). The half-redox and the global reactions are:

$$NAD^+ + H^+ + 2e^- \rightleftharpoons NADH \ (E_2'° = -0,32V)$$

$$CH_3CHO \ (acetaldehyde) + 2H^+ + 2e- \rightleftharpoons C_2H_5OH \quad (E_1'° = -0,18V)$$

$$NADH + acetaldehyde + H^+ \rightleftharpoons NAD^+ + ethanol \qquad (global \ reaction)$$

At equilibrium, the potential of the solution is given by one of the two following relations. (Both grouped are simply equivalent of Nernst relation).

$$E°(Ox_1/Red_1) - (RT/nF) \ln [red_{1eq}]/[Ox_{1eq}] = E°(Ox_2/Red_2) - (RT/nF) \ln [red_{2eq}]/[Ox_{2eq}] \tag{183}$$

The equilibrium constant K of the reaction is, hence, defined by the expression:

$$K = [NAD^+_{eq}][C_2H_5OH_{eq}]/[NADH_{eq}][CH_3CHO_{eq}][H^+_{eq}]$$

Let us reason in terms of concentrations rather than in term of activities for the sake of simplicity and apply relation (180) above. We find:

$$-0,18 - (RT/2F) \ln[C_2H_5OH]/[CH_3CHO][H^+]^2 = -0,32 - (RT/2F) \ln[NADH]/[NAD^+][H^+]$$

Rearranging, we obtain the equation:

$-0,14 = \{(RT/2F) \ln \{[CH_3CHO][H^+][NADH]/[C_2H_5OH] [NAD^+]\}$

Introducing the values of the constants R and F at 298 K and using decimal logarithms, the equation becomes:

$-0,140 = 0,0296 \log \{[C_2H_5OH] [NAD^+]/[CH_3CHO][H^+][NADH]\}$

and the equilibrium constant is:

$K' = 1,8 \ 10^{-5}$

Remark: Actually, this value is obtained with the standard biochemical potentials by taking for pH = 1 : a_H = 1 since by definition, in the standard state, the activity of the species is equal to unity. In other words, with the biological standard states, the K value quantifies the following equilibrium at pH = 7. With the chemical standard states (pH = 0), the equilibrium constant K of the reaction:

$C_2H_5OH + NAD^+ \rightleftharpoons CH_3CHO + NADH + H^+$

would be:

$K = 1,8 \ 10^{-12}$

12) Formal potentials

Most of the time, the ionic strength of a medium, together with some other parameters defining it (such as the presence of other substances, their concentrations, etc.) in which we want to perform a redox reaction, are unknown. In these conditions, it is difficult to forecast the possibilities of the reaction. To partially overcome these difficulties, the concept of formal potentials E°' has been devised. (Unfortunately, their symbols are the same as the standard biological potentials). The formal potentials are those measured with solutions containing both Ox and Red forms of the couple at the unit concentration and that contain some other species the concentrations of which are specified. They take into account the variations in the activity coefficients with the ionic strength, the acid-base equilibria involving the forms Ox and Red and their possible complexation with other solution species.

There may exist a considerable difference between the standard potential of a couple and its formal one in particular conditions. A well-known example is that of the couple hexacyanoferrate (III)/hexacyanoferrate (II) (ferricyanure/ferrocyanure) whose standard potential is E° = 0,36V. When the couple is dissolved at equal concentrations, its formal potential is about 0,71V.

Unfortunately, the systematic use of formal potentials is impossible, owing to the innumerable possible experimental conditions.

Chapter **28**

Other Equilibria in Solutions

In this chapter, we briefly mention some other equilibria in solutions which are of interest for our purpose. We retain those involving the formation of complexes, the partition of solutes between two non-miscible solvents and also the so-called osmotic work in biological systems.

1) Complexation equilibria

According to IUPAC, a *complex* or "a coordination entity" is composed of a central atom, usually a metal atom, to which is attached a surrounding array of other atoms or groups of atoms, each of which is called a *ligand*. The central atom is called the nucleus. Numerous comments can be made about the complexes. For our purpose, we confine ourselves to mentioning some of them. They concern their physico-chemical behavior in aqueous solutions, in particular the quantitative features of their formation and dissociation. Many biochemical reactions indeed involve the formation of complexes in quantitative way, thus making difficult the foreseeing of the course of some of their reactions. Perhaps, in this perspective, the theory formulated by the French school in analytical chemistry is the most judicious to adopt.*

According to this theory, a complex can be defined as being a species which is able to give "a particle" p to an acceptor. It is a donor of a particle p, according to the reaction:

donor $\rightleftharpoons$ acceptor + p   (184)

The term particle must not be understood according to the meaning given by the physicists, that is to say the meaning of an elementary particle. Here, the particle is a chemical species which may be a molecule, an ion, etc. As simple examples, let us mention the following complexes:

– the argentomonoammine ion $[AgNH_3^+]$, which dissociates according to:

$[AgNH_3^+] \rightleftharpoons Ag^+ + NH_3$

NH_3 being the particle,

– the dichloromercureII (mercuric chloride) $[HgCl_2]$ which dissociates (hardly) according to:

$[HgCl_2] \rightleftharpoons [HgCl^+] + Cl^-$

Here, the chloride ion is the particle. (A very known particle in analytical chemistry is the ethylenediaminotetraacetic acid, edta, which is more or less ionized).

---

* G. Charlot, J.P. Wolff and S. Lacroix. Analytica Chimica Acta, 1947, 9, 73.

A given particle may be exchanged between two different couples donor/acceptor according to:

$$donor_1 \rightleftharpoons acceptor_1 + p \tag{185}$$

$$p + acceptor_2 \rightleftharpoons donor_2 \tag{186}$$

The global reaction is:

$$donor_1 + acceptor_2 \rightleftharpoons acceptor_1 + donor_2 \tag{187}$$

Reaction (184) is analogous to the global reactions encountered in the acid-base and redox phenomena, reactions (182) and (183) appearing, thus, as being complexation half reactions. This viewpoint of complexation reactions appears to be an attempt to generalize the treatment of acid-base and redox reactions. (Two great differences with these cases, however, do exist. One is the fact that the exchanged particles in complexation reactions are multiple and, the second, that these particles exist! Recall, for example, that in redox processes, the only exchanged particle is the electron and the exchange of electrons is not directly visible).

From the quantitative standpoint, half reactions (182) and (183) are governed by dissociation constants K_c. They are introduced to maintain the similarity with the redox and acido-basic equilibria:

$$K_c = a_{(acceptor)} \, a_{(particle)} / a_{(donor)}$$

They are written in terms of activities. When the solutions are sufficiently diluted, one can define the equilibria in terms of concentrations:

$$Kc \approx [acceptor][particle]/[donor]$$

Remark: In other aspects of the chemistry of complexes, it is recommended by the IUPAC to handle formation constants of complexes rather their dissociation constants.

The rules prevailing in the prediction of complexation reactions are analogous to those governing the acid-base and redox phenomena. One may use the dissociation constants K_c of the complexes and introduce the values pX defined by the equations:

$$pX = p\chi - \log (donor/acceptor)$$

where pX plays the part of pH (it is the decimal cologarithm of the activity of the exchanged particle X) and $p\chi$ the decimal cologarithm of the dissociation constant of the half dissociation equilibrium.

It must also be known that the rate of formation or dissociation of complexes is variable. The complexes for which these reactions are fast are said to be labile, while others are inert.

Complexation reactions can be foreseen as are, for example, the acid-base ones. Notice that the latter are exchange reactions of protons whereas the former ones are exchange reactions of particules. For doing such foreseeings, it is necessary to know the dissociation constants of each particle exchanged. Scales related to the exchanged particles, analogous to that of pH, can be and have been established.

2) Partition equilibria between two non-miscible solvents

This kind of equilibria certainly occurs in cells, owing to the presence of several phases. To be convinced by this fact, it suffices to recall the structure and properties of cell membranes.

Let's consider a substance A being soluble (at least somewhat) in an organic solvent and also in water, both solvents being non-miscible. The substance spontaneously partitions between both phases until the following partition is attained:

$$A_w \rightleftharpoons A_{org}$$

At equilibrium, the activities of the solute in the two solvents do not change further. At constant temperature, they are in a constant ratio P, called the "partition coefficient P":

$$P = (a_{Aorg}/a_{Aw}) \quad \text{(at equilibrium)} \tag{188}$$

$$p = constant \quad (dT = 0)$$

From the thermodynamic standpoint, this relation is found as follows:

At equilibrium, there is equality of the chemical potentials of the solute μ_{org} and μ_w in each solvent. This is the condition of the equilibrium of partition of the solute:

$$\mu_{org} = \mu_w$$

In both phases, the chemical potentials are given by the relations:

$$\mu_w = \mu^\circ_w + RT \ln a_{Aw}$$

$$\mu_{org} = \mu^\circ_{org} + RT \ln a_{Aorg}$$

The standard chemical potentials in both phases are not the same but are constant. This is just because the two solvents are chemically different. At equilibrium, the following equation is satisfied:

$$\mu^\circ_{org} + RT \ln a_{Aorg} = \mu^\circ_w + RT \ln a_{Aw}$$

The standard chemical potentials being constant at a given temperature, Equation (185) is immediately found. When both phases are sufficiently diluted at equilibrium, the activities can be replaced by the concentrations:

$$P \approx [A]_{org}/[A]_w \quad \text{(solutions sufficiently diluted)} \tag{189}$$

It can be said that, in these conditions of equilibrium, the concentrations in both phases are in a constant ratio. Of course, the numerical value of P depends on the standard states chosen for the definitions of activities in both solvents and also of temperature.

3) The concentration work

The other name of this work is the osmotic work.

It is known that there cannot subsist gradients (at a first approximation: the word gradient means a difference—see appendix II-3) of concentrations of a solute within a solution, provided the time to reach the equilibrium has elapsed. This is a consequence of the second principle. If it would subsist a gradient of concentrations, it would be in contradistinction with the principle of the maximum disorder (see Chapter 13). However, cells are capable to do the work necessary to accumulate substances into some point, even against an unfavourable gradient of concentrations. The subject of this paragraph is to determine the energy necessary to sustain a gradient of concentrations. The problem can be schematized as follows.

The system is constituted by a solution containing one solute and the solvent at constant temperature and pressure. It is contained in a vessel. The solution is not at equilibrium, that is to say the concentration of the solute is not uniform in the whole container. Let's suppose that its concentration is C_1 at point A and C_2 at point B and that $C_2 > C_1$. The problem is to determine the exchanged work when one mole of the solute is transferred from point A to point B. To simplify the reasoning, we assimilate activities to the concentrations.

Since the process is carried out at constant pressure and temperature, it is judicious to reason in terms of Gibbs energies. Let μ_2 and μ_1 be the chemical potentials of the solute in the final and initial states 2 and 1. They are given by the relations:

$$\mu_2 = \mu° + RT \ln C_2$$

$$\mu_1 = \mu° + RT \ln C_1$$

Quite evidently, the standard potential $\mu°$ (in which the concentration is usually $C_0 = 1$ mol L^{-1}—see Chapter 19) is the same, the solute, the solvent, the pressure and the temperature also being the same in both states. The Gibbs energy change $\Delta G_{1 \to 2}$ accompanying the process is

$$\Delta G_{1 \to 2} = \mu_2 - \mu_1$$

This is because of the fact that a chemical potential is a (partial) molar Gibbs energy. Hence

$$\Delta G_{1 \to 2} = RT \ln C_2/C_1$$

We notice that the change in Gibbs energy accompanying the process is positive.

Thus, as the useful work of interest w' is positive, the system must receive work to maintain the concentration gradient. (This point will be reconsidered in Chapter 40).

Chapter 29

The "Natural Trick" for Bioenergetics to Function

It is a well-known fact that the direction of a chemical reaction in solution is not obligatorily easy to predict. Often, this is due to the fact that there exist several kinds of equilibria occurring simultaneously. The same problems exist for biochemical equilibria. Their resolution is still more complicated to achieve. The "reason-why" is simple: biochemical molecules are larger and more complex than chemical ones. Thereby, they give rise to a greater number of simultaneous equilibria than the chemical ones. In turn, the supplementary equilibria give rise to mutual interferences by the coupling of several kinds of reactions and may promote the reactions of interest to occur in the "wrong or in the good" direction, that is to say that which is too naively foreseen. The occurring of reactions in the wrong or the good direction is purely and simply a consequence of what the chemists name "displacement of equilibrium". We have already evoked these difficulties (see Chapter 21). Owing their importance in bioenergetics, we consider them again but under the viewpoint of the displacement of equilibria.

One can say that the "natural trick" for biochemical reactions of bioenergetics to evolve in the right direction, despite the fact that several of them do exhibit unfavorable Gibbs energies, is the occurrence of coupled reactions. Therefore, it would not be astonishing that the master word for the functioning of bioenergetics could be the word: *coupling.*

The phenomenon of the coupling of reactions occupies a pivotal place in the multiple biochemical reactions which take a part during the whole phenomena of bioenergetics.

In this chapter, by introduction, we begin by giving some examples of couplings which displace chemical equilibria.

1) Displacements of chemical equilibria by coupling reactions

   1-1) Coupling between redox and acid-base reactions

   There exist numerous examples of this kind. A well-known one is that in which the redox couple permanganate ion MnO_4^-/manganous ions Mn^{2+} evolves in media of different acidities. The half-reaction redox is:

   +VII   +II
   $$MnO_4^- + 8H^+ + 5e- \rightleftharpoons Mn^{2+} + 4H_2O \qquad (190)$$

   An exchange of five electrons with another redox pair is possible. There is a change of oxidation number of manganese from the state +VII to +II. The potential of the corresponding electrode (a platinum cable dipping in a mixture of permanganate MnO_4^- and Mn^{2+} ions) is given by the Nernst equation:

$$E(MnO_4^-/Mn^{2+}) \approx E°(MnO_4^-/Mn^{2+}) + (RT/5F) \ln \{[MnO_4^-][H+]8/[Mn^{2+}]\} \qquad (191)$$

by assimilating in a first approximation, activities to concentrations to simplify the reasoning. We see that if we want to carry out the oxidation reaction by the permanganate ion in a sufficiently basic medium (rich in hydroxide ions OH^-), a second reaction will evolve simultaneously with the preceding. It is:

$$H^+ + OH^- \rightleftharpoons H_2O \qquad (192)$$

Hence, there will be a superimposition of the equilibria (187) and (189).

The consideration of Equation (188) shows that the redox potential $E(MnO_4^-/Mn^{2+})$ *(not the standard one: $E°(MnO_4^-/Mn^{2+})$)* decreases when the acidity of the medium itself $[H^+]$ decreases. It is sufficient to consider the logarithmic term to be convinced by this assertion. There is a displacement of the position of the equilibrium of the redox reaction between the permanganate ion with the reduced form of the antagonist redox pair. In these conditions, the permanganate ion appears to be less oxidizing than awaited after consideration of its standard potential.

1-2) Interference between complexation and redox reactions

As another example, let us consider the following half redox reaction between ferric Fe^{3+} and ferrous Fe^{2+} ions:

$$Fe^{3+} + 1e- \rightleftharpoons Fe^{2+}$$

Let us add fluoride ions F^- to a solution already containing ferric and ferrous ions. Fluoride ions give a complex with ferric ions, the ion complex "ferrifluoride" $[FeF^{2+}]$. The two following reactions may evolve simultaneously:

$$Fe^{3+} + 1e- \rightleftharpoons Fe^{2+}$$

$$Fe^{3+} + F^- \rightleftharpoons [FeF^{2+}]$$

As a consequence of the complexation of ferric ions, the activity (concentration) of ferric ions decreases and Nernst's equation related to the pair Fe^{3+}/Fe^{2+} shows that the corresponding electrode potential $E (Fe^{3+}/Fe^{2+})$, not the standard one, is less high than awaited. The redox couple Fe^{3+}/Fe^{2+} is a weaker oxidant than it is awaited.

1-3) Interferences between acid-base and complexation reactions

Now, let us consider the complexation reaction, the complexed particle being the fluoride ion:

$$[FeF^{2+}] \rightleftharpoons Fe^{3+} + F^-$$

The fluoride ion F^- has a basic character in water, since it captures a proton to give hydrofluoric acid HF:

$$F^- + H^+ \rightleftharpoons HF$$

Both equilibria may evolve simultaneously, according to:

$$[FeF^{2+}] \rightleftharpoons Fe^{3+} + F^-$$

$$F^- + H^+ \rightleftharpoons HF$$

The dissociation of the complex ion "ferrifluorure" is favored by formation of hydrofluoric acid. The dissociation equilibrium is displaced towards the right. The complex appears to be less stable as awaited. Reciprocally, if we regard the acidic character of hydrofluoric acid, we see that its dissociation is favored by the complexation of fluoride ions. In these conditions, it appears to be a stronger acid as awaited.

1-4) Interferences between an acido-basic reaction and a partitioning process

Let us now consider a carboxylic acid RCOOH. It dissociates in water according to:

$$RCOOH_w \rightleftharpoons RCOO^-_w + H^+_w$$

whereas the formed ions remain only in water, the acidic form RCOOH partitions between water and an organic non miscible solvent, according to:

$$RCOOH_w \rightleftharpoons RCOOH_{solv}$$

Moreover, in the organic solvent, the acid dimerizes according to:

$$2\ RCOOH_{solv} \rightleftharpoons (RCOOH)_{2\ solv}$$

The whole processes may be schematized by the three following equilibria:

$$RCOOH_w \rightleftharpoons RCOO^-_w + H^+_w$$

$$RCOOH_w \rightleftharpoons RCOOH_{solv}$$

$$1/2\ RCOOH_{solv} + 1/2\ RCOOH_{solv} \rightleftharpoons \tfrac{1}{2}\ (RCOOH)_{2\ solv}$$

The acid is extracted from the aqueous phase by the organic solvent. The fact that it dimerizes in the latter strengthens the extraction. The consequence is that the acid appears to be less strong as awaited in water, since there are less H^+_w ions (in water). There is a displacement of the ionization equilibrium.

Of course, there is plenty of other examples of coupled reactions and of displacements of equilibria.

2) Inversion of the direction of a reaction

These examples of displacements of equilibria immediately permit to conceive that a displacement of equilibrium by a coupling may be sufficient to inverse the direction of a reaction which it was awaited to follow at first glance. Therefore, a reaction, which as a rule appears to be impossible to evolve owing to its Gibbs energies, may become possible after a judicious coupling.

An interesting example is that of:

– oxidation of iodide ions by vanadate ions VO_2^+ giving iodine and vanadyl ions VO^{2+} according to the reaction:

$$VO_2^+ + I^- + 2H^+ \rightarrow VO^{2+} + \tfrac{1}{2} I_2 + H_2O$$

The reaction evolves in this direction for pH < 2;

– oxidation of vanadyl ions by iodine to give vanadate ions and iodide ions

$$VO^{2+} + \tfrac{1}{2} I_2 + H_2O \rightarrow VO_2^+ + I^- + 2H^+$$

This reaction occurs for pH > 2. Evidently, about this pH value, a frank equilibrium occurs. The first reaction transforms the vanadate ions into vanadyl ones. It is a coupling reaction which permits the inversion of this reaction. These results are summarized in Figure 47 in which are mentioned the redox potentials of couples V(+v)/V(iv) and I_2/I^- as a function of the pH.

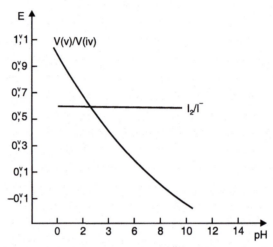

Figure 47. Redox potentials of the couples V(+v)/V(iv) and I_2/I^- as a function of the pH.

3) Coupling of reactions

The problem is all the more complicated with bioenergetics as it often involves reactions occurring in chains, whose steps themselves result from the superimposition of several equilibria. In several cases, an endergonic process may be coupled with an exergonic one with the result that the latter delivers energy to the endergonic process. In such coupled systems, the endergonic process takes place only if the decrease of free energy of the exergonic process is larger than the gain in free energy of the endergonic process. More precisely, the algebraic sum of the free energy changes in the two processes must be negative in sign, corresponding to a net decline of free energy, in order for a coupled reaction to occur.

This condition is necessary but by no means sufficient for this goal. In order to mention the second condition, let us first study the formation of sucrose from glucose plus fructose. It is a reaction which occurs in biological system. Sucrose is a disaccharide formed from 1 mole of glucose and 1 mole of fructose. It is a fairly strong endergonic reaction since $\Delta G° = 23$ kJ mol^{-1}. (Further details concerning the chemistry of sugars will be given later).

To occur, the reaction must be coupled to another reaction which must be more exergonic than that of synthesis of sucrose endergonic is. This is the first condition for the coupling to work. In the chosen example, the synthesis is achieved by coupling its reaction to the breakdown of ATP into ADP and phosphate. The sequential occurring reactions are:

$$ATP + glucose \rightarrow ADP + \textit{glucose-1-phosphate} \tag{193}$$

$$\textit{glucose-1-phosphate} + fructose \rightarrow sucrose + phosphate \tag{194}$$

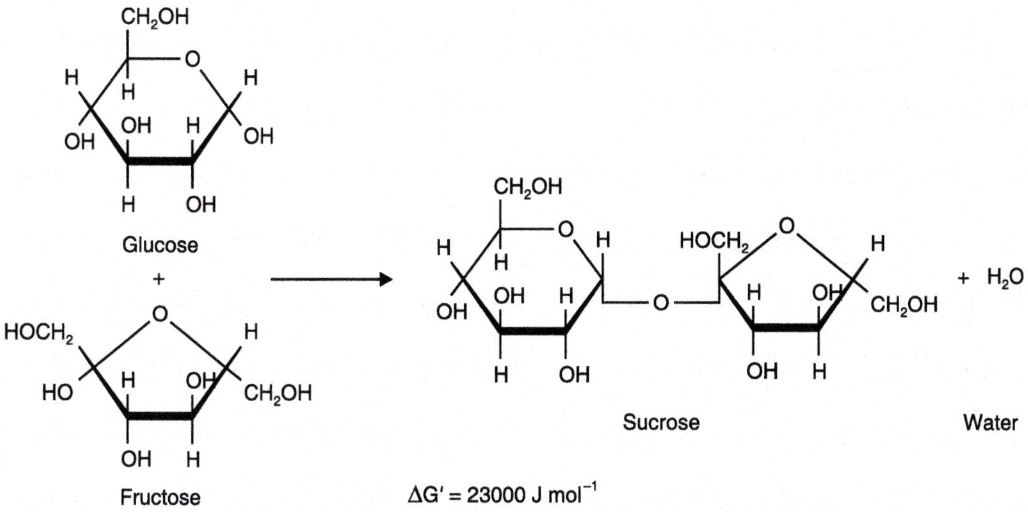

Figure 48. Synthesis of sucrose in some cells starting from glucose and fructose.

We notice that there is a common intermediate to the two coupled reactions. It is the glucose-1-phosphate. *This is the general result. For a coupling to occur, there must be a common chemical intermediate. We can remark that in the chemical examples of displacements of equilibria given above, there also existed a common intermediate.*

It is very interesting to also notice that the coupling aid does not function by a direct release of energy to the reactants of the reaction which will evolve thanks to the coupling reaction. The release of energy is done by formation of a transitory chemical derivative which has a higher energy than the starting molecule. This higher energy is conferred by the formation of a particular bond between the reactant molecule and the intermediate. From a simplified viewpoint, the preceding schema (190, 191) would be conceived as being the result of the two following reactions:

$$ATP^{4-} + H_2O \rightarrow ADP^{3-} + HPO_4^{2-} + H^+$$

$\Delta G' = -29,3$ kJ mol^{-1}

glucose + Fructose $\rightarrow$ sucrose + H_2O

$\Delta G' = +23$ kJ mol^{-1}

According to what we have said, this presentation is fallacious because it does not take into account the part played by the common intermediate.

Part III
Thermodynamics of Biological Cells

Chapter **30**

Enzymes–Kinetics of Enzymatic Reactions

Enzymes are biological catalysts. They are capable of the most complex chemistry. The part they play in every biochemical process and hence in bioenergetics is of utmost importance. It may be put forward that the two great features of biological reactions, that is to say their extremely high reaction velocities at low temperatures and their high stereospecificities, are due to them. There is no doubt that life depends on the catalytic power of enzymes. About 3000 enzymes, at least, are known and the International Union of Biochemistry puts forward the number of 25000 enzymes existing in nature. Each of them is capable of catalysing some specific chemical reaction.

Hence, the study of enzymes is of extreme importance. In this book, we focus ourselves essentially on their exceptional catalytic power.

1) The structure of enzymes

Enzymes are *protein* molecules of definite molecular structures. Their primary, secondary, tertiary and quaternary structures are essential to their catalytic activity. They have molecular weights ranging from about 12000 to more than 1000000 Da.*

Some enzymes require an additional chemical component to exert their catalytic activity. It is named a *cofactor*. Some of them may be either one or more inorganic ions or an organic substance or a complex metalloorganic molecule, called a *coenzyme*. When a metal ion or a coenzyme is tightly bound to the enzyme protein, it is called a *prosthetic group*. When the enzymes are associated with a cofactor, the latter ones are essential to their action. (The nature of the inorganic ions serving as cofactors and that of coenzymes will be given bit by bit in this book, when the part played by them will be explained).

The molecular structures of enzymes are chains of linear poly [α-amino acids] bearing side-chains. The whole primary structure is constituted of about 20 essential amino-acids (appendix 1–10). (There also exist few uncommon amino-acids). The enzymatic activity also arises from their intra-molecular bonding (secondary structure). The consequence of their occurrence is that local regions of the polymer are associated (through mainly hydrogen bonding) into helicidal or other conformations. The tertiary structure, which is a three-dimensional configuration, is ensured by a combination of many weak interactions together with some covalent linking through disulfides -S- S- bridges. They are formed from two cysteine thiol groups by oxidation:

---

* Da: Dalton, unified atomic mass unit, 1 Da = 1,660 540 10^{-27} kg.

$$
\begin{array}{ccc}
\begin{array}{c}
\text{COO}^- \\
| \\
\text{H}_3\overset{+}{\text{N}} - \text{CH} \\
| \\
\text{CH}_2 \\
| \\
\text{SH}
\end{array}
&
\rightleftharpoons
&
\begin{array}{c}
\text{COO}^- \\
| \\
\text{H}_3\overset{+}{\text{N}} - \text{CH} \\
| \\
\text{CH}_2 \\
| \\
\text{S} \\
| \\
\text{S} \\
| \\
\text{CH}_2 \\
| \\
\text{CH} - \overset{+}{\text{N}}\text{H}_3 \\
| \\
\text{COO}^-
\end{array}
\end{array}
$$

schema: cystein oxidation.

Finally, some enzyme molecules are known to associate in groups of two, four or more units. Then, one speaks of quaternary structure.

For a number of enzymes, the evidence is that the catalytic activity is due to a relatively small region of the protein molecule, region called *active site* or *active center.*

Due to their aqueous environment, the polar hydrophilic groups ($-COOH$, $-OH$, $-NH_2$, $-CONH_2$) of the molecules of enzymes are located at their outer surface, whereas their lipophilic substituents (alkyl and aryl chains) stay inside. As a consequence, the surface of an enzyme is covered by a layer of water which exhibits some particular properties. It is named "structural water". The term of "biowater" has even been used by some authors (Bockris).*

The complexity of enzyme structures can be enormous. Their structural determination poses great problems. Their peptide chain may be split into smaller fragments by careful hydrolysis and identified by chromatographic techniques and the amino-acids sequence deduced. The three-dimensional structure can only be obtained from X-ray crystallography which requires the enzyme to be isolated and obtained in pure crystalline form. In addition, many enzymes are too unstable for isolation.

2) Classification of enzymes

There exists an international classification of enzymes. It is mentioned in Table 14. We confine ourselves to give the main types of reactions in which they intervene. They are numbered from 1 (oxidoreductases) up to 6 (ligases).

Table 14. Classification of enzymes.

oxidoreductases	:	oxidation-reduction, oxygenation of C-H, C-C, C = C bonds, addition or removal of hydrogen atoms.
transferases	:	transfer of groups; aldehydic, ketonic, acyl, sugar, phosphoryl or methyl.
hydrolases	:	hydrolysis –formation of esters, amides, lactones, lactams, epoxides, nitriles, anhydrides, glycosides, organohalides.
Lyases	:	addition-elimination of small molecules on C = C, C = N, C = O bonds.
Isomerases	:	Isomerizations such as racemization, epimerisation, rearrangements.
Ligases	:	Formation-cleavage of C-O, C-S, C-N, C-C bonds with concomitant triphosphate cleavage.

---

* J.O'M. Bockris and A.K.N. Reddy, "Modern Electrochemistry" 2nd edition, T.1., general bibliography.

Remark: In this book, a group of enzymes, the generic name of which is kinases, is often mentioned. Kinases are a subclass of transferases. They catalyse the transfer of the terminal phosphoryl group of ATP into a nucleophilic acceptor.

As a comment, let us notice that some reactions mentioned in this table are not easy to carry out in the synthetic laboratory.

3) Some properties of enzymes

- Enzymes are biocatalysors. As all the catalysts, they increase reaction rates but they do not change the location of the equilibrium of the reaction they mediate.

- Enzymes are very powerful catalysts. The rates of the reactions mediated by enzymes are accelerated by a factor of $10^8 - 10^{10}$ (and even 10^{12}) compared to the same reactions carried out non-enzymatically. Their power of catalysis is very highly explained by two kinds of theories:
    - the first one is of mechanistic order (it is mentioned in the paragraph 5),
    - the second takes into account pure chemical aspects which are a consequence of the configuration and conformation of the transition state of the enzymatic reaction.

- The specific substance acted upon by an enzyme is named *substrate*. Catalysis by enzymes is much more specific than that carried out by other kinds of catalysts. Some enzymes even show absolute specificity.

    Recall that if any reaction leads predominantly or exclusively to only a set of stereoiomers, it is named stereoselective. In a stereospecific reaction, a given isomer leads to one product, while another stereoisomer leads to the opposite product. While all stereospecific reactions are stereoselective, the converse is not true.

    - Enzymes, in principle, react with only a single type of functional group. Hence, they show *chemoselectivity*;
    - They also exhibit *regioselectivity* and *diastereoselectivity*. This is due to their three-dimensional structure (see under). *When a reaction can potentially give rise to two or more structural isomers but actually produces only one, the reaction is said to be regioselective. Any reaction in which only one of a set of stereoisomers is formed, exclusively or predominantly, it is named stereoselective.*
    - Almost all enzymes are chiral. They are chiral catalysts. This is because they are constituted by L-amino acids (see appendix I-4). The consequence is that any kind of chirality present in the substrate molecule is recognized when the intermediary "complex" enzyme-substrate is formed. Hence, as example, a prochiral substrate may be transformed into an optically active product and both enantiomers of a racemic may react at different rates offering the possibility of kinetic resolution. This property is one of the most remarkable features of enzymes. Most of the time, enzymes are *enantioselective*.

Notice that a solution containing an enzyme constitutes a chiral medium in itself. Thus, their property of enantioselectivity is, in no case, an exception to the "iron rule" saying that "enantiomers have identical properties in a symmetrical environment, but have differing properties in an unsymmetrical environment" (see appendixes I-4 and I-5). Hence, the solution containing an enzyme constitutes an unsymmetrical environment.

In quasi-all cases, the stereoselectivity of enzymes originates from the energy differences between the enzyme transition state complexes. For example, let us consider the two enantiomeric substrates A and B. Because of the chiral environment of the active site of the enzyme, diastereomeric enzyme-substrate complexes E_A and E_B are temporarily formed. They possess different activation Gibbs energies, hence different individual reaction rates

v_A and v_B. As a result, there is a kinetic resolution. The process is referred to as "chiral recognition".

- Enzymes are delicate structures. They can be deactivated easily. Thus, they are said to be denaturated. The denaturation can be caused:
  - by an increase of temperature. It is not necessary that the temperature should be too great so that it would be the case. A temperature of about 40°C may be sufficient. At greater temperatures, the hydrolysis of the peptides bonds is possible. It is interesting to notice that enzymes work the best at about 30°C;
  - an extreme pH value. Typically, enzymes act in the pH range 5–8;
  - by the presence of a high ionic strength medium;
  - by the occurrence of parasitic chemical reactions, such as, for example, the crossed reactions between free thiol groups and disulfides or those of elimination and oxidation, for example reactions acid-bases also.
- Enzymes can catalyze a lot of chemical reactions. Table 14 is a mark of this assertion.
- An enzyme action can be inhibited.

  Many reagents can slow down reactions that are catalyzed by enzymes. They are called inhibitors. This point is considered in the paragraph 7.

- Regulatory enzymes.

  A kind of enzymes that merits further comments for our purpose. They are *regulatory enzymes*.

- The chemical mechanisms of enzymatic reactions are often complicated.

  In particular, enzymes may exhibit a *vectorial* action. This is a particular and interesting notion. Such an action is described in the appendix I-7.

4) A diversion on the origin of the L configuration of the amino-acids

Let us first recall that chains of L amino-acids constitute the primary structure of proteins and, hence, of enzymes.

Concerning the chirality of enzymes there is still a thought provoking issue: In fact the configuration of natural amino-acids are systematically of L configuration. It is well established, indeed, that the physical and chemical properties of two enantiomers are identical except in a chiral medium. One example of chiral medium is that of a medium submitted to the polarized light. In this condition, one knows that both enantiomers exhibit a different property, that is to say in the occurrence, a rotatory power of their plane of polarized light. Another case in which they can be distinguished is when one allows them to chemically react with a third substance, already optically active. Let A(+) and A(–) be the racemate, which is the mixture in equal quantities of the A enantiomers. They show identical properties in an a chiral environment. If the mixture is put in the presence of B(+), a third optically active product, the medium becomes chiral. Both products A(+)B(+) and A(–)B(+) are formed:

$$A(+) + B(+) \rightarrow A(+)B(+)$$

$$A(–) + B(+) \rightarrow A(–)B(+)$$

They have different chemical properties. They are diastereoisomers. (This experiment constitutes the principle of a well-known means to resolve a racemate).

As a consequence of these considerations, it is taken for granted that, in order to distinguish two enantiomers, the medium (in which the attempt is made) must be chiral. Hence, chiral, once understood that pure nonracemic and enantiomeric compounds found in nature arise mainly from chemical reactions catalyzed by enantioselective catalysts (i.e., enzymes). But, the original source of the latter compounds remains *finally mysterious*.

This question may be fascinating because it stems from that of life (at least on earth) which appears to be related to the presence of enantiomerically pure substances at the origin. This question may even be a metaphysical problem. Some theories have been advanced. Let us only mention that, according to one, absolute asymmetric synthesis would occur at the origin under the influence of a circularly polarized light.

The problem does not set up only in the case of amino-acids. For example, it sets up with hexoses which are, in majority, of the series D.

5) Catalysis

A catalyst, here the enzyme, takes part in the reaction but it emerges unscathed.

– The origin of the catalytic power is attributed to the stabilization of the transition state of the reaction by the enzyme. The hypothesis is that the catalyst *binds* more strongly to the transition state than to the ground state of the substrate by a factor approximately equal to the rate acceleration. The deep origin of the powerful activity of catalysis of enzymes is thus this binding energy.

Let us suppose that the uncatalysed reaction is:

$A \rightleftharpoons B$

The catalysed one may be written as:

$A + E \rightleftharpoons EA \rightleftharpoons EB \rightleftharpoons B + E$

where E is the enzyme and EA and EB are the intermediate complexes between the substrate and the enzyme and between the enzyme and the product. Figure 49 summarizes these considerations.

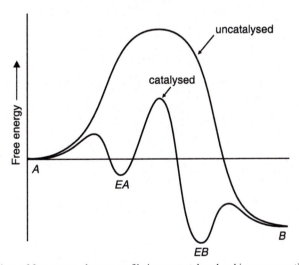

Figure 49. Comparison of free energy changes profile in an uncatalysed and in an enzymatic catalysed reaction.

We can notice that the intermediate complexes EA and EB are more stable than the reactant, EB being more stable than EA. This is the reason why the reaction is governed towards the right. We can also notice that the free energy of activation is weaker in the catalysed case. Finally, one can admit that the enzyme provides an easier way up to the product.

– Concerning now the mechanistic explanation of this catalytic power, three theories are put forward:

* the first one is that named the "Lock-and-Key" mechanism (E. Fisher). According to it, the enzyme and its substrate are in interaction like a lock and a key, both together constituting a rigid structure (Figure 50).

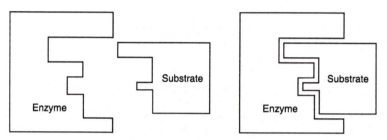

Figure 50. The "lock-and-key" model.

The principal drawback of this model is that it cannot explain why many enzymes can convert non-natural substrates, exhibiting different structures from that of their natural substrate, owing to its rigidity.

* The "induced-fit" mechanism supposes that upon approach of the substrate, that is to say during the formation of the enzyme-substrate complex, the enzyme can change its conformation, of course, under the influence of the structure of the substrate. In a way, the enzyme wraps the substrate. The induced deformation explains the large number of substances of quite different structures amenable to transformation under the action of the same enzyme.

* The "desolvatation theory" is based on the hypothesis that the kinetics of enzymatic reactions looks, in a certain manner, like gas-phase reactions. When the substrate enters into the active site of the enzyme, it replaces all its water molecules initially solvating it.

There are still discussions upon this theory.

6) Kinetics of the catalysis by enzymes—The Michaelis-Menten equation

The study of the influence of substrate concentrations (when there is a single substrate) leads to the equation of Michaelis-Menten.

The dependence of the rates on substrate concentrations [S] frequently obeys the curve drawn in Figure 51.

The mechanism suggested by Michaelis and Menten comes from the hypothesis of the occurrence of the two following reactional steps:

$$E + S \underset{k_{-1}}{\overset{k_1}{\rightleftharpoons}} ES$$

$$ES \overset{k_2}{\rightarrow} E + P$$

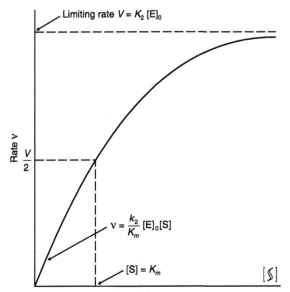

Figure 51. Variation of rates with substrate concentrations for an enzyme-catalyzed reaction obeying the Michaelis-Menten equation.

E and S are the enzyme and the substrate, P is the product and ES is the intermediate complex. The steady-state treatment gives the following equation (see appendix I-3):

$$k_1[E][S] - k_{-1}[ES] - k_2[ES] = 0$$

Usually, the molar concentration of substrate is much greater than that of the enzyme. The total concentration of the enzyme $[E]_0$ is:

$$[E]_0 = [E] + [ES]$$

With the aid of this relation, the steady state equation becomes:

$$k_1([E]_0 - [ES])[S] - (k_{-1} + k_2)[ES] = 0$$

Therefore,

$$[ES] = k_1[E]_0[S]/\{k_{-1} + k_2 + k_1[S]\}$$

With the starting hypothesis, the rate of reaction is:

$$v = k_2[ES]$$

$$v = k_1 k_2[E]_0[S]/\{k_{-1} + k_2 + k_1[S]\}$$

$$v = k_2[E]_0[S]/\{(k_{-1} + k_2)/k_1 + [S]\}$$

$$v = k_2[E]_0[S]/\{K_M + [S]\} \tag{195}$$

This relation is referred to as being the Michaelis-Menten equation. The constant $K_M = (k_{-1} + k_2)/k_1$ is named Michaelis constant.

At this point, two hypothesis can be done:

– when [S] is sufficiently small, it may be neglected in the denominator and:

$v = (k_2/K_M)[E]_0[S]$

Kinetics becomes first order in substrate concentration;

when $[S] \gg K_M$,

$v = k_2[E]_0$ (196)

Kinetics becomes zero order in it. Let us set up:

$V = k_2[E]_0$

V is the limiting rate at high substrate concentrations. Then (192) becomes:

$v = V[S]/\{K_M + [S]\}$ (197)

When $[S] = K_M$,

$v = V/2$

This relation is the basis of the determination of the Michaelis constant. By plotting v as a function of [S], it is sufficient to find the concentration of substrate giving one half of the maximal rate.

Relation (194) can be transformed into another one which is linear:

$1/v = K_M/V[S] + 1/V$

The plot of $1/v$ as a function of $1/[S]$ gives a straight line permitting to obtain the parameters V, K_M and k_2 (the latter if the concentration $[E]_0$ is known) from the slope and the x-intercept. This straight line is called the *Lineweaver-Burk plot*. Plotting the Lineweaver-Burk lines is useful to detect the phenomenon of inhibition.

Another linear variant of the Michaelis-Menten equation is:

$v K_M + v[S] = V[S]$

Many enzyme–catalyzed reactions obey the Michaelis-Menten equation. However, it is important to notice that a nice fit of the experimental data to the Michaelis-Menten equation does not absolutely imply that the Michaelis-Menten is the true one in the occurrence, since other mechanisms may give the same kinetic law.

It is important to notice that the pH of the solution in which the enzymatic reaction occurs may have a great effect on its rate. Firstly, the rates of enzymatic reactions pass through a maximum at a given pH named optimum pH. Secondly, effects of pH are irreversible when the pH value becomes by far too low or too high with respect to the optimum pH. The great changes in the rates are probably due to the acid-base reactions affecting the free carboxylic and amino rests remaining at the surfaces of the protein. The statistical values of the pk_a of aliphatic carboxylic acids ($\approx 3, 0$) and of protonated aliphatic amines (≈ 10) are in agreement with this hypothesis.

Concerning now the influence of the temperature on the enzymatic reactions, it must be known that it is difficult to establish it firmly because at temperatures about 35°C enzymes may undergo some deactivation. As a result, there is an optimum temperature at which the rate is at its maximum. Its value depends on the conditions of the reaction.

Finally, it is interesting to note that many enzymatic reactions may also be under the dependence of cooperative binding processes. This point is now briefly mentioned from the standpoint of kinetics. In such cases, initial rates of the enzymatic reactions are usually measured. Plots of initial velocities versus the concentrations of the substrates may deceal cooperativity. In many cases, these plots are identical in form with those of the binding isotherms. This fact may be the proof that the binding steps, which are before the rate determining steps, are fast, reversible and that the catalytic power of all the binding sites is identical.

7) Reversible and irreversible inhibitors of enzymes

One distinguishes reversible and irreversible inhibitions of enzymes.

- Reversible inhibition implies that the enzyme activity can be recovered, once the action of the inhibitor is finished. There exist several kinds of reversible inhibition.
  - *The competitive inhibition.* It is due to the fact that a substance, the competitive inhibitor, competes with the substrate for the active site of the enzyme. It is not a surprising fact that the structure of the competitive inhibitor is similar to that of the substrate. The inhibitor combines with the enzyme to form the intermediate complex but there is no catalysis;
  - *The uncompetitive inhibition.* It can be only observed with enzymes having two or more substrates. The uncompetitive inhibitor binds at a site distinct from the substrate active site;
  - *The mixed inhibition.* The "mixed inhibitor" also binds at a site distinct from the substrate active site but it binds to either E or ES.
- Irreversible inhibition corresponds to the covalent binding of an irreversible inhibitor with a functional group located on the enzyme that is essential for its activity. The action of the inhibitor may also be due to the destruction of the functional group it induces.

The inhibitions can be detected by a careful study of the kinetics of the studied reactions.

8) Regulatory enzymes—Allosterism of enzymes

In the study of bioenergetics, one frequently encounters the case in which groups of enzymes work together in sequential reactions in order that a metabolic process can be carried out. In such sequences, the reaction product of one enzyme becomes the substrate of the next. It is an experimental fact that each sequential reaction involves one or more enzymes that have a great effect on the rate of the whole sequence. These enzymes can increase or decrease the catalytic activity in response to certain signals. Hence, they permit the cell to change its immediate needs in energy, for example. Their behavior may be considered as that of an adjusting variable. Such enzymes are named *regulatory enzymes*.

The activities of regulatory enzymes can be modified by a variety of manners. Some regulatory enzymes may be allosteric, that is to say, as some proteins, they may exhibit changes in their conformations under the induction of compounds named *modulators* or *effectors*.

9) Coenzymes

Certain enzymes react with their substrates only when they are combined with another substance called a coenzyme. A coenzyme is not usually a protein. It is a much simpler organic molecule than an enzyme and the enzyme-coenzyme complex is formed reversibly. A given coenzyme may function with more than one enzyme to operate on different substrates.

An important example of cofactor we shall encounter later is that of the couple $NAD^+/NADH$.

Chapter **31**

The Flow of Energy
in the Biological World

This chapter is an overview of what we are developing in the following ones. It begins by a recalling of the origin of biological energy, that is to say, the radiant energy coming from the sunlight. The content of the chapter is an introduction of the photosynthesis, of the respiration and of the fermentation. Then, it introduces the biological work. The flow of matter in the biological world is also briefly investigated.

The chapter essentially regards phenomena occurring in a single cell.

1) The flow of energy in the biological world

At first glance, it seems that the sources of energy of the human organism come from the components of its diet. This sentence is too short. Further considerations point out the fact that our major foodstuffs derive directly both from the plant world and, also, from the animal world. Moreover, after studies on the foods of animals, it clearly appears that, in turn, the latter ones derive from the plant world.

This is not the whole story. Two questions remain to be answered. The first one is to know from what does the plant world extract its energy? The answer is from the radiant energy in the form of sunlight. Solar energy is hence the ultimate source of all the biological energy. The second question can no more be avoided. Certainly, it is not lacking of interest! What is the origin of this energy? The answer is the thermonuclear reactions arising in the interior of the sun.

Finally, solar energy is dispersed according to different manners. One of them is due to the phenomena occurring in the biological world. Therefore, it is interesting to notice that even if one only considers the latter one, the entropy of the isolated system constituted by the sun and the earth (and more probably by the whole Universe) have obligatorily increased (second principle), provided they are constituting an isolated system. Figure 52 summarizes the different steps of the energy flow in "our world".

Of course, the plant world not only requires energy to be constituted but, also, it requires matter. They are inorganic nutrients.

2) Sunlight, the ultimate origin of the biological energy

Where does solar energy come from? The energy of sunlight comes from nuclear energy. At the huge temperature of the interior of the sun (about 6000 K), a part of the enormous energy confined in the nucleus of hydrogen atoms (of the sun) is released by their conversion into several

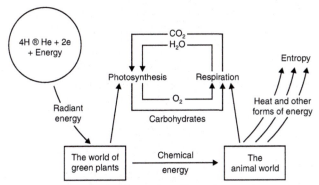

Figure 52. Different steps of the biological energy flow from the sunlight to the remaining of the Universe and the corresponding displacements of matter.

particles: helium atoms, positive electrons (positions e^+) and neutrinos v_e. (A neutrino, also called "the small neutral molecule", is an elementary particle of null mass and of null energy at rest. Its spin is ½). The global reaction of formation of helium is a reaction of *nuclear fusion*. (Do not confuse fusion and fission. Nuclear fusion reaction is at the base of the H-bomb whereas a nuclear fission reaction is at the origin of the A-bomb). The reaction of fusion in question can be written as:

$$4^1H \rightarrow 4He + 2e^+ + 2v_e \quad Q = 26{,}72 \text{ MeV}$$

In the equation above, Q is the energetic effect accompanying it. (MeV—a mega electronvolt—is an energy unit. 1 MeV $= 1{,}6 \ 10^{-13}$ J; 1 eV $= 1{,}6 \ 10^{-19}$ J). By substracting the energetic effect carried away by the two neutrinos ($2v_e$ term) ($2 \times 0{,}25$ MeV), this leaves the value 26,22 MeV for the reaction above and for the radiation which follows. This value is strictly equivalent to 4,20 pJ (p; pico; 10^{-12}) per helium atom and *not per the Avogadro number of atoms*, that is to say $2{,}53 \ 10^{12}$ J mol^{-1}. This is a huge value! It is released from deep in the sun's interior as high-energy γ-rays of energies $E = hv$, where h is Planck's constant and v the frequency of the gamma radiation. (γ-rays are photons of the electromagnetic spectrum. They have no mass and no charge and travel at the speed of light. They are very energetic. They are emitted by the excited nuclei of atoms. As for a photon, they are "grains" of light of energy $E = hv$). γ-rays interact with stellar material and are gradually transformed into photons of longer wavelengths and become less energetic. After a complex series of reactions in which the γ-rays are absorbed by the electrons, the major part of gamma radiations are emitted again in the form of photons of weaker energies than before.

In passing, it is interesting to devote some comments to the above reaction. Firstly, its release of energy is very important. It arises mainly from the difference between the rest mass of the helium nucleus and the 4 protons from which it is formed according to Einstein's law of mass–energy equivalence. Despite the huge energy released by the reaction, only 0,7% of the mass is lost during the transformation, so that the star remains approximately constant in mass. For example, in the sun, during each second, some 600 10^6 tonnes of hydrogen are processed into 595,5 10^6 tonnes of helium. The remaining 4,5 10^6 tonnes are transformed into energy. From this viewpoint, we can hope to have an appreciable survival time before us. If the nuclear reactions of fusion would be domesticated, the energetic future of the humanity would be probably definitively assured.

3) Photosynthesis

Photosynthesis begins with the absorption of the radiant energy by chlorophyll. Chlorophyll is a pigment of green plant cells. It achieves the conversion of the absorbed light energy into chemical energy and the use of the latter for the reduction of carbon dioxide of the atmosphere to form glucose. The reaction involves the reduction of carbon dioxide by water with formation of molecular oxygen together with glucose. The overall reaction is:

$$6CO_2 + 6H_2O \rightarrow C_6H_{12}O_6 + 6O_2 \tag{198}$$

The standard thermodynamic parameters of the reaction are at 273 K:

$\Delta G° = 2867\ 480$ J mol^{-1}

$\Delta H° = 2813\ 140$ J mol^{-1}

$\Delta S° = -182,3$ J K^{-1} mol^{-1}

Clearly, the reaction does not evolve spontaneously from the left to the right as it is shown by the Gibbs energy change accompanying the reaction which is markedly positive. Besides, we notice that the change in entropy of the system is negative and is not counterbalanced by the enthalpy change which always remains possible by virtue of the fundamental equation $\Delta G = \Delta H - T\Delta S$. Reaction (195) is endergonic. It is an "uphill" process.

More on photosynthesis will be given in Chapter 36.

It is sufficient, now, to know that there is formation of glucose from carbon dioxide with the aid of light. The glucose which is formed in photosynthesis may be subsequently converted in other carbon containing components of the plant cell which are cellulose, lipids, proteins. The types of cells which are capable of making all these complex molecular components from very simple small molecules such as CO_2 and NH_3 are called *autotrophic* cells.

A large amount of energy input is necessary to the system in order for the "uphill" reaction to take place. It is supplied by the light energy which is captured by the chlorophyll. Hence, a better representation of the reaction (195) would be:

$$6CO_2 + 6H_2O + nh\nu \rightarrow C_6H_{12}O_6 + 6O_2$$

where nhv represents the light energy under the form of quanta which is necessary to promote the reaction. The gain by the system of the light energy to promote reaction (195) obeys the same principle as the assistance of a second reaction coupled with the first one brought to an "uphill" reaction (see Chapters 21 and 29).

As it will be seen later (see Chapter 36), the photosynthetic process is very complex. However, Equation (195) is an accurate balance-sheet of the phenomenon. It is important to notice that there exist many kinds of organisms in the plant world, but not all plant cells, which can participate in photosynthesis. Only those containing chlorophyll can do it.

4) The great stages (metabolic pathways) of the flow of biological energy

We are interested here in the formation and the origin of the necessary Gibbs energy in order to achieve the metabolisms of multienzyme systems. These metabolisms are the sum of the chemical transformations taking place in a cell or organism through a series of enzyme-catalyzed reactions constituting the metabolic pathways.

We shall successively study:

–   the glycolysis and fermentation,
–   the citric acid cycle or Krebs' cycle,
–   the oxidative phosphorylation,
–   the pathway of pentoses.

5) Respiration

The name "respiration" is also found in literature. One of its possible definitions is "the oxidative breakdown and release of energy from fuel molecules by reaction with dioxygen in aerobic cells".

Actually, after the photosynthesis, the next great stage in the flow of biological energy is this process.

Somewhat surprisingly, at first glance, is the fact that the newly formed glucose may be oxidized to CO_2 and H_2O according to the reverse reaction of the preceding one. The difference between both is that the oxidization reaction has no need to be coupled to another process in order to spontaneously evolve as it is indicated by its markedly negative Gibbs energy change. This is an *exergonic* or "*downhill*" reaction. It is a regulatory process of the production of carbonic anhydride.

$$\text{glucose} + 6 \; O_2 \rightarrow 6 \; CO_2 + 6 \; H_2O$$

Of course, its parameters are:

$\Delta G^\circ = -2867\,480 \; J \; mol^{-1}$

$\Delta H^\circ = -2813\,140 \; J \; mol^{-1}$

$\Delta S^\circ = + 182,3 \; J \; K^{-1} \; mol^{-1}$

Actually, the respiration process is the combustion of carbohydrates, fats, and proteins. It is carried out by cells of the animal world. To work, the process requires the existence of energy-rich products of photosynthesis, named *fuel*, because some cells are unable to use simple molecules such as CO_2 as either fuel or as building blocks for synthesis of cell macromolecular components. Such cells are called *heterotrophic cells*. Heterotrophic cells include not only almost all the cells of the animal but also some of the plant world, those of most of bacteria and fungi. Heterotrophic cells thus require the complex organic molecules such as glucose, lipids, and amino acids fabricated during the photosynthesis. Thus, heterotrophic and autotrophic cells' lives depend on each other.

As an example, we already know that glucose is oxidized by most heterotrophic cells at the expense of dioxygen coming from the atmosphere giving carbonic anhydride and water. Its energy is conserved in a chemical form as is most of the energy gained through respiration. Despite the fact that the equation of respiration looks simple, it is not actually the case. It is carried out through numerous, sequential enzymatic steps, as it will be seen (see Chapters 34–36).

The oxidation of complex organic fuel molecules is the most important process yielding *chemical energy* in heterophic cells. These cells using dioxygen are called aerobic cells and the process is aerobic.

There also exist *anaerobic cells* and *anaerobic organisms* (see Chapter 34).

6) Biological work

We shall also be interested in the works that can be done by living organisms thanks to the occurrence of the flow of biological energy. It concerns the utilization of the chemical energy released during the combustion of foodstuffs.

A first point to stress is that all living organisms do some kinds of work to stay alive in an environment which, at first sight, is essentially hostile. In response to this fact, some organisms make work on their environment whereas others overcome the effect of their environment by multiplying themselves very rapidly.

One can consider that there are three kinds of work carried out by them: the *chemical work*, the *work of transport and concentration* and the *mechanical work*.

– The chemical work is done by all cells during their growth and after it, in order to keep themselves alive. The major chemical components of cells such as proteins, nucleic acids, lipids, and polysaccharides are continuously synthesized from small building-blocks molecules by the action of enzymes. This process is called *biosynthesis*. It requires input of energy. To maintain the cells alive, their carbohydrates, proteins and lipids are contantly synthetized and degraded according to a dynamic steady state (see Chapter 24). Then, the rate of formation of new molecules is exactly balanced by that of degradation of the old.

– The work of transport and concentration is that required to transport and concentrate substances. All cells are capable of accumulating certain essential substances from the environment. For example, it is the case of K^+ ions or of the necessary fuel molecules such as glucose. The result is that the intracellular concentration of the substance may be much higher than in the medium outside the cell. Conversely, unwanted and deleterious substances may be pumped out of the cell, even if their external concentrations are much higher than the internal. Such movements of molecules against gradients of concentrations cannot occur spontaneously (for the definition of a gradient see appendix II-3). It is sufficient to consider the corresponding Gibbs energies of transport to be convinced by this fact. Considering the same viewpoint, let us notice that such displacements would be accompanied by a decrease in the entropy of the system as a result. One can admit, indeed, that the system cell plus surroundings is an isolated one.

The energy-dependent movement of solute molecules against a concentration gradient is called *active-transport* or *active translocation*. The work of transport and concentration is sometimes rather badly named *osmotic work*.

– It is a well-known fact that *mechanic work* is done by most kinds of cells. Perhaps, the most famous example is the contraction of skeletal muscles in higher animals. Moreover, actually, nearly all cells exert intra-cellular pulling forces by means of contractile filaments. The mechanical work done by cells is directly empowered by chemical one.

– Energy: From the thermodynamic standpoint, the flow of energy in the biological world leads to the dissipation of energy into the system and into the surroundings. Finally, it leads to the

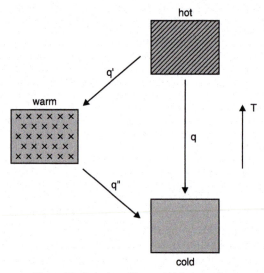

Figure 53. Energies of low and high entropies.

increase of the entropy of the Universe. During the flow of energy in the biological world, there is a constant degradation of energy. The high-grade energy of the sun (energy of low entropy: energy at high temperature) becomes, in the first stage, the medium-grade energy of organic molecules of the intermediary steps of the flow and, afterwards, is dissipated as the low-grade energy, that is to say heat dissipated with an increase of the entropy.

According to these processes and the second law, it is evident that the flow of biological energy is irreversible. Moreover, there is a supplementary reason for the occurrence of irreversibility. There exist unavoidable losses of energy by friction at each of the many sequential steps of the energy conversion.

7) The flow of matter in the biological world

Evidently, while there is a flow of energy between the plant and animal worlds, there is also a flow of matter. We have seen that, during respiration, animal cells take dioxygen from the atmosphere whose action on glucose gives carbon dioxide and water which go back into the atmosphere. Conversely, the green plants extract carbon dioxide from the atmosphere to give glucose and dioxygen back. Hence, there exist cycles of dioxygen, carbon dioxide and water between the animal and plant worlds.

8) Transformation of energy in heterotrophic anaerobic cells—Fermentation

We are continuing to quickly investigate energy processes which permits the function and the survival of living cells to occur. Recall that, as we have just seen yet, these vital processes have the "so-called" osmotic, mechanical and chemical works as the final steps. We already know that the most important process of oxidation of the fuel such as glucose is carried out at the expense of molecular dioxygen. What is of interest for us now is the oxidation of complex organic molecules and the recovering of the corresponding liberated energy as chemical energy through another way than the aerobic one, i.e., the recovering by what is called "fermentation".

There also exist heterotrophic cells, especially some bacteria and other simple organisms which do not use dioxygen. They are called *anaerobic organisms* or *anaerobes*. They obtain their energy from the oxidation of complex foodstuff molecules but instead of using dioxygen, they employ other kinds of molecules as oxidizing agents.

Recall (see Chapter 27) that dioxygen may not be necessarily the reactant in order to carry out an oxidation reaction. The part played by dioxygen in an oxidation reaction is nothing other than a particular case of a general group of chemical reactions, precisely those named "oxidation reactions". Oxidizing agents are substances which are electron acceptors whereas reducing agents are electron donors (Cf Chapter 27).

Anaerobic cells exhibit a remarkable series of processes permitting the oxidation of their fuel without using dioxygen. The whole process is called *fermentation*. It consists in the breakdown of the glucose molecule (possessing six carbon-atoms) into two three-carbon fragments. One of the three-carbon fragments plays the part of a reductor. It reduces the other three-carbon fragment which accepts the electrons coming from the former. Hence, the second fragment plays the part of the oxidant. (Fermentation will be studied in Chapter 34 devoted to glycolysis.)

9) The fate of the energy coming from the fuel: A first view on the part played by ATP

In both aerobic and anaerobic cells, the energy coming from the oxidation of the foodstuff molecules is not conserved as heat but as *chemical energy*. Actually, it is essentially conserved in the compound named adenosine triphosphate (ATP). A brief overview of the part played by ATP is given now. It is further developed in Chapter 33.

It is formed from adenosine diphosphate (ADP) and one molecule of phosphate (P) according to the highly endergonic reaction (their formula are given in the next chapter):

$$ADP + P \rightarrow ATP$$

The fact that ATP is formed is due to its coupling with exergonic reactions of oxidation of foodstuffs.

The many chemical reactions intervening in the formation of ATP are catalyzed by several enzyme systems. It can be said that the energy coming from the oxidation of foodstuffs is saved thanks to the ATP/ADP system.. It is recovered after the "saving step" when it is at work during the chemical, mechanical and osmotic works carried out by the cell. Many more comments concerning these processes are given in the next chapters.

10) The machinery of cells

R. Hooke was the first to discover the structure called a cell. This is a central fact of biology. A cell is the basic unit of structure and function in living organisms. All cells are endowed with extremely complex, efficient features and are near-miraculous devices in the realm of our interest.

Cells exhibit some similarities with manufactories. They possess varied subcellular compartments called *organelle*s. They can be seen in electron microscopes. They have some specific part to play as in the case of manufactories which usually are divided into several divisions, each of them being devoted to a specific burden. However, there exists a great difference between them. The different divisions of a manufactory obey a master plan of consistency; it is also the case for cells as is indicated by their mervellous working. Their great difference lies in the following question: what governs the functioning of a cell?

Here, we confine ourselves to mentioning some compartments of a cell which are endowed with a particularly great part to play in bioenergetics. Let us mention:

– mitochondria. They are often described as floating power stations. They are small membrane-surrounded structures located in the cytoplasm of aerobic cells. They have two membranes. The outer membrane is permeable to small molecules. The inner one bears the components of the respiratory chain. It encloses the mitochondrial matrix. It is pickered inward in a series of folds called cristae. They extend the whole body of the mitochondrion. It contains the enzymes of several pathways. They are the sites of the enzyme systems which participate in the oxidation of foodstuffs by dioxygen and to the recovery of energy as ATP. The Figure 54 schematically represents a mitochondria.

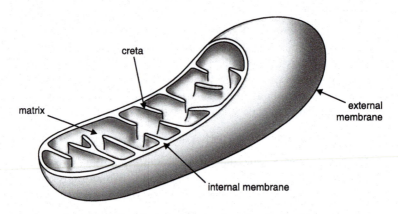

Figure 54. Schematic representation of a mitochondria.

- the plasma, membrane where the osmotic work is carried out;

- the ribosomes, "the protein factories" which are the sites of most protein synthesis. They are frequently located on the surface of the endoplasmic reticulum which itself contains important enzymes required in biosynthesis of lipids—the cell nucleus which is the site of replication of deoxyribonucleic acid (DNA). The transcription of genetic information is also carried out in the nucleus since the messenger ribonucleic acid (mRNA) is synthetized in it at the expense of ATP energy;

- the membranes in which the cells themselves are held inside. They consist of a layer of phospholipids;

- the chloroplasts are the organites of the photosynthesis (Figure 55). As mitochondria, chloroplasts possess an external and internal membrane with an intermembranar space. The internal membrane surrounds the stroma containing soluble enzymes and other membranar structures called thylacoids. The latter ones contain a machinery which is able to perform the transduction of the energy (see Chapter 36).

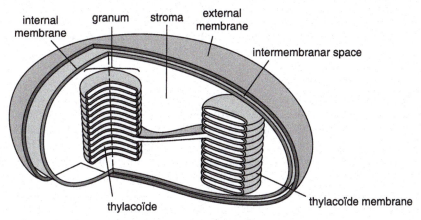

Figure 55. Structure of a chloroplast.

Chapter **32**

Adenosine Triphosphate, Adenosine Diphosphate, Monophosphate and Derivatives–NAD⁺

Some Physico-Chemical Properties

This chapter is devoted to some physico-chemical properties of the molecule named adenosine triphosphate (ATP) and to some of its derivatives-adenosine diphosphate (ADP) and adenosine monophosphate (AMP). It also talks about some properties of the coenzyme NAD⁺ and some properties of phosphate and pyrophosphate ions of interest for us. The part played by ATP in bioenergetics is very important. It is the basis of one of the most useful concepts in the domain of biochemical changes occurring in the intermediary metabolism—the concept of the "high-energy bond". Of course, before tackling these bioenergetic aspects, some physico-chemical properties of ATP and those of some of its derivatives must be recalled. It will be the same for NAD⁺, NADH and some of their derivatives.

ATP occurs in all types of cells, animals, plants and microbial ones.

1) Chemical structures of adenosine triphosphoric acid and derivatives

    1-1) Mononucleotides

        Let us begin by mentioning that adenosine triphosphoric acid and derivatives (ATP, ADP and AMP—see just below for the adopted nomenclature here) are examples of *mononucleotides*. The structures of mononucleotides contain a *single* purine or pyrimidine base, a single five-carbon sugar such as D-ribose (D-ribofuranose) fixed to the previous one and a triphosphoryl (or a di-or-monophosphoryl) rest fixed to the sugar (Figure 56).

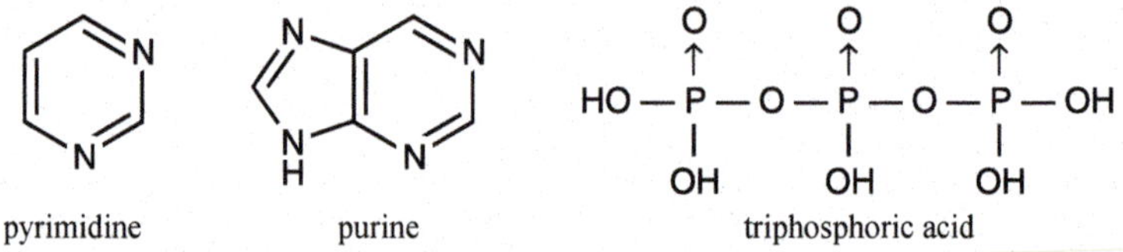

pyrimidine   purine   triphosphoric acid

Figure 56. Some building-blocks of mononucleotides.

(From the pure chemical standpoint, purine and pyrimidine are aromatic nuclei. They are, indeed, planar and possess 10 and 6 electrons π, respectively. They obey Hückel's rule).

1-2) Adenosine triphosphoric acid

There is no doubt about the chemical structure of adenosine triphosphoric acid. Among other arguments which establish it, let us cite its direct synthesis. However, using the symbol ATP to designate it is somewhat ambiguous because of its multiple possible ionizations (see paragraph 2). It is preferable to symbolize the acid (strictly speaking) by $ATPH_4$ owing to the fact that under this form, it is not at all ionized in water—see later).

$ATPH_4$ is comprised of several kinds of building blocks. A first block has the structure of adenine which is a derivative of the aromatic nucleus named purine. Adenine is the 6-amino purine (Figure 58).

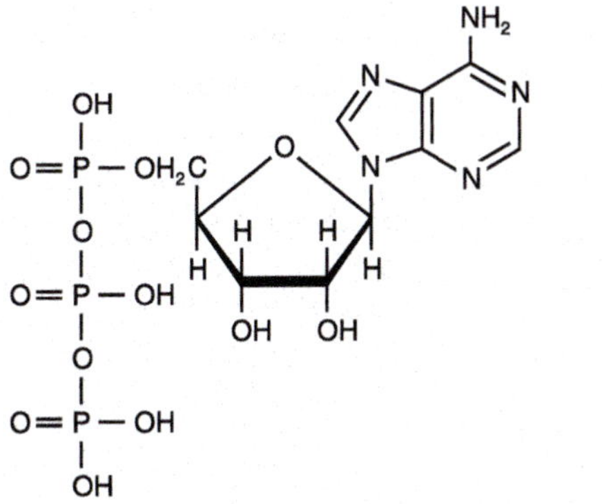

Figure 57. Structure of adenosine triphosphoric acid $ATPH_4$.

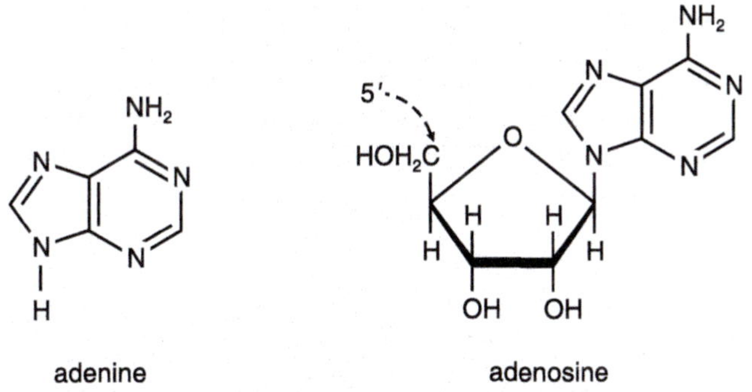

adenine   adenosine

Figure 58. Structures of adenine and adenosine.

Adenosine results from the attachment of adenine to the five-carbon sugar D-ribose through a bond which may be considered as being an extension of a glycosidic linkage. (In principle, a glycosidic linkage is formed when a hydroxyl group of one sugar molecule reacts with the anomeric hydroxyl of another sugar with formation of a water molecule. Sometimes, it is more accurate to represent an carbohydrate by a cyclic structure—appendix I-5 and

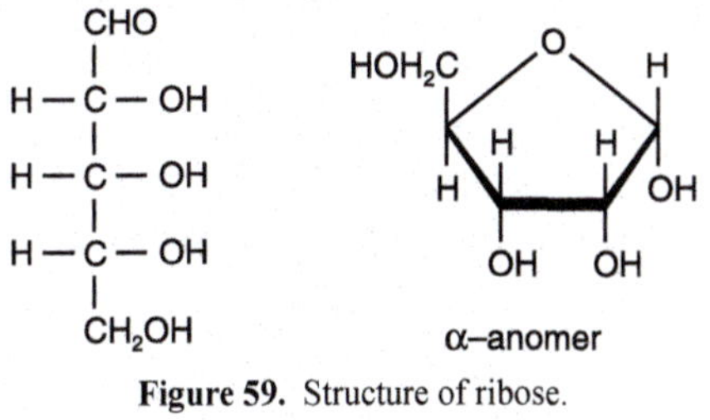

α–anomer

Figure 59. Structure of ribose.

below). In the case of adenosine, a water molecule is formed from the anomeric hydroxyl of the β-D-ribofuranose and the hydrogen atom brought by the nitrogen 9 of adenine (for definitions of anomers and carbohydrates, see appendix I-5).

The last block is constituted by a group, diphosphoric acid or ortophosphoric acid whose structures are:

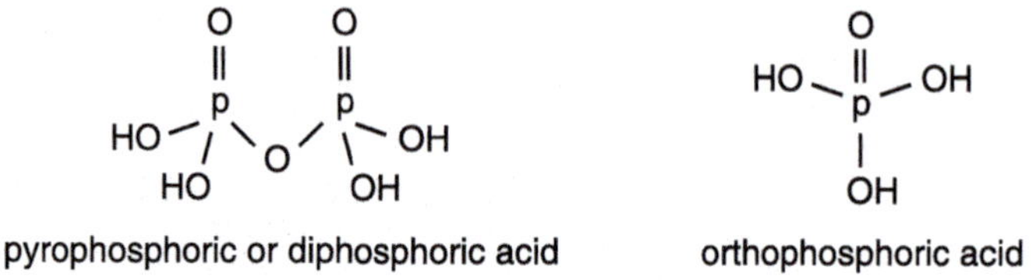

pyrophosphoric or diphosphoric acid   orthophosphoric acid

Figure 60. Structures of diphosphoric and orthophosphoric acids.

The formula of orthophosphoric acid with a double bond $P = O$ between phosphorus and oxygen atoms is not fully satisfactory. A better representation is probably that which contains a semi-polar bond. Nevertheless, we shall only use the representation with the double bond for the sake of simplicity. It will be the same for all the phosphate derivatives encountered in this book.

In the triphosphoric acid, the three atoms of phosphorus form a linear chain and they are linked to each other through an oxygen atom. Both oxygen atoms of the linear chain come from the formation of an anhydride between two molecules of orthophosphoric acid, and more precisely between two hydroxyl groups.

1-3) Adenosine 5'-monophosphoric and diphosphoric acids

Another name of adenosine monophosphoric acid is *adenylic acid*. As it is the case for adenosine triphosphoric acid, using the symbol AMP (adenosine monophosphate) is ambiguous (see paragraph 2). It is preferable to symbolize it by $AMPH_2$. Its structure is given below (Figure 61):

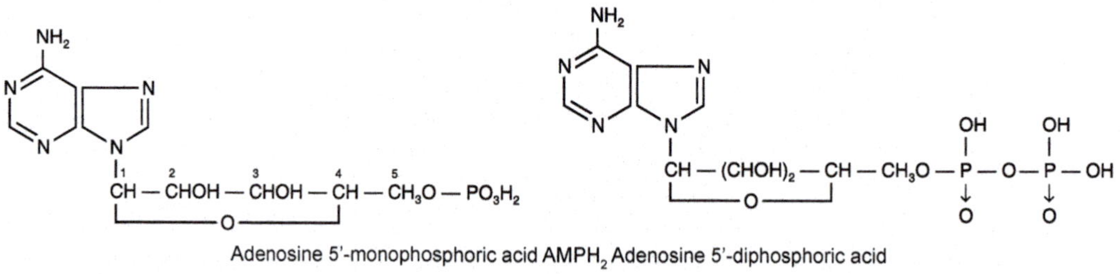

Adenosine 5'-monophosphoric acid $AMPH_2$ Adenosine 5'-diphosphoric acid

Figure 61. Structures of adenosine-5-diphosphoric acid and of adenosine-5-monophosphoric acid.

Its structure is very close to that of adenosine triphosphoric acid. The only difference is that adenosine is esterified by only one molecule of orthophosphoric acid in position 5' of the ribose rest.

Adenosine 5'-diphosphoric acid has an analogous structure to both preceding acids except the fact that it is esterified in the position 5' of the rest ribose by the diphosphoric acid. The symbol ADP is also somewhat ambiguous. We symbolize the Adenosine 5'-diphosphoric acid by $ADPH_3$.

2) Some physico-chemical properties of adenosine triphosphoric acid and derivatives

Oxoacids of phosphorus are numerous. From a general standpoint, all the phosphorus atoms in the oxoacids and in all the oxoanions are 4-coordinate and contain at least one P=O unit. All P atoms in the oxoacids also possess at least one P-OH group.

2-1) Acid dissociation

All the hydroxyl rests of groups P-OH are ionizable in water. Oxoacids are proton donors.

- The pka values of adenosine 5'-triphosphoric acid $ATPH_4$ in water are 0,9 –1,5 –4,1 –6,95. It is quite impossible to attribute these values to a defined group of the molecule because of the problem of the overlapping of its microscopic constants (see Chapter 26). However, according to the approximate rule given in the same chapter, at pH ≈ 7 and owing to the above values of the macroscopic constants, adenosine 5'-triphosphoric acid is certainly trionized and, furthermore, its fourth acidity is about half-ionized. In order to facilitate the explanations, we make the hypothesis that the pH value of the cell is such that $ATPH_4$ is wholly ionized, that is to say it is under the form ATP^{4-}. This hypothesis locates the pH value of the medium at about 9. Some authors have adopted the fact that the molecule is tetraionized in water. It is to the tetraionized structure that the symbol ATP is attributed (Figures 62 and 63).

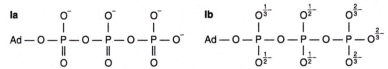

Figure 62. Structure of ATP^{4-} Ia and of one of its mesomeric forms Ib.

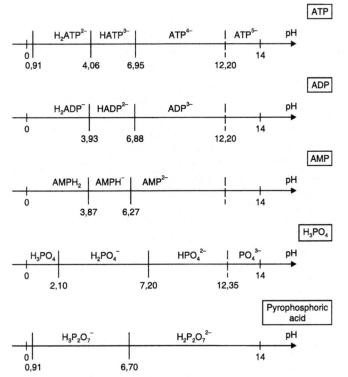

Figure 63. Predominance areas of acido-basic species of ATP, ADP, AMP, H_3PO_4 and $H_4P_2O_7$ as a function of pH.

It is interesting to notice in passing that ATP^{4-} is mesomeric and that among the different possible representations, formula Ib has probably the greatest weight. The four negative charges of ATP are concentrated along the linear polyphosphate structure. This is an important feature of ATP. It is closely related to its "high-energy" nature (see below). (Notice that the prefix "tri" does not indicate the number of charges after total ionization but indicates the number of rests phosphoryl $-PO_3^{2-}$ linked to the ribose moiety).

- Concerning adenosine 5'-diphosphoric acid, pk_a values are 0,9 –3,9 –6,9. The same comments as above are valuable. In particular, at pH about 7, probably, two acidities are fully ionized and the third one is about one half ionized. As above, we adopt the hypothesis that the acid is wholly ionized at the pH of the cell and we name ADP the form triionized ADP^{3-}. It is interesting to notice that at the same pH, both acids $ATPH_4$ and $ADPH_3$ are fully ionized. It will be also the case for $AMPH_2$ and H_3PO_4 (see below). (This fact greatly simplifies the writing of the chemical reactions involving them).

- pK_a values of adenylic acid $AMPH_2$ are 3,9 and 6,3. According to what is preceding, one can infer that at the same pH as that chosen for the two preceding acids, it is the species biionized AMP^{2-} that we name AMP.

Remark. It must be recalled that the blocks ribose of ATP, ADP and AMP (together with those of other ribonucleotides) possess another acidic rest located in the positions 2' or 3' of the sugar. Their pKa values stand in the range of about 12,2. These values are far too great to play a part in bioenergetics and will not be considered further in the book.

- In passing, let us recall that orthophosphoric acid exhibit the pK_a values 2,10 –7,20 –12,35. Pyrophosphoric acid (diphosphoric acid) $H_4P_2O_7$, which we shall encounter later, behaves in water as a diacid, whose pK_a values are 0,91 and 6,70 (see Chapter 38).

2-2) Formation of complexes

ATP and ADP form stable soluble complexes with some bivalent cations existing in a cell such as Ca^{2+} and Mg^{2+}. It also forms complexes with K^+. (From the strict chemical standpoint, it is interesting to notice that ATP and derivatives, including orthophosphoric acid derivatives, give complexes with potassium and sodium ions, even though alkali ions are known to have a very weak coordinating ability). The association constants are great, of the order of ln K_{ass} changing from 3,5 to 4,5 for Mg^{2+}, according to the phosphate derivative (ATP or ADP). The affinity of the nucleotide for the cation increases in the order $K^+ < Na^+ < Ca^{2+} < Mg^{2+}$, the association constants with Na^+ and K^+ remaining weak. The consequence is that very little ATP or ADP exists under the form of a pure anion in the cell. They principally exist under the form of Mg^{2+} complexes.

Of course, the formation of complexes implies the occurrence of plenty of supplementary chemical equilibria in the cells. Now, we mention some of them (the list below being non exhaustive):

$ATP^{4-} + Mg^{2+} \rightleftharpoons ATPMg^{2-}$

$ADP^{3-} + Mg^{2+} \rightleftharpoons ADPMg^-$

$HPO_4^{2-} + Mg^{2+} \rightleftharpoons HPO_4Mg$

$ATP^{4-} + K^+ \rightleftharpoons ATPK^{3-}$

$$ADP^{3-} + K^+ \rightleftharpoons ADPK^{2-}$$

$$HPO_4^{2-} + K^+ \rightleftharpoons HPO_4K^-$$

Furthermore, these complexes also exhibit acido-basic properties. For example:

$$ATPHMg^- \rightleftharpoons ATPMg^{2-} + H^+$$

$$ADPHMg \rightleftharpoons ADPMg^- + H^+$$

and so forth.

These complexation equilibria displace the equilibria obtained with other species in which ATP and ADP are engaged. Such species are notably organic molecules participating in some intermediary metabolisms of which we shall see examples later. Of course, these supplementary equilibria complicate the calculations of the positions of the studied ones. This is another manifestation of the pivotal chemical phenomenon highlighted in this book, that is to say the coupling of several equilibria. This is all the more true here. There are more than two equilibria to superpose, owing to the number of reactants: the targeted organic molecule, the more or less ionized ATP, ADP, the occurrence of H^+ and of metallic ions.

Some structures of these complexes have been studied, at the solid state, by X-ray methods. Concerning the Mg^{2+} complexes of ADP and ATP, it seems that the metal ion is bonded only to the terminal adjacent phosphate group without any further interaction with a nitrogenous basic group of adenine.

It is evident that the knowledge of the structural geometry of ATP molecules is important since enzymes involving them have active sites with which the ATP sites must exactly fit.

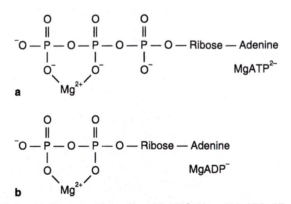

Figure 64. Structures of complexes MgATP²⁻ 64a and MgADP⁻ 64b.

3) The reaction of hydrolysis of ATP

This paragraph may also be entitled as the reaction of donor of phosphoryl groups of ATP.

3-1) Some generalities

The matter of this paragraph is the determination of the standard Gibbs energy ΔG_p° of the following reaction of hydrolysis:

$$ATP + H_2O \rightleftharpoons ADP + P \qquad (K_p) \tag{199}$$

Actually, this reaction (1) has no clear chemical meaning. It is simply a simplification of writing of the following two true reactions (197) and (198)

$$ATPH^{3-} + H_2O \rightleftharpoons ADPH^{2-} + H_2PO_4^- \tag{200}$$

$$ATP^{4-} + OH^- \rightleftharpoons ADP^{3-} + HPO_4^{2-} \tag{201}$$

Some other reactions of hydrolysis are conceivable but at other pH values. It must not be forgotten that reactions in living cells occur at pH about 7. This is the reason why the only retained reactions are (197) and (198).

- Both reactions differ from each other only by the fact that they occur at different pH. (197) occurs at a pH value of about 5,5 whereas (198) occurs at pH of about 9,0. Finally both reactions, globally for our purpose, can be considered as being equivalent if we consider a group under the forms of dihydrogenophosphate $H_2PO_4^-$ or monohydrogenophosphate HPO_4^{2-} ions. (Notice that, from a structural standpoint, a phosphoryl rest must be distinguished from the dihydrogenophosphate and monohydrogenophosphate groups).

  In any case, whatever the reaction is, it exhibits a strong Gibbs energy decline. That is to say, the reaction is strongly displaced towards the right. Because of this property, ATP has been named a *high-energy phosphate compound*. It is also said to possess a *high-energy phosphate bond*. (This term is somewhat misleading—see the next chapter). This only means that ATP (in the conditions of the reaction) possesses a strong tendency to give a phosphoryl rest to another molecule. This is the reason why ATP is also named a *phosphate donor* system whereas the molecule to which the phosphate rest is transferred is called a *phosphate-acceptor* (see the following chapter).

- The best means to obtain the standard Gibbs energy of reaction (1) is probably to determine its equilibrium constant K and to use the general relation (see Chapter 22):

$$\Delta G_p^\circ = -RT \ln K_p$$

where:

$$K_p = [ADP][P]/[ATP]$$

The difficulty of determination lies in the fact that reaction (196), as it is considered, is a composite reaction. (The different reactants and products are mixtures). Moreover, there may exist several equilibria which superpose to that of hydrolysis, such as those of complexation and also the acido-basic ones. It has been possible, however, to overcome the difficulty (see appendix I-6). The searched for physico-chemical parameters are extracted from the experimental data with the aid of (relatively modern) mathematical techniques (see appendix I-6). The latter ones show how superposing equilibria are now studied from the quantitative standpoint.

The result is:

$$\Delta G_p^\circ = -30 \text{ kJ mol}^{-1}$$

and

$$K_p = 10^5$$

Obtaining the value of K_p actually offers a supplementary difficulty, this time of practical order. Its value is so high that equilibrium state is reached at vanishingly small concentrations of remaining ATP, thus precluding its direct measurement. It has been, however, overcome by combining data of an ATP-driven reaction with another, the equilibrium constant of it being known. This is also a good example of a coupled reaction.

It has been possible to overcome the difficulty inherent in the fact that the equilibrium constant of hydrolysis of ATP is too great, by combining data for an ATP-driven reaction with another compound, the equilibrium constant of it being known. The determination is carrying out for known values of pH (about 7) and of the total concentration of Mg²⁺ ions.

4) The reaction of hydrolysis of ATP and complexation with magnesium ions

We have already said that numerous overlapping equilibria greatly complicate the determination of quantitative data. The occurrence of multiple equilibria, indeed, induces displacements of equilibria (see appendix I-6).

In this paragraph, at first sight, we study a simple example of the variation of the Gibbs energy of a chemical reaction when the initial and the final products are complexed. It is compared with the case where the same products are not complexed. We study the hydrolysis reaction ATP → ADP when both the reactant and the product are simultaneously complexed by Mg²⁺ or not, given the values of the formation constants together with those of pH and of the total concentration of Mg²⁺. It is probably the reaction between ATPMg²⁻ and ADPMg⁻ which occurs in priority in the course of hydrolysis. The reasoning is based on the additive property of Gibbs energy (Figure 64').

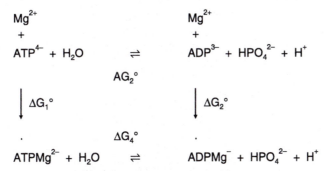

Figure 64'. Determination of the Gibbs energy of hydrolysis of ATP in presence of Mg²⁺ ions.

Attributing the Gibbs energies according to the directions indicated below:

$$\text{ATPMg}^{2-} \rightarrow \text{ATP}^{4-} + \text{Mg}^{2+} \qquad \Delta G_1°$$

$$\text{ATP}^{4-} + \text{H}_2\text{O} \rightarrow \text{ADP}^{3-} + \text{HPO}_4^{2-} + \text{H}^+ \qquad \Delta G_2°$$

$$\text{ADP}^{3-} + \text{Mg}^{2+} \rightarrow \text{ADPMg}^- \qquad \Delta G_3°$$

permits to conclude that:

$$\Delta G_4° - \Delta G_2° = \Delta G_1° + \Delta G_3°$$

The determination is qualified as being apparently simple. Actually, it is not so simple as it appears because it remains to determine the different Gibbs energies intervening in the preceding calculation! Moreover, not only there exist *multiple* kinds of equilibria, but also the problem of the *ionic strength* of the aqueous phase of the cell. It must not be forgotten that its influence is more important, the more polycharged the species of the medium are (see Chapter 20).

*In an indicative way, let us mention that the activity coefficient of the orthophosphate ion PO_4^{3-}, that is the ratio of its activity to its concentration, is only 0,4 for an ionic strength of 10^{-2} mol L^{-1}!. The activity of a species may be assimilated to the fraction of its concentration which actually takes part in the reaction or process. **It** is the activity which must be taken into account for the calculations (We shall not consider this problem further in this book).*

The way the conditions of determination are presented, the determination seems to be a fantastic task to solve! However, an elegant strategy does exist. It is postponed to appendix I-6.

- Many biosynthetic reactions for which ATP provides the "driving force" do not proceed by loss of a single terminal phosphate group of ATP but rather by loss of two terminal phosphate groups, grouped in one piece named a pyrophosphate group with concomitant formation of AMP:

  adenine – ribose – P – P – P → adenine – ribose – P (AMP) + P – P

  Such a metabolic way is mentioned in chapter 38

5) Coenzymes NAD⁺, NADP⁺, NADPH

  5-1) Structures

   NAD⁺ is nicotinamide-adenine nucleotide. This substance has been called "diphosphopyridine nucleotide or DPN⁺" and also "coenzyme I". Its structure is given under (R = H). NADP⁺ is its phosphorylated analogue (R = $-PO_3H_2$) (Figure 65). It is also named triphosphopyridine nucleotide or coenzyme II (TPN⁺).

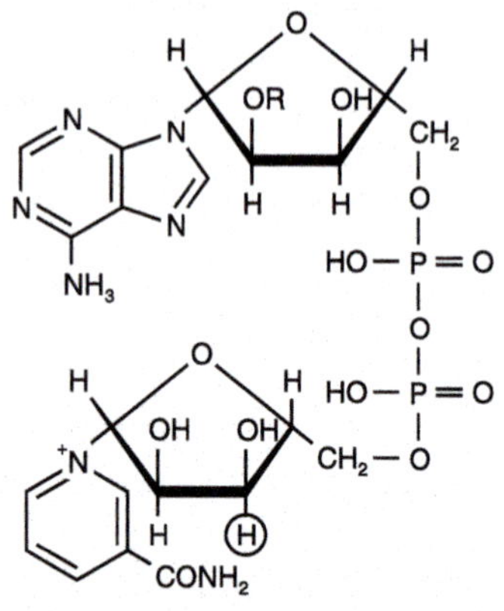

Figure 65. Structures of NAD⁺ and NADP⁺.

They are composed of two nucleotides joined through their phosphate groups by a phosphoanhydride bond. One nucleotide contains the substance *nicotinamide*—Figure 66 —as one of its building block together with a molecule of D-ribose and a rest phosphoryl bound to an identical one belonging to the other nucleotide.

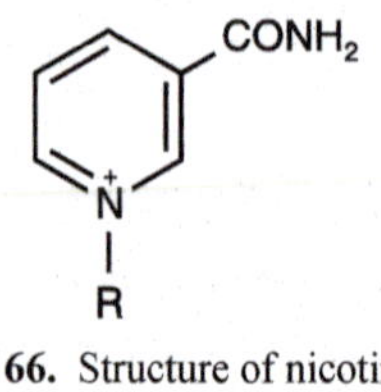

Figure 66. Structure of nicotinamide.

The other mononucleotide contains a rest adenine in place of nicotinamide.

The couple $NAD^+/NADH$ is a couple redox. NAD^+ is the form Ox. It is also symbolized by NAD^+ and NAD_{ox}. The charge positive is justified by the presence of the function quaternary ammonium on the nitrogen atom of nicotinamide. The other symbol NAD_{ox} only recalls that this form is the oxidant of the couple. The form NADH is the reduced form of the couple. It is sometimes symbolized by NAD_{red}. The redox half-reaction is:

$$NAD^+ + H+ + 2e^- \rightarrow NADH \qquad E'^\circ = -0,320V$$

It is the portion nicotinamide of NAD^+ which can accept electrons and become reduced. From the structural point of view, it is interesting to notice that, in the oxidized member, the pyridine ring of the nicotinamide block even with "quaternarized" nitrogen is quasi-planar; this is no longer the case in the reduced form. Then, it is the pyridine ring which is reduced and it is a derivative of a dihydropyridine which is formed. A dihydropyridine is no planar Figure 67.

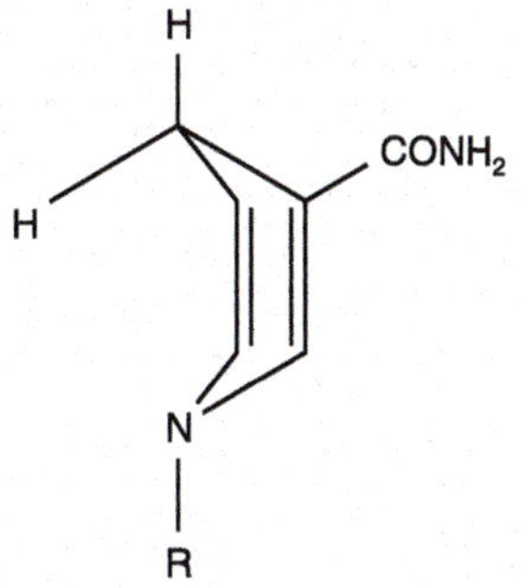

Figure 67. Representation of the block dihydropyridine of NAD_{red}.

NAD^+ is the coenzyme of the enzyme alcohol dehydrogenase (ADH).

Analogous considerations concerning $NADP^+$ can be given. It belongs to the couple redox $NADP^+/NADPH$, the redox equilibrium of which is:

$$NADP^+ + H^+ + 2e- \rightarrow NADPH \qquad E'^\circ = -0,324V$$

For both forms NAD^+ and $NADP^+$, it is quasi-certain that their reduction is carried out with the aid of an hydride ion H^-.

Chapter 33

The Transfer of Chemical Energy with the Aid of ATP

We shall see in this chapter how the terminal phosphate group of ATP may be transferred to a second molecule which is a phosphate-acceptor. During the course of this reaction, ATP is transformed into ADP. The latter, in turn, can "recapture" a phosphate group to give ATP after transfer of a phosphate rest from a phosphate-donor species. This is an illustration of the previously named "high energy bond" concept. From a very general standpoint, it can be said that it deals, indeed, with changes in Gibbs energies when some groups are transferred from one molecule to another.

In brief, ATP is a carrier of chemical Gibbs energy.

1) Come back to the free energy of hydrolysis of ATP

Let us recall that the reaction of hydrolysis, depending on the pH value, may be written:

in some pH conditions:

$$ATP^{4-} + H_2O \rightarrow ADP^{3-} + HPO_4^{2-} + H^+ \tag{202}$$

It is now known that it is a nucleophilic substitution reaction SN, the nucleophilic reactant being either H_2O or OH^- ion according to the pH. With H_2O as reactant, the reaction is:

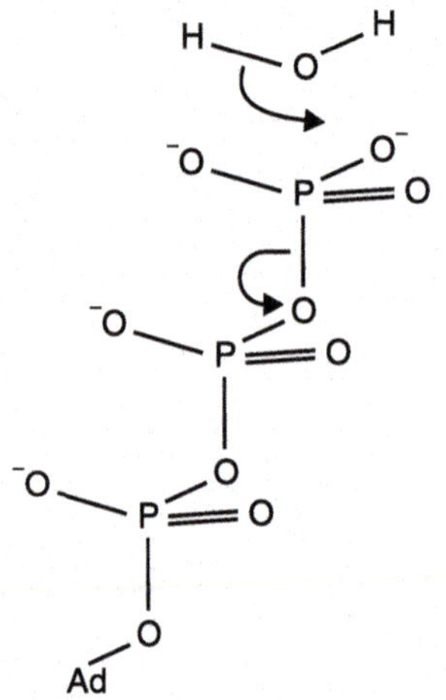

Figure 68. Mechanism of the reaction of hydrolysis of ATP into ADP.

This scheme shows that actually the group which is transferred is the phosphoryl rest: $-PO_3^{2-}$.

Reaction (199) occurs with a large liberation of heat. Therefore, it is not surprising that it is accompanied by a large decrease of Gibbs energy. We know that:

$\Delta G^{\circ'} \approx -30$ kJ mol^{-1} at 25°C

This value is that corresponding to the changes: biochemical standard states/chemical standard states (see chapter 21). As a result, using the mass action law, it is easy to find that the hydrolysis Gibbs energy of ATP may be markedly higher than the standard one. It is likely that it is in the order of -50 kJ mol^{-1}.

The Gibbs energy of hydrolysis of ATP is clearly higher than that of simple esters, glycosides and amids. There are two good chemical reasons for which ATP is endowed with a high hydrolysis enthalpy and Gibbs energy.

– the first one is that its triphosphoryl rest is tetracharged, that is to say it is highly charged and its charges are very close to each other (see the preceding chapter). They repel each other very strongly. After hydrolysis of the last phosphoryl group, a part of the preceding electrostatic stress is relieved. Moreover, the two formed products tend to separate from each other because they are both negatively charged;

– the second reason is that the two products formed by hydrolysis (ADP and P) are stabilized by resonance. It is particularly the case of the ion monohydrogenophosphate HPO_4^{2-}. Certainly, there also exists possibility of mesomerism in the ATP^{4-} but it is more than counterbalanced by the electrostatic stress.

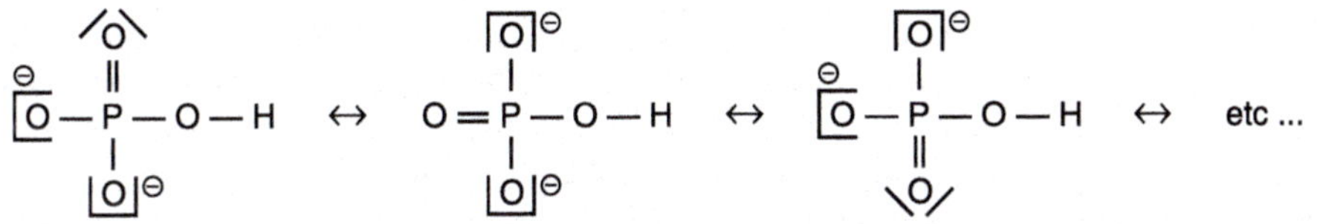

Figure 69. Explanations of the high hydrolysis enthalpies.

2) Gibbs energies of hydrolysis of some phosphorylated compounds

Even if the hydrolysis of ATP^{4-} liberates much heat, given the part played by ATP in the intermediary metabolism, we are more interested in the Gibbs energy change during the hydrolysis than by the quantity of heat liberated in the course.

In Table 14 are given Gibbs energies of hydrolysis of some phosphorylated derivatives.

The values of the Gibbs energies of hydrolysis permit to classify the phosphorylated compounds as being endowed with *high phosphate group transfer potential* or with *low phosphate group transfer potential*. (We continue to speak of high and low *phosphate* group transfer, even if it would be better to use the word *phosphoryl* group rather than phosphate group). The transfer potential is equal to the Gibbs energy of hydrolysis with its sign inverted.

Compounds possessing the highest transfer potentials can spontaneously transfer phosphoryl group to another located lower than it in the above scale. Clearly, ATP has an intermediate position in this scale. As a result, it is able to donate a phosphoryl group as it is able to accept a phosphoryl group, according to the value of the transfer potential of the antagonist molecule. Its position is somewhat analogous to that of the couple I_2/I^- in the scale of redox standard potentials.

Table 15. Hydrolysis Gibbs energy of some phosphorylated compounds
(according to A.L. Lehninger—see general bibliography).

	$\Delta G°'$ kJ mol^{-1}	phosphate transfer potential $-\Delta G°'$
Phosphoenolpyruvate	−53,5	53,5
1,3-diphosphoglycerate	−49,3	49,3
ATP ($\rightarrow$ AMP + PP)	−45,6	45,6
Phosphocreatine	−43;9	43,9
Acetylphosphate	−42,2	42,2
ADP ($\rightarrow$ AMP + P)	−32,8	32,8
Phosphoarginine	−32,2	32,2
ATP	−30,5	30,5
Glucose 1-phosphate	−20,9	20,9
PP (P + P)	−19,2	19,2
Fructose 6-phosphate	−15,9	15,9
AMP ($\rightarrow$ adenosine + P)	−14,2	14,2
Glucose 6-phosphate	−13,8	13,8
3-phosphoglycerate	−13,0	13,0
Glycerol 1-phosphate	−9,6	9,6

3) An unfortunate qualifier

In the biochemical literature, we still often encounter the unfortunate terms *high energy phosphate bonds* and *low energy phosphate bonds* to qualify the compounds having a high or low transfer potential. These terms must be avoided. They are misleading. No bond energy is released in phosphate-transfer processes. There is only the transfer of a group, that is to say a rearrangement of bonds when two new equilibria are attained. The free energy of hydrolysis is not localized in only chemical bond as it must be the case in pure physical-chemistry, by definition.

4) ATP provider of energy by group transfers

ATP is a carrier of chemical energy. It transports chemical energy from high-energy donors to low-energy phosphate acceptors. But, there is an important point to highlight: it is not the energy, that is to say the heat liberated by the hydrolysis reaction, which permits ATP to induce numerous biochemical reactions of the intermediary metabolism to occur although they are not possible as it is indicated by their Gibbs energy. In other words, reaction (199) is coupled with a reaction which is in principle forbidden. We have seen that there should be coupling if the product of the first reaction must be a reactant of the second (See Chapters 21 and 29).

ATP can not solely be a phosphoryl group transfer but, is also a pyrophosphoryl and an adenylyl group provider. The nature of the transferred group depends on the location of the nucleophilic attack of the triphosphoryl group of ATP (see Figure 70).

These results have been proved by using an alcohol marked by ^{18}O on the hydroxylic group R^{18}OH as a reactant. The attack on the phosphor γ leads to a phosphoryltransfer, that on phosphor β to the pyrophosphoryl transfer and that of phosphor α to the transfer of the group adenylyl. The rest adenylyl exhibits the structure given in the Figure 70.

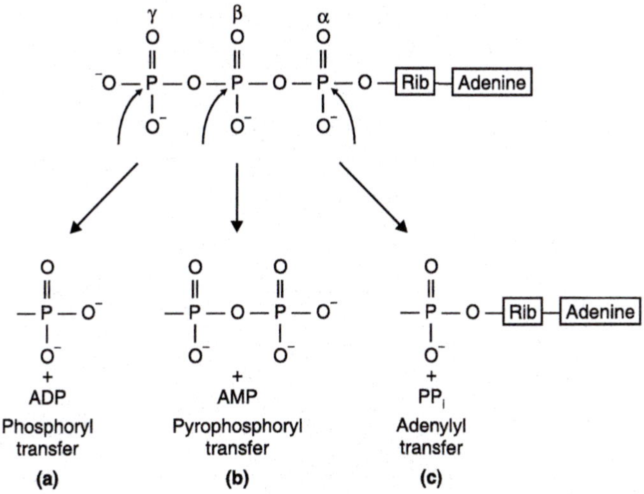

Figure 70. Nature of the transferred group according to the location of the nucleophilic attack of ATP by water.

5) An example of utilization of ATP free energy to do chemical work

First, let us recall that an polysaccharides results from the union of a variable number of molecules of simple carbohydrates. Holosides are exclusively formed by the union of carbohydrates. Sucrose is a diholoside (see Chapter 29). It is composed by one molecule of D(+) glucose and D(−) fructose. Glucose is under the pyran form whereas fructose is under the furan form. Another name of sucrose is saccharose (see Chapter 29).

It is interesting to study this example more thoroughly as a case of the multiple parts that can be played by ATP. Let us, hence, consider the "thermodynamic mechanism" by which sucrose is formed from component oses. The mechanism is enzymatic. The synthesis obeys the following global scheme:

ATP + glucose + fructose → sucrose + ADP + phosphate

The formation reaction is an "uphill" one. It is endergonic. It exhibits the positive free energy change $\Delta G^{\circ\prime} = + 23,0$ kJ mol^{-1}. However, it is accomplished by coupling it to the reaction ATP/(ADP + P) according to:

ATP + Glucose → ADP + glucose-1-phosphate

glucose – 1-phosphate + fructose → sucrose + phosphate

Again, we can notice that there is a common intermediate between the two coupled reactions. It is the glucose-1-phosphate. The global coupled reaction is a "downhill" one: $\Delta G^{\circ\prime} = -6,3$ kJ mol^{-1}.

6) Steps in the extraction of energy from foodstuffs

One can consider that the mechanism of the formation of energy by oxidation, at least for superior animals, proceeds in three steps. In the first one, the great molecules of the foodstuffs are destroyed in small molecules. Hence, proteins are transformed into the twenty amino-acids constituting them, polysaccharides are hydrolyzed in simple sugars and fats into glycerol and fatty acids. No Gibbs energy is recuperated in this step.

In the second step, these small molecules are degraded into small simple chemical unities which play a pivotal part in the metabolism. Actually, they are essentially transformed in acetyl-coenzymeA (see Chapter 35). Few ATP is generated in this step.

The third step is that of Kreb's cycle and of oxydative phosphorylation. The most part of the formed ATP is generated in this last term. The Figure 71 summarizes these points.

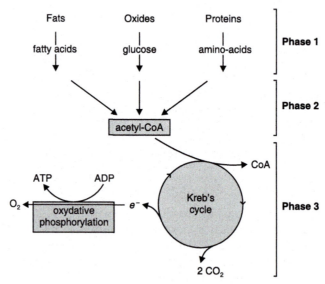

Figure 71. Different steps in the extraction of energy from foodstuffs.

Chapter 34

Glycolysis and Fermentation

Glycolysis is a sequence of reactions which transform the glucose in pyruvate ions with simultaneous formation of ATP. In the aerobic conditions, the glycolysis is the prelude of the citric acid cycle. If the conditions are not sufficiently aerobic, the pyruvate ion does not enter into the citric acid cycle. It is transformed into the lactate ion. This is the first step towards the phenomenon of fermentation.

Glycolysis is one of the major pathways of glucose utilization. Glycolysis also happens, in part, in anaerobic conditions in cells. In the course of glycolysis, the fate of a molecule of glucose is actually to be degraded into two molecules of pyruvic acid, objectivated as pyruvate ions. It evolves through a series of enzyme-catalyzed reactions during which a part of the Gibbs energy released from glucose is conserved in the form of ATP and NADH. We examine the different steps of glycolysis and, later, those of fermentation from the point of view of bioenergetics, but before, for the sake of clarity, we present an overview of the cycle.

1) An overview of the glycolytic chain

   In Figure 72, we give the names of the successive intermediary compounds which mark the ends of the different steps of the glycolytic chain together with the names of the enzymes which govern their transformations in each of them.

   The chain of reactions constituting the glycolysis process is also named the *Emden-Meyerhof* cycle.

   In Figure 73, we give the structures of the intermediary products.

2) Structures of intermediary products

   Some comments above the different steps of the chain

   2-1) In the first step is formed glucose 6-phosphate I' from glucose:

   $$\text{glucose} \xrightarrow{\quad \textit{hexokinase} \quad} \text{glucose-6-phosphate 1'}$$

   This outline does not represent the reaction which is:

   $$\text{ATP} + \text{glucose} \rightarrow \text{glucose-6-phosphate} + \text{ADP}$$

   For the calculation of its Gibbs energy, the reaction can be considered as resulting from the coupling of the two following reactions:

   $$\text{ATP} + \text{H}_2\text{O} \rightarrow \text{ADP} + \text{P} \qquad \Delta G^{\circ\prime} = -30{,}5 \text{ kJ mol}^{-1}$$

   $$\text{glucose} + \text{P} \rightarrow \text{glucose-6-phosphate} + \text{H}_2\text{O} \quad \Delta G^{\circ\prime} = 13{,}8 \text{ kJ mol}^{-1}$$

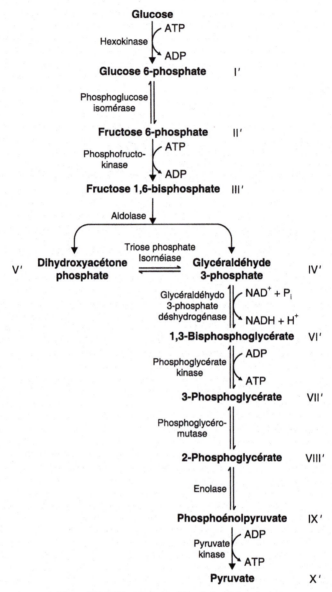

Figure 72. Different steps of the chain of glycolysis.

It is puzzling that glycolysis, through which energy is recuperated, begins by the destruction of a molecule of ATP which, *in fine*, permits to stock it.

(Notice that the writing ATP and ADP avoids to have to specify the pH. Assigning electrical charges to species ATP, ADP and P should require the knowledge of the pH of the medium if it could be exactly known). Hexokinase, however, requires the presence of Mg^{2+} ions in order to function because it is the complex $[MgATP]^{2-}$ which is the true substrate of the enzyme. The global reaction occurs because of its strong decline of Gibbs energy (about $-16,8$ kJ mol^{-1}). As we shall see, ATP is regenerated later:

The actual mechanism of the reaction of ATP with glucose is a nucleophilic substitution. The glucose functions as a nucleophilic reagent by virtue of the unshared electrons of the oxygen atom of the primary hydroxyl group (see Chapter 33).

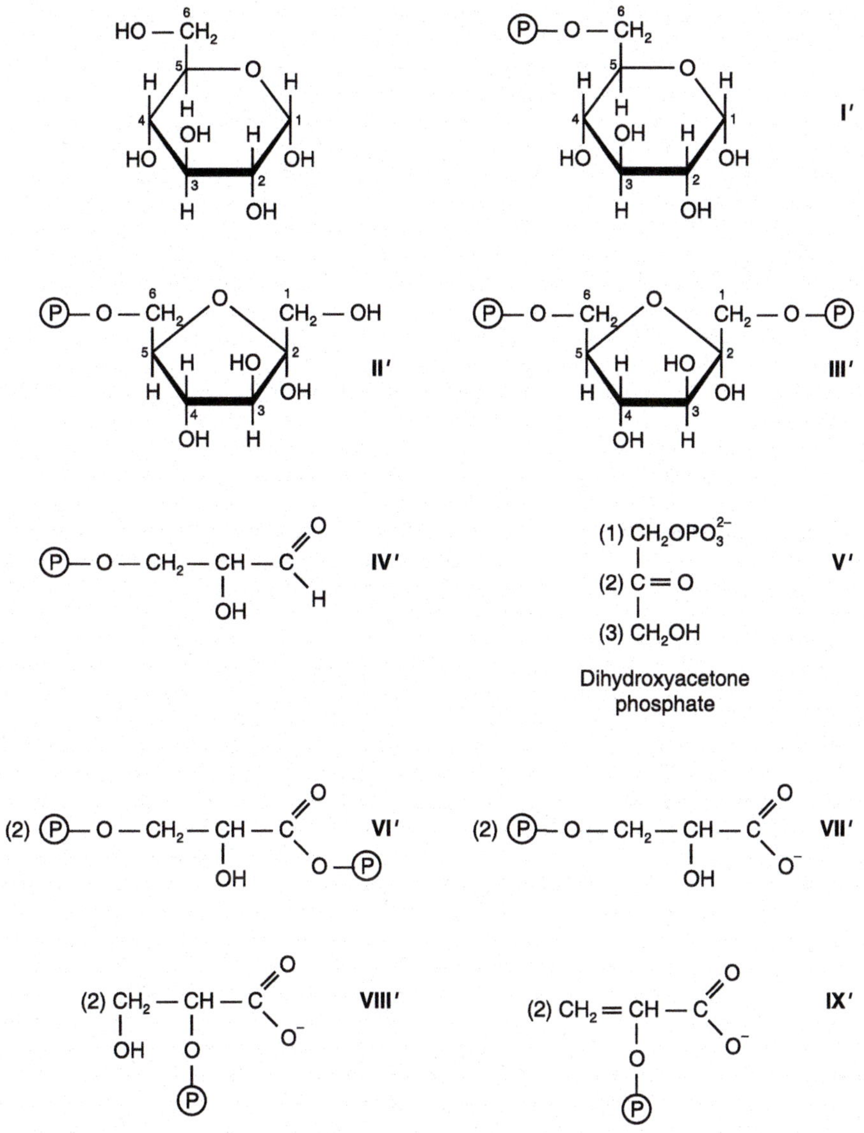

Figure 73. Structures of the intermediary products.

2-2) In the second step, the glucose-6-phosphate is transformed into the fructose-6-phosphate II':

$$\text{glucose-6-phosphate} \xrightarrow{\quad \text{phosphohexoseisomerase} \quad} \text{fructose-6-phosphate II'}$$

The working enzyme is the phosphohexose isomerase. The reaction evolves in the presence of magnesium ions. The Gibbs energy of the transformation ($\Delta G^{\circ\prime} = 1{,}7$ kJ mol^{-1}) is slightly positive. Nevertheless, this value does not pose any problem from the Gibbs energy standpoint, owing to the concentrations of the reactants and products in the cell. Recall that concentrations of reactants and products may change the locations of equilibria. By example, if we take for the initial state of the reaction the concentrations [glucose-6-phosphate] $= 0{,}083\ 10^{-3}$ mol L^{-1} and [fructose-6-phosphate] $= 0{,}014\ 10^{-3}$ mol L^{-1} (these data are those encountered in erythrocytes in some conditions), we obtain for the reactional quotient Q

Q = (0,014/0,083)

The corresponding energetic term, RT ln Q is: (see Chapter 20)

RT ln Q = –4,41 kJ mol^{-1} (at 298 K)

The Gibbs energy change of the reaction is under these conditions:

$\Delta_r G = \Delta_r G° + RTlnQ$

where $\Delta_r G°$ is the standard Gibbs energy change accompanying the reaction ($\Delta_r G° = 1,7$ kJ mol^{-1}):

$\Delta_r G = –2,7$ kJ mol^{-1}

Despite the positive value of the standard Gibbs energy change, the isomerisation spontaneously evolves in the indicated direction. (Taking the temperature equal to 337 K would not markedly change this conclusion. Standard states are as usual for biochemical reactions).

The mechanism of chemical reaction of transformation involves a pathway through an enediol (Figure 74) which results from prototropic exchanges. There is formation of a cis-enediol intermediate. It results from the abstraction of a proton by the basic nitrogen of a molecule of histidine which in turn acts as a proton-donor. The histidine molecule acts as a proton relay because of the occurrence of its basic and acidic sites =N— and —NH$^+$= of its diazole 1–3 nucleus (Figure 75).

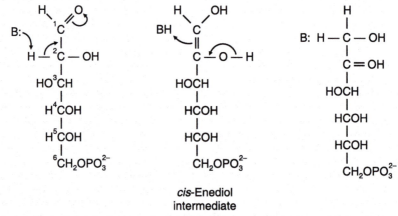

Figure 74. Intermediate enediol in the isomerisation glucose-6-phosphate into fructose-6-phosphate and structure of histidine.

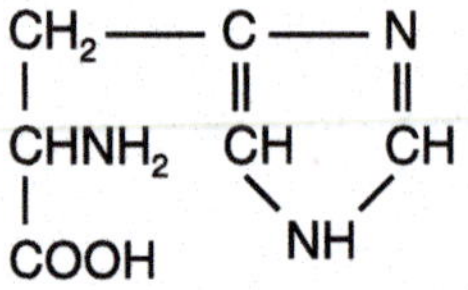

Figure 75. Structure of histidine.

2-3) In the third step, there is formation of fructose-1,6-bisphosphate III':

$$\text{Fructose-6-phosphate} \xrightarrow{\textit{phosphofructokinase}} \text{fructose-1-6-diphosphate III'}$$

(By convention, compounds that contain two phosphate or phosphoryl groups attached at different positions of the molecule are named bisphosphates or biphosphocompounds). The enzyme is the phosphofructokinase-1 (PFK-1). It must be distinguished from the phosphofructokinase-2 (PFK-2). (The latter catalyzes the formation of fructose-2,6-bisphosphate from fructose-6-phosphate). The reaction evolves in presence of magnesium ions. From the bioenergetic standpoint, the reaction necessitates the aid of the couple ATP/ADP. The global reaction is:

$$\text{Fructose-6-phosphate} + \text{ATP} \rightarrow \text{fructose-1,6-bisphosphate} + \text{ADP}$$

$\Delta G^{\circ\prime} = -14{,}2$ kJ mol^{-1} whereas for the reaction:

$$\text{fructose-1,6-bisphosphate} + H_2O \rightarrow \text{fructose-6-phosphate} + P$$

$\Delta G^{\circ\prime} = +16{,}3$ kJ mol^{-1}.

Notice again that in this reaction there is a consumption of a second molecule of ATP.

2-4 and 2-5) These steps actually constitute the same one. It consists in the transformation of fructose-1,6-bisphosphate into a mixture of glyceraldehyde-3-phosphate IV' and of dihydroxyacetone phosphate V':

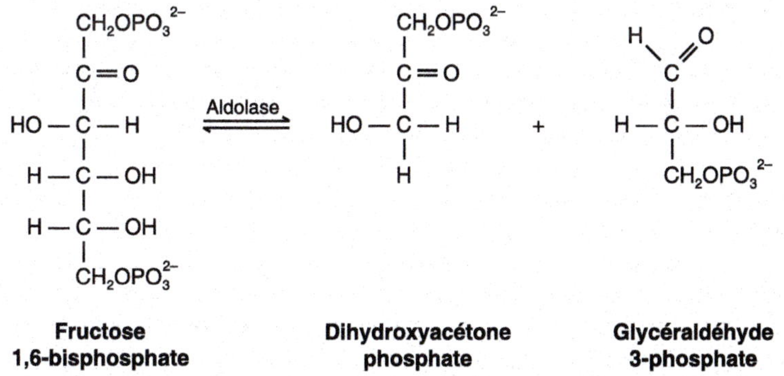

Figure 76. Formation of the dihydroxyacetone phosphate and of glyceraldehyde-3-phosphate.

The breakdown of the six-carbons chain of glucose into two three–carbons chains may be surprising at first sight. Actually, the reaction is simply the inverse of a reaction of aldolisation. The enzyme is aldolase. It is also named fructose-1,6-bisphosphate aldolase. There is a number of enzymatic reactions that can be classed as aldol additions. Another example is the reaction studied below. It is catalyzed by aldolase itself in which D-glyceraldehyde-3-phosphate and dihydroxyacetone phosphate combine to give fructose-1,6-diphosphate and sorbose-1-6-diphosphate:

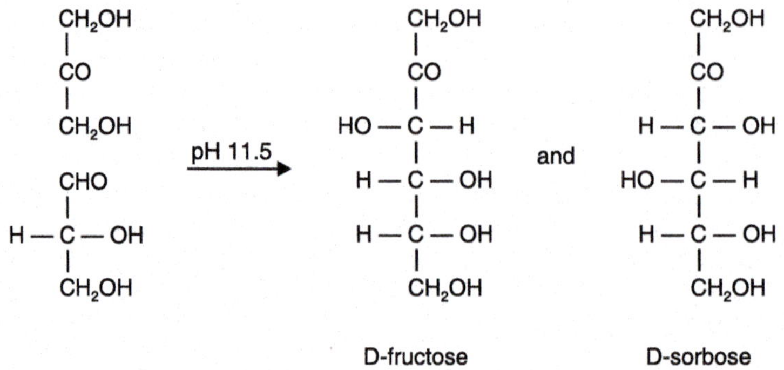

Figure 77. Formation by aldolisation of fructose-1,6-diphosphate and sorbose-1,6-diphosphate.

This aldolisation reaction is the inverse of that studied. As a result, the latter is catalyzed by the same enzyme. From the bioenergetic standpoint, the standard Gibbs energy is positive:

aldolase

fructose-1,6-bisphosphate $\longrightarrow$ dihydroxyacetone phosphate
+ Glyceraldehyde-3-Phosphate $\Delta G°' = +23,8$ kJ mol^{-1}

In principle, the reaction cannot evolve spontaneously in the standard conditions. Notwithstanding, at the low concentrations of reactants and products in the cells, the actual Gibbs energy change accompanying the reaction is small and the aldolisation reaction is reversible.

Remark: Now, it is known that there are two classes of aldolases, but in the context of this book, we do not study this point further.

2-6) This step completes the transformation V' → IV', that is to say the transformation of the dihydroxyacetone phosphate into glyceraldehyde-3-phosphate. The enzyme is the triosephosphate isomerase:

triosephosphate isomerase
V' $\longrightarrow$ IV'

The enzyme is widespread. The standard Gibbs energy of the reaction is $\Delta G°' = + 7,5$ kJ mol^{-1}. Actually, with the initial concentrations [dihydroxyacetone-phosphate] = $0,14 \; 10^{-3}$ mol L^{-1} and [glyceraldehyde-3-phosphate] = $0,019 \; 10^{-3}$ mol L^{-1}, a reasoning conducted as before gives the value $+ 2,6$ kJ mol^{-1} for the reactional Gibbs energy change in these conditions. Despite the standard Gibbs energy change, one can conceive that the equilibrium term of the reaction may remain in favor of the aldehyde according to the cell concentrations. *Moreover, it must not be forgotten that the multiple equilibria in the chains of reactions such as that of glycolysis are displaced by other reactions of the chain, whatever the nature of the reaction considered.*

2-7) The next step is the formation of 1,3-biphosphoglycerate VI':

glyceraldehyde-3-phosphatedeshydrogenase

glyceraldehyde-3-phosphate $\longrightarrow$ 1,3-bisphosphorylglycerate VI'

Each molecule of glyceraldehyde-3-phosphate is oxidized and phosphorylated to form 1,3 bisphosphoglycerate.

- The oxidation of 3-phosphoglyceraldehyde is realized by NAD^+ with an uptake of one molecule of inorganic phosphate under the influence of the enzyme. The 1,3-bisphosphorylglycerate VI' is a product of high energy. The oxidation reaction is:

3-phosphoglyceraldehyde $+ HPO_4^{2-} + NAD^+ \rightleftharpoons$

1,3-bisphosphoglycerate $+ NADH + H^+$ $\Delta G'^\circ = 6,3$ kJmol^{-1}

One molecule of NAD^+ oxidizes one molecule of glyceraldehyde-3-phosphate with an exchange of two electrons. The two half oxydo-reductions are:

$NAD^+ + H+ + 2e- \rightarrow NADH$

$RCHO + H_2O \rightarrow RCOOH + 2H^+ + 2e-$

(RCHO represents the glyceraldehyde-3-phosphate and RCOOH the 1,3-bisphosphorylglycerate). We notice that the global reaction is a redox one. Whereas NAD^+ is reduced into NADH, RCHO is oxidized into the acid RCOOH which is phosphoryled.

2-8) Then, the formed 1,3-bisphosphoglycerate VI' reacts with ADP to give 3-phosphoglycerate VII' according to:

phosphoglyceratekinase

1,3-bisphosphoglycerate $+ ADP \longrightarrow$ P-O-CH$_2$ CHOH COO$^-$ + ATP
                                                        3-phosphoglycerate

$\Delta G'^\circ = -18,8$ kJmol^{-1}

We notice that the oxidation of one mole of 1,3-bisphosphoglycerate is accompanied by the formation of one mole of ATP. But, according to the preceding steps of the chain, one molecule of glucose gives two molecules of glyceraldehyde-3-phosphate (one directly, the other after isomerisation of dihydroxyacetone phosphate). As a result, one molecule of glucose has already given back two molecules of ATP at the end of this step.

2-9) The next step consists in the transformation of 3-phosphoglycerate VII' to 2-phosphoglycerate VIII'

phosphoglyceratemutase

VII ' $\longrightarrow$ 2-phosphoglycerate VIII'

$\Delta G'^\circ = 4,6$ kJmol^{-1}

The reaction is catalyzed by the enzyme phosphoglyceratemutase. *The mechanism of its action is complex. It involves a transfer of a phosphoryl group primarily attached to a histidine residue of the enzyme. It is transferred to the hydroxyl group at C2 of the 3-phosphoglycerate. Transitorily, there is the existence of a 2,3-bisphosphoglycerate. The phosphoryl group at C3 of the bisphosphate is then transferred to the initial histidine residue in the presence of histidine.*

2-10) The following step consists in the action of enolase on IX'

$$\text{2-phosphoglycerate VIII'} \xrightarrow{\text{enolase}} \underset{\textit{phosphoenolpyruvate}}{\text{I X'}}$$

This reaction is a reaction of dehydration:

$$\text{VIII'} \xrightarrow{\text{enolase}} \text{IX'} + H_2O$$

It is reversible and involves a magnesium complex as intermediate. From the energetic standpoint, the standard Gibbs energy of the reaction is $\Delta G^{\circ\prime} = +7{,}5$ kJ mol^{-1}. Beyond this result, let us mention that this reaction transforms a compound with a relatively low Gibbs energy of hydrolysis (2-phosphoglycerate: $-17{,}6$ kJ mol^{-1}) into another of high Gibbs energy of hydrolysis (2-phosphoenolpyruvate: $-61{,}9$ kJ mol^{-1}). For these reasons, the 2-phosphoglycerate and the 2-phosphoenolpyruvate are respectively classified as low-energy and as high-energy phosphate bonds. Undoubtedly, the high hydrolysis Gibbs energy of 2-phosphoenolpyruvate is related to the fact that pyruvic acid exhibits two tautomeric structures, the enol and the ketone ones. The latter is predominant, at least in aqueous medium and for this reason, it displaces the studied equilibrium in its favor. The step strongly increases the transfer potential of the phosphoryl group.

2-11) The last step of glycolysis corresponds to the transfer of the phosphoryl group from the phosphoenolpyruvate I X' to ADP with recuperation of ATP and pyruvic acid ($pK_a = 2{,}30$) under the form of pyruvate X': CH_3COCOO^-. The reaction is:

$$\text{I X'} + \text{ADP} \xrightarrow{\textit{pyruvate kinase}} CH_3COCOO^- + \text{ATP}$$

$$\Delta G^{\prime\circ} = -31{,}3 \text{ kJ mol}^{-1}$$

The reaction is catalyzed by the pyruvate kinase in presence of ions K^+ and Mg^{2+} or Mn^{2+}. Hence, two moles of ATP are formed again since, before, there were already two moles of phosphoenolpyruvate (see above).

Pyruvate ions may have different fates according to the experimental conditions of the process, in particular aerobic or anaerobic ones.

3) Fermentation

We are speaking now of anaerobic glycolysis. Anaerobic glycolysis is the sequence of reactions that metabolizes glucose into lactate and also produces ATP.

When there is a lack of dioxygen for animal tissues, NAD^+, which is an essential reactant in glycolysis, is regenerated from NADH by the reduction of pyruvate to lactate $CH_3CHOHCOO^-$. The corresponding half-redox reactions are:

$$CH_3COCOO^- + 2H^+ + 2e- \rightleftharpoons CH_3CHOHCOO^- \quad E^\circ = -0{,}19V$$

$$NADH \rightleftharpoons NAD^+ + H^+ + 2e- \quad E^\circ = -0{,}32V$$

The oxidized form CH_3COCOO^- of the couple which possesses the highest standard potential (of reduction) must spontaneously react with the reduced form of the couple possessing the lowest value of the standard value. The global redox reaction is:

$$CH_3COCOO^- + NADH + H^+ \rightarrow CH_3CHOHCOO^- + NAD^+$$

It must also be mentioned that some tissues and cells (such as erythrocytes which have no mitochondria and thus cannot oxidize pyruvate to CO_2—see oxidative phosphorylation—Chapter 36) produce lactate from glucose under anaerobic conditions.

Fermentation is defined as the energy-yielding enzymatic breakdown of fuel molecules that takes place in certain cells under anaerobic conditions. Dioxygen is not required in the process. Fuel molecules are amino-acids, fatty acids and glucoids.

An example is furnished by the alcoholic fermentation. The global reaction is:

glucose + 2P + 2ADP + 2H$^+$ → 2 ethanol + 2CO$_2$ + 2ATP + 2H$_2$O

It is interesting to notice that, on one hand, neither NAD$^+$ nor NADH appear in this reaction.

These examples nicely illustrate the fact, already mentioned (see Chapter 27), that oxidations can be performed without using dioxygen. Cells which do not use dioxygen for the oxidations they perform are called *anaerobic organisms* or *anaerobes*. In anaerobic cells, it may be an organic molecule which is the oxidant.

4) Glycolysis and fermentation

In both aerobic and anaerobic cells, the energy of foodstuff molecules is conserved during their oxidation not as heat but as chemical energy, more precisely as in ATP molecules. ATP is formed from ADP through an endergonic reaction, which, of course, must be coupled with an oxidation one proceeding with a large decline in Gibbs energy.

ATP is the carrier of chemical energy coming from the oxidation of foodstuff molecules whether the oxidation conditions are aerobic or anaerobic. The chemical energy stocked as ATP is then used to perform the chemical, mechanical and osmotic works of the cell.

There exist *facultative* cells which can live under aerobic or anaerobic conditions. In the second case, glucose is broken down until lactic acid is formed. At this point, the process may stop. When dioxygen is present, oxidation continues further until CO_2 and H_2O are formed. Therefore, the fermentation reactions are common in both the aerobic and anaerobic breakdowns of glucose in facultative organisms, at least until the formation of pyruvate anions is achieved.

5) A balance-sheet of glycolysis

From the strict chemical standpoint, when we consider the glycolytic chain of glucose in aerobic condition plus the step of formation of lactic acid, the global equilibrium reaction is:

$$C_6H_{12}O_6 \rightarrow 2\ CH_3\ CHOH\ COOH \qquad \Delta_r G' = -217{,}4\ kJ\ mol^{-1} \qquad (203)$$

In this scheme, it appears as *no net oxido-reduction reaction*. However, the anaerobic breakdown of glucose to lactate does not take place according to this global scheme and it is convenient to introduce light and shade into this assertion. We are now going back on this point.

(Notice first that, here again, we find a difficulty to classify organic reactions as being redox ones). However, several remarkable features appear:

– No oxygen is required. We have already noticed that there is no net reduction nor oxidation;

– The reaction may evolve in principle with a large decline in Gibbs energy ($\Delta G' = -217{,}4$ kJ mol^{-1}). Actually, this reaction does not occur directly in living cells. It proceeds through a series of enzymatic reactions in which phosphate, ADP and ATP molecules participate. An attentive look at the successive steps of the anaerobic glycolysis, indeed, shows that its course can be divided into two successive ones of different kinds;

- The first part begins with the formation of glucose-6-phosphate and ADP and finishes with the isomerisation dihydroxyacetone-P → glyceraldehyde-3-P included. The overall reaction to the first part is:

glucose + 2ATP $\rightleftharpoons$ 2 glyceraldehyde-3-phosphate + 2 ADP   (204)

It corresponds to a borrowing of energy from the reactant ATP.

- The second part is the pay off. It begins with the formation of 3-phosphoglycerate until that of lactate ion. The overall reaction is:

2 glyceraldehyde-3-phosphate + 4 ADP + 2 P $\rightleftharpoons$ 2 lactate + 4 ATP + 2 H$_2$O   (205)

The overall equation of the anaerobic glycolysis is:

glucose + 2HPO4^{2-} + 2ADP^{3-} → 2lactate$^-$ + 2ATP^{4-} + 2H$_2$O

$$\Delta G' = -159 \text{ kJ mol}^{-1} \qquad (206)$$

Equation (203) is not the same as (200) as it is shown notably by the values of the reactional standard Gibbs energies.

The balance-sheet of glycolysis calls for the following comments:

- the most important point concerning the glycolysis lies in the fact that it permits the conservation of the energy liberated by the glucose molecule. The conservation is carried out by the regeneration of molecules of ATP from ADP. Two molecules of ATP are formed for one molecule of glucose entered in the process of glycolysis. From the thermodynamic standpoint, since the actual process liberates $-158{,}8$ kJ mol^{-1} by molecule of glucose and since the direct transformation glucose to molecule of lactic acid is supposed to liberate $-217{,}4$ kJ mol^{-1}, the formation of two molecules of ATP permits to save:

$217{,}4 - 158{,}8 = 58{,}6$ kJ mol^{-1}

Moreover, some free energy is also saved by the process of uptake of phosphate during the enzymatic oxidation of 3-phosphoglyceraldehyde in the presence of NAD$^+$.

- all the intermediate products are phosphoric esters. Not only do they play an important part in the working of kinases and hence in the regeneration of ATP from ADP, but they also play a part in the confinement of these intermediates inside the cells. They cannot, indeed, go through their membranes for solubility reasons. In contrast, glucose and lactate ions are freely soluble in them. If the intermediates could escape from the cells, the rate of glycolysis would be too small for a simple question of kinetics.

6) Fructose and galactose can enter into the glycolytic chain

Fructose and galactose are abundant sugars (Figure 78). Let us recall first that the hydrolysis of saccharose gives a mixture of fructose and glucose and that of lactose gives a mixture of galactose and glucose.

Fructose and galactose can enter into the glycolytic chain.

- fructose enters into glycolytic chain through the formation of fructose-1-phosphate with the aid of fructokinase. Then, the fructose-1-phosphate is cut into two parts: the glyceraldehyde plus the dihydroxyacetonephosphate. Here, again, there is a cleavage by retroaldolisation catalysed

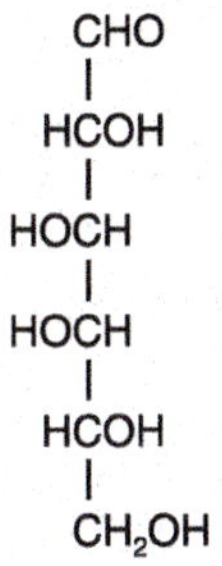

$$
\begin{array}{c}
\text{CHO} \\
| \\
\text{HCOH} \\
| \\
\text{HOCH} \\
| \\
\text{HOCH} \\
| \\
\text{HCOH} \\
| \\
\text{CH}_2\text{OH}
\end{array}
$$

D-Galactose

Figure 78. Linear structure of galactose.

by a specific fructose-1-phosphate aldolase. The glyceraldehyde is then phosphorylated in glyceraldehyde-3-phosphate by a triose kinase. Hence, it can enter into the glycolysis:

$$\text{fructose} \xrightarrow[\text{ATP} \rightarrow \text{ADP}]{\text{fructokinase}} \text{fructose-1-phosphate} \xrightarrow[\text{kinase}]{\text{fructose-1-phosphate}} \begin{array}{c}\text{Glyceraldehyde}\\+\\\text{dihydroxyacetone}\\\text{phosphate}\end{array}$$

$$\xrightarrow[\text{ATP} \rightarrow \text{ADP}]{} \text{Glyceraldehyde} - \text{3-phosphate}$$

Figure 79. Entry of fructose into glycolysis.

• galactose enters through the glycolysis chain once it is transformed into glucose-6-phosphate by a process in four steps. There is first the transformation galactose → galactose-1-phosphate:

$$\text{galactose} + \text{ATP} \xrightarrow{\text{galactokinase}} \text{galactose-1-phosphate} + \text{ADP} + \text{H}^+$$

Secondly, the galactose-1-phosphate reacts with the uridine diphospho-glucose (UDP-glucose) and gives the UDP-galactose and the glucose-1-phosphate. The reaction is catalyzed by the galactose-1-phosphate uridyl transferase.

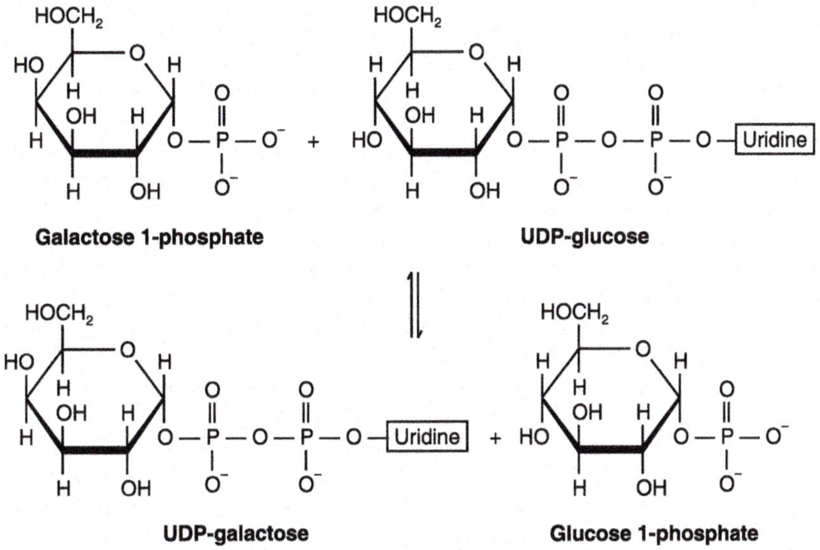

Galactose 1-phosphate   **UDP-glucose**

UDP-galactose   **Glucose 1-phosphate**

Figure 80. Transformation of galactose-1-phosphate into glucose-1-phosphate.

The galactose is actually epimerized during the time it is linked to the UDP. It is the configuration of the hydroxyl group in C4 which is inverted by the UDP galactose-4-epimerase which is linked to NAD^+. NAD^+ is reduced in NADH during the catalysis. NAD^+ probably accepts the hydrogen atom linked to C_4 and a 4-keto intermediary is formed. Then NAD^+ is regenerated while UDP glucose is formed.

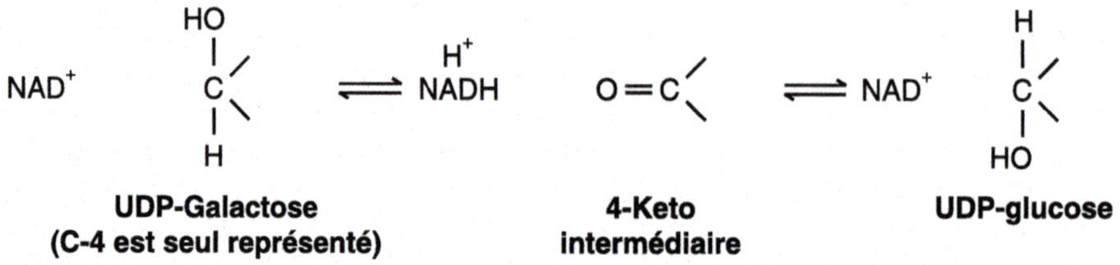

Figure 81. Epimerization UDP galactose → UDP glucose.

Finally, the whole process can be written:

galactose + ATP → Glucose-1-phosphate + ADP + H^+

Finally, the glucose-1-phosphate is isomerized into glucose-6-phosphate by the phosphoglucomutase and so forth.

Chapter 35

The Citric Acid Cycle

In the aerobic glycolysis, the metabolic way was ordered to be stopped when pyruvate ions were formed. We said that, in the aerobic conditions, glycolysis was the prelude of the citric acid cycle. Actually, the entry of pyruvate ions into this metabolic way is its beginning. The citric acid cycle is the final and general way of oxidation of molecules of fuel. It is also named *Krebs' cycle*.

But the energy recovered by oxidation does not stop here. It can be already said that the energy of oxidation is made available during another kind of metabolism involving electron transport and is conserved as phosphate bond energy by the process of *oxidative phosphorylation* (see Chapter 36). The latter comes after the citric cycle.

For the eucaryotes, the reactions of Krebs' cycle occur inside the mitochondries whereas glycolysis occurs in the cytosol.

1) General features of the cycle

The part played by Krebs' cycle is to completely oxidize the acetyl coenzyme A (acetyl-CoA) into CO_2. Before, acetyl-CoA was formed by oxidation and decarboxylation of the pyruvate ion. Krebs' cycle is the final common way of oxidation of the varied molecules of fuel (glucoids, amino-acids, fatty acids) which enter into the cycle through the acetyl-CoA.

There are four dehydrogenation steps in the cycle. As a consequence, there are four pairs of electrons which can be extracted from the intermediary compounds of the cycle.

Describing the process of oxidation of acetyl-CoA as being a cycle is justified by the fact that an ion belonging to the cycle, the oxaloacetate ion COO^-COCH_2COO- (which permits the entry of the fuel into the cycle), is regenerated at the end of the latter.

Krebs' cycle can only accept acetic acid under its "activated" derivative "acetyl coenzyme A: acetyl-CoA" as fuel. Fatty acids, amino-acids and pyruvate-ions (for glucoids) must be converted into acetyl-coenzyme A first. We begin by considering the transformation of ions pyruvate into acetyl-CoA and later by detailing the Krebs' cycle. Later, we shall investigate the transformation of fatty acids and of (some) amino-acid in acetyl-CoA. But, before that, we present a schema of the Krebs' cycle together with some involved structures.

2) Formation of acetyl coenzyme A by starting from pyruvate

Coenzyme A has the structure (Figure 82):

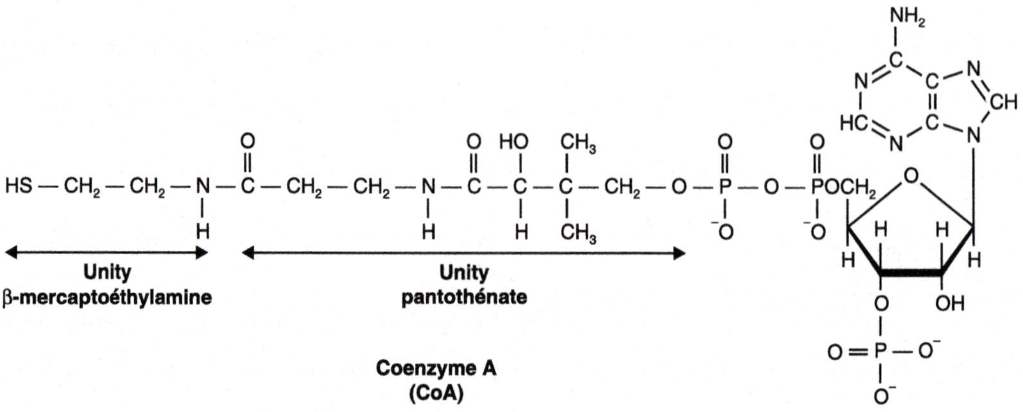

Figure 82. Structure of coenzyme A (HSCoA).

It plays the part of a cofactor in several reactions of acetylation catalyzed by enzymes. Its reactive site is its thiol rest. The group acetyl as well as other acyl groups are linked to HSCoA by a group thioester (see below):

CH_3CO –S - CoA RCO – S - CoA

The standard Gibbs energy of the reaction:

$CH_3COO^- + CoA + H^+ \rightarrow$ acetyl-CoA + H_2O

is:

$\Delta G'^\circ = -31,4$ kJ mol^{-1}

The over-all reaction of formation of acetylcoenzyme A from pyruvate ions is:

pyruvate + CoA + $NAD^+ \rightarrow$ acetyl-CoA + CO_2 + NADH $\Delta G'^\circ = -33,4$ kJ mol^{-1}

It is a redox reaction. NAD^+ oxidizes the pyruvate ion whereas it is reduced itself in NADH. More precisely, it is an oxidative decarboxylation reaction which evolves under the enzymatic action of the *pyruvate dehydrogenase*. The pyruvate dehydrogenase is a complex of three enzyme components (We shall not describe further the mechanism of action mechanism of this enzymatic complex) formed by three kinds of enzymes.

3) The Krebs' cycle

The general scheme of the Krebs' cycle is given in the Figure 83.

4) Some comments

4-1) The first step of the Krebs' cycle—The formation of citrate ion

Citrate ion results from the condensation of oxaloacetate with acetyl-CoA. Recall that the first and the last steps of the Krebs' cycle involve the oxaloacetate ion. Its structure is $COO^-COCH_2COO^-$.

The reaction is (Figure 84).

It is an union of a molecule possessing four carbons (oxaloacetate) with a group possessing two carbons, the rest acetyl, which is brought by acetyl-CoA. *It is an aldol reaction in which there is a nucleophilic addition of the enolate ion derivating from the acetyl group of*

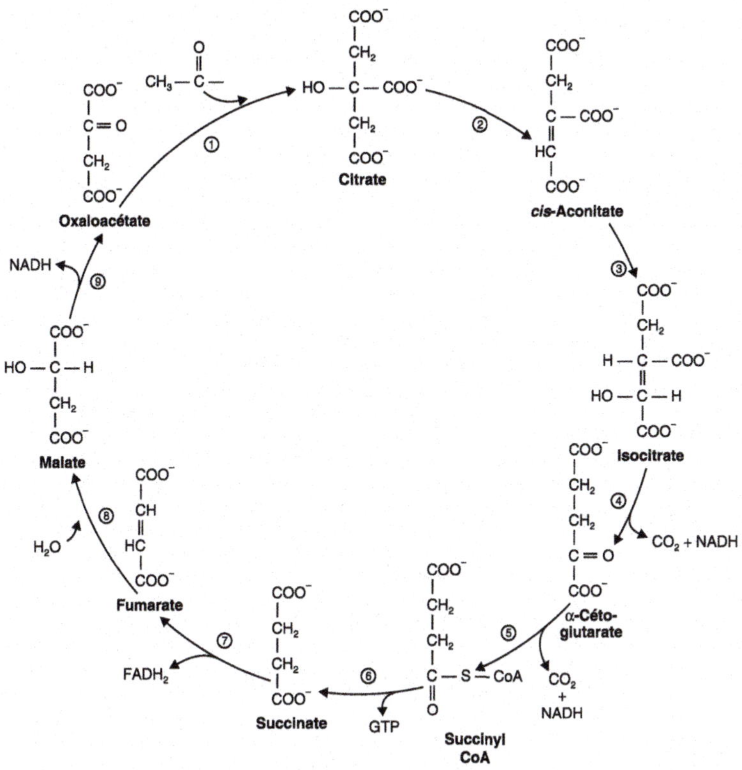

Figure 83. General scheme of the Krebs' cycle.

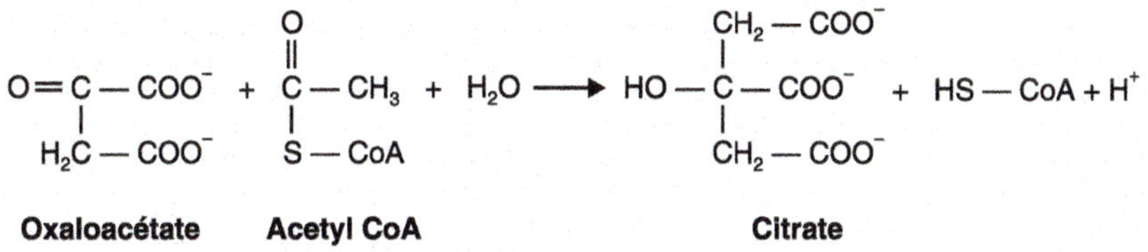

Oxaloacétate   **Acetyl CoA**   **Citrate**

Figure 84. Condensation of oxaloacetate with acetylcoenzyme A.

acetyl-CoA, on the carbonyl of the keto group of oxaloacetate. The reaction is catalyzed by the enzyme *citrate synthase*. This reaction evolves spontaneously: $\Delta G'° = -32,2$ kJ mol^{-1}.

4-2) The isomerization citrate-isocitrate

The next step is the transformation of citrate → isocitrate. The isomerization evolves in two steps: the first is a deshydratation and the second one a hydratation (Figure 85).

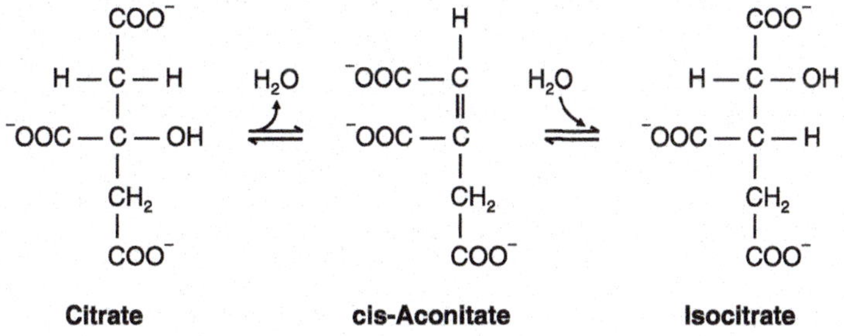

Citrate   **cis-Aconitate**   **Isocitrate**

Figure 85. Isomerization citrate → isocitrate.

The enzyme catalysing the isomerization is the *aconitase* and the reaction involves the *cis-aconitate* as intermediary. The aconitase does contain Fe atoms which are not linked to a heme rest. The mechanism of this deshydratation-hydratation is interesting to study.

The cis-aconitase catalyzes the following reactions:

$$\text{citrate} \quad \underset{H_2O}{\overset{-H_2O}{\rightleftharpoons}} \quad \text{cis-aconitate} \quad \underset{-H_2O}{\overset{H_2O}{\rightleftharpoons}} \quad \text{isocitrate}$$

The cis-aconitate is an unsymmetrical olefine. Therefore, there are two possible orientations for the addition of water. The interesting point is that the configuration of the formed isocitrate (OH and COOH rests placed in threo—see appendix I-4) shows that the elements of water can be added in a trans fashion to the cis-olefine. The equilibrium mixture at pH = 7,4 and at 298 K contains less than 10% isocitrate, but in the cell, the reaction is pulled to the right because isocitrate quickly reacts according the next step. As indicated, the overall-reaction is equilibrated: $\Delta G'^\circ = 6{,}7$ kJ mol L^{-1}.

4-3) Transformation isocitrate $\rightarrow$ α-ketoglutarate

The reaction is an oxidative decarboxylation one. It is (Figure 86):

isocitrate + NAD$^+$ $\rightleftharpoons$ α-ketoglutarate + CO$_2$ + NADH

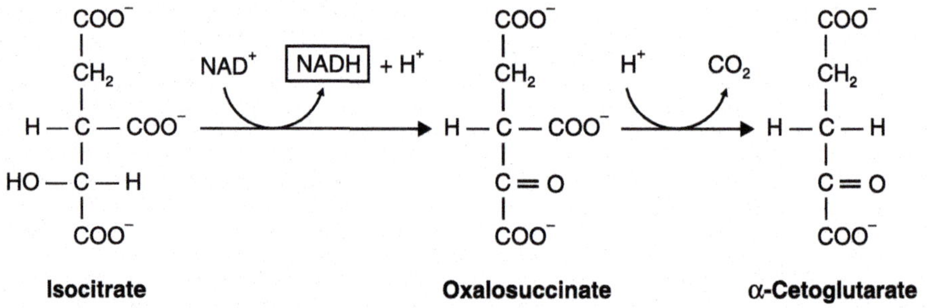

Figure 86. Transformation isocitrate $\rightarrow$ α-ketoglutarate.

The intermediary derivative is the *oxalosuccinate*. As all the other β-ketonic acids, it is unstable because of decarboxylation. It loses a molecule of carbonic anhydride while it is still linked to the reactional enzyme called the *isocitrate deshydrogenase*. We notice that the whole reaction consists in two successive ones. The first is the oxidation of the rest alcohol in a keto group. The second is the decarboxylation. Overall, we notice that through the decarboxylation, there is elimination of a first molecule of CO$_2$. That is, it is already possible to say from the pure balance-sheet viewpoint that one of both carbon atoms of the acetyl group has been eliminated. The reaction is downhill: $\Delta G'^\circ = -8{,}4$ kJ mol l^{-1}.

4-4) Oxidative decarboxylation of α-ketoglutarate in succinylcoenzyme A

This is a second reaction of oxidative decarboxylation of the cycle. The reaction is:

α-ketoglutarate + NAD$^+$ + CoA $\rightarrow$ Succinyl-CoA + CO$_2$ + NADH

The structure of succinyl-CoA is the following one:

$COO^- - CH_2 - CH_2 - CO - S - CoA$

The oxidant is, as usually in this kind of reaction, NAD^+. The reaction is catalyzed by a complex of *α-ketoglutarate deshydrogenase*. The mechanism of this reaction is close to that commanding the transformation pyruvate → acetyl-CoA. The reaction is markedly exergonic: $\Delta G'^\circ = -37,1$ kJ mol^{-1}.

4-5) Transformation of succinyl-CoA into succinate and guanosine triphosphate

The reaction is:

$$\text{succinyl-CoA} + P + GDP \rightleftharpoons \text{succinate} + GTP + CoA \tag{207}$$

P represents a phosphate rest. GDP and GTP represent the guanosine di and triphosphate (Figure 87).

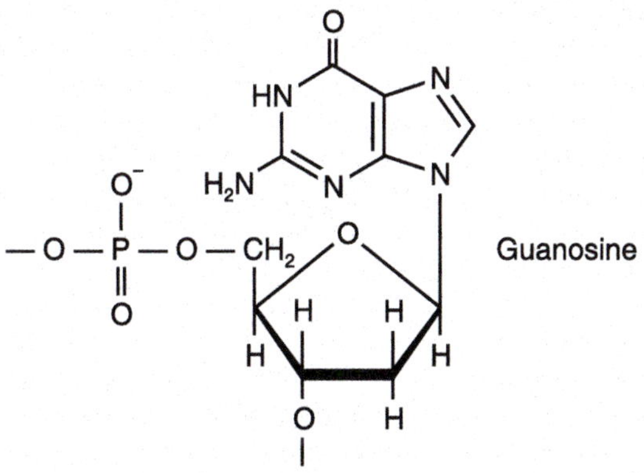

Figure 87. Structures of guanosine di and triphosphate.

The succinylthioester of coenzyme A possesses a rich-energy bond. We have just seen that its Gibbs energy of formation according to the above conditions is of the order of 37 kJ mol^{-1}. The cleavage of the bond thioester of succinyl-coenzyme A is coupled to the phosphorylation of guanosine diphosphate (GDP). Reaction (204) is the sole step of the Krebs' cycle which directly gives a rich-energy phosphate bond. Besides, the following reaction is possible:

$$GTP + ADP \rightleftharpoons GDP + ATP$$

It is catalyzed by the nucleoside diphosphokinase.

4-6) Transformation of succinate to fumarate

The succinate is oxidized in fumarate with the aid of the enzyme succinate deshydrogenase. The acceptor of hydrogen is FAD in place of NAD^+ which is used in the other oxidation reactions of the cycle. FAD is the acceptor of hydrogen when the change of Gibbs energy is not sufficient to reduce NAD^+. FAD is quasi-systematically the acceptor of electrons when the oxidization gets out two hydrogen atoms from a substrate. FAD and $FADH_2$ have the following simplified structures (Figure 88):

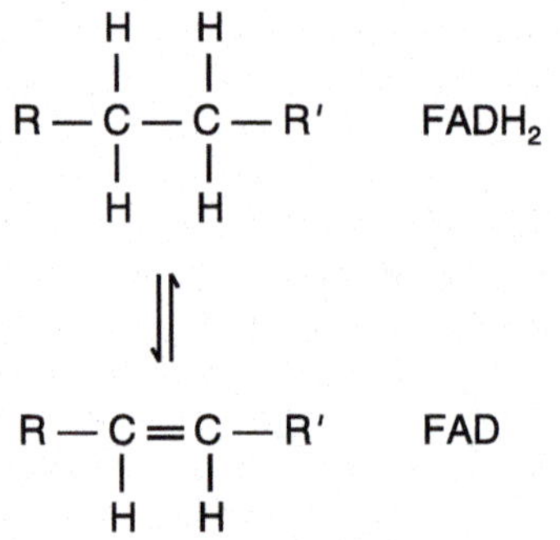

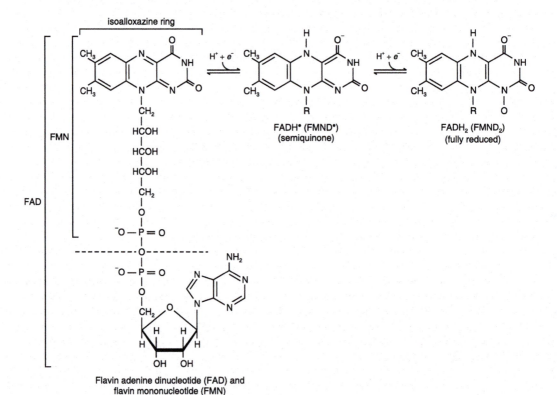

Figure 88. Simplified structures of FAD and of FADH$_2$.

The structure of isoalloxazine is shown in the general formula of FAD (Figure 89):

Figure 89. Structures of alloisoxazine, FMN and FAD.

$$R = -CH_2 (CHOH)_3 CH_2 O PO_3^- AMP$$

In the succinate dehydrogenase itself, the isoalloxazine nucleus of FAD is bond to the lateral chain of an histidine component of the enzyme. The reaction is:

$$\text{enzyme} - \text{FAD} + \text{succinate} \rightleftharpoons \text{enzyme} - \text{FADH}_2 + \text{fumarate} \qquad \Delta G'^{\circ} = 0 \text{ kJ mol}^{-1}$$

The structure of fumaric acid is given in Chapter 26.

4-7) Transformation fumarate → L malate

This is a hydratation reaction.

fumarate + H_2O ⇌ L malate

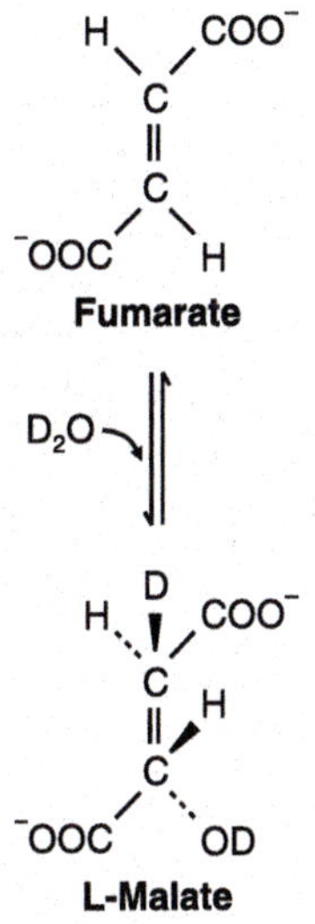

Figure 90. Transformation fumarate → L malate.

The enzyme fumarase catalyzes the stereospecific addition trans of the groups H and OH. The Gibbs energy or the reaction is $\Delta G'^\circ = -3,6$ kJ mol^{-1}.

4-8) Transformation malate → oxaloacetate

The last step of the Krebs' cycle is the regeneration of oxaloacetate by oxidation of malate by NAD^+. The reaction is:

malate + NAD^+ ⇌ oxaloacetate + NADH + H^+

The occurring enzyme is the *malate hydrogenase*. The Gibbs energy is $\Delta G'^\circ = 28,8$ kJ mol^{-1}.

5) The balance-sheet of the citric acid cycle

The balance-sheet of the cycle is given by the reaction:

acetyl-CoA + 3 NAD^+ + FAD + GDP + P + $2H_2O$

→ $2CO_2$ + 3NADH + $FADH_2$ + GTP + $2H^+$ + CoA

It appears, therefore, that:

− two carbon atoms enter into the cycle under the form of a rest acetyl bound to CoA. Acetyl-CoA is condensed with oxaloacetate. But, two carbon atoms leave the cycle, both by decarboxylation. Both decarboxylations correspond to two oxydations;

− the energy released by the latter changes is conserved in the reduction of three NAD^+ and one FAD and there is production of one molecule of ATP (GTP) from the thioester bond, a rich-energy bond of succinyl-CoA;

− two water molecules are also used.

NADH and $FADH_2$ molecules, formed in the citric cycle, are oxidized by the chain of electrons transport (see chapter on oxidative phosphorylation—Chapter 36).

6) Slightly more about citric acid cycle

– The citric acid cycle can provide intermediaries for biosynthesis. Let's confine ourselves to saying that:

* the majority of carbons of porphyrines come from succinyl-CoA,

* that of amino-acids come from α-ketoglutarate and from oxaloacetate.

– the citric acid cycle is controlled. Its rate is regulated in order to be matched to the needs in ATP. All along the cycle, there exist check-points permitting to deceal if the energetic charge is weak or not. Means of regulation are based on allosteric inhibitions of some enzymes and by covalent modifications. The required rates are those granting a stable steady state of cells.

Chapter **36**

Oxidative Phosphorylation–Photosynthesis

The oxidative phosphorylation is the process by which ATP is formed when electrons are transferred from NADH and from $FADH_2$ to dioxygen by a series of electrons carriers. It can be considered as being the last step of the wider process called respiration, the latter being the oxidative breakdown and release of energy from fuel molecules by reaction with dioxygen in aerobic cells. Hence, the oxidative phosphorylation is the principal source of ATP of aerobic organisms.

There are several points in common in the process of oxidative phosphorylation and that of photosynthesis. This is the reason why they are treated in the same chapter.

1) Brief overview

Let us recall that NADH and $FADH_2$ are formed by glycolysis and by the citric cycle. They are also formed by oxidation of fatty acids (see Chapter 39).

The oxidative phosphorylation is carried out in respiratory assemblies located in the internal membrane of the mitochondrion, whereas the citric acid cycle and the oxidization pathway of fatty acids which bring the most part of NADH and $FADH_2$, also treated in the course of the oxidative phosphorylation, are located in the adjacent matrice of the mitochondrion.

We shall see that the oxidation of NADH supplies three molecules of ATP whereas that of $FADH_2$ supplies two ATP. We shall also see that oxidization and phosphorylation are two coupled processes.

The respiratory assemblies contain numerous electrons-carriers such as, for example, the cytochromes.

Oxidative phosphorylation and photophosphorylation exhibit some similarities, although the former takes place in mitochondria and the latter in the chloroplasts. The understanding of the ATP synthesis in both mitochondria and chloroplasts is based on the *chemiosmotic* theory given by P. Mitchell in 1961.

2) Redox potentials and oxidative phosphorylation

The reducing or oxidising power of a redox couple is quantified by its reducing potential measured in volts (see Chapter 27). Its value refers to the following half-redox reaction written according to:

$Oxidant + ne^- \rightleftharpoons Reductant$

When two couple redox are face to face, a global reaction redox may evolve (the term global being quasi-systematically omitted in literature). For its forecasting, we know that the approximative (and not absolute) used rule is the following one (Chapter 27): the direction of the resultant spontaneous redox reaction is such that the oxidant of the couple possessing the highest standard redox potential oxidises the reduced form of the couple which possesses the weakest redox potential. *(The values of the standard redox potentials to consider must be read as algebraic quantities. That is to say for example: the value of the couple NAD$^+$/NADH E'$^\circ$ = –0,32 V is higher than that of the couple acetate/acetaldehyde E'$^\circ$ = –0,60V, although the absolute value of the latter is higher than the other).*

We have already mentioned in Tables 10–12 and appendix I-10 the standard reduction potentials of some biochemical couples.

The standard Gibbs energy change $\Delta G'^\circ$ accompanying a redox reaction can be readily calculated from the values of the standard potentials of both half reduction redox couples E'°_1 and E'°_2 participating in the global reaction. The used equation is:

$$\Delta G'^\circ = -nF\Delta E'^\circ$$

n is the number of exchanged electrons between both couples, F is the faraday and $\Delta E'^\circ$ the difference of standard biological potentials of both reacting couples (see Chapter 27):

$$\Delta E'^\circ = E'^\circ_2 - E'^\circ_1$$

when E'°_2 is higher than E'°_1. The oxidant of couple 2 Ox_2 spontaneously oxidizes the reduced species of couple 1 Red_1. Thus, *in standard conditions*, the spontaneously evolving reaction is:

$$Ox_2 + Red_1 \rightarrow Red_2 + Ox_1$$

We can immediately verify that the reaction is exergonic ($\Delta G'^\circ < 0$).

As an example, let us consider the reaction of pyruvate with NADH. (This is the reaction of the lactic acid fermentation). The biological standard potentials of reduction of the couples are: E'$^\circ$(NAD$^+$/ NADH) = –0,32V and E'$^\circ$ (pyruvate/lactate) = –0,19 V.

$$\Delta E'^\circ = -0,19 - (-0,32) \; volts$$

$$\Delta E'^\circ = 0,13 \; V$$

$$\Delta G'^\circ = -2 \; x \; 0,13 \; x \; 96480 \; J \; mol^{-1}$$

$$= -25,08 \; kJ \; mol^{-1}$$

3) The respiratory chain—the global Gibbs energy

In the respiratory chain, electrons are transferred through three proteic complexes called *NADH-Q reductase, cytochrome reductase* and *cytochrome oxydase* from NADH, succinate or some other primary electrons donors through flavoproteins, ubiquinone, iron-sulfur proteins cytochromes and ultimately until dioxygen (see under—paragraph 5). The respiratory chain is the final common pathway by which all electrons derived from different fuels finally flow to dioxygen. Hence, this flow has several origins. They are the degradations of carbohydrates, fats and amino acids (see Chapter 39).

The thermodynamic cause (origin) of the occurrence of the oxidative phosphorylation is the decline in the Gibbs energy accompanying the whole process. The respiratory chain seems to correspond *globally* to the reaction:

$$NADH + ½ O_2 + H^+ \rightarrow NAD^+ + H_2O \tag{208}$$

It is the oxidation by the dioxygen of the reduced nicotinamide adenine dinucleotide NADH to give the oxidised form NAD^+. One can notice, according to the simple theory of redox reactions, that NADH is the carrier of electrons in the respiratory chain and that dioxygen is their ultimate acceptor. (Actually, the Equation (205) is not accurate—see below). Nevertheless, it is interesting to develop it. The corresponding half redox reactions are:

$$½ O_2 + 2H^+ + 2 e^- \rightarrow H_2O \qquad E'^\circ = +0,82 \ V$$

$$NAD^+ + H^+ + 2 e^- \rightarrow NADH \qquad E'^\circ = -0,32 \ V$$

The standard Gibbs energy accompanying the whole respiratory chain is:

$$\Delta G'^\circ = -2 \times 96480 \times 1,14$$

1,14 is the difference measured in volts between the standard biological reduction potentials of both couples.

$$\Delta G'^\circ = -220 \ kJ \ mol^{-1}$$

The reaction is largely exergonic.

4) The enzymatic complexes and the mobile carriers of electrons involved in the respiratory chain

The electrons are transferred from NADH to dioxygen through three proteic complexes called *NADH-Q reductase*, *cytochrome reductase* and *cytochrome oxydase* (Figure 91).

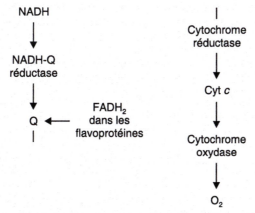

Figure 91. Steps of the electrons' carriers in the respiratory chain.

The electronic flux inside these complexes goes through the internal mitochondrial membrane.

The respiratory chain consists of a series of cytochromes which are electron-transferring enzyme molecules containing colored active groups, called *hemes*. Hemes are complexes of porphyrins and iron. The iron atom of each cytochrome molecule can exist in the ferrous Fe^{2+} or ferric form Fe^{3+} form. Cytochromes differ somewhat chemically. Each cytochrome in its oxidized form can accept an electron and become reduced. This, in turn, can give an electron to the next carrier and so on. With simplification, the chain consists in the following members which occur successively. They are:

- NADH + flavoprotein ox → flavoprotein red + NAD^+,
- a flavoprotein ox,
- the cytochrome b red,
- the cytochrome c red,
- the cytochrome a red.

The electron flow down the chain can be represented by the series of reactions:

NADH + FMN (flavoprotein ox) + H^+ → NAD^+ + FMN H_2 (flavoprotein red)

flavoprotein red + 2 cyt b ox → flavoprotein ox + 2 cyt b red

2 cyt b red + 2 cyt c ox → 2 cyt b ox + 2 cyt c red

2 cyt c red + 2 cyt a ox → 2 cyt c ox + 2 cyt a red

2 cyt a red + 1/2 O_2 → 2 cyt a ox + H_2O

(Notice that cytochromes can carry only one electron at a time).

Electrons enter the chain of cytochromes only *via* one flavoprotein which can accept the electrons from NADH.

5) The last step of the respiratory chain

The stepwise transport of electrons from NADH to O_2 leads to a pumping of protons from the mitochondrial matrice towards its exterior.

The pumping of protons occurs from the matrice of the mitochondria to the "cytosolic face" of the internal mitochondrial membrane. (The term "cytosolic face" names the face of the internal membrane opposite to the matricial border).

The transfers have, for consequence, the pumping of protons towards the outside of the mitochondrial matrice. Transmembranar pH gradient and electrical potential are hence generated. The ATP is synthesized when protons come back into the mitochondrial matrice. They come back through an enzymatic complex.

6) The different steps of the respiratory chain

* The flavine mononucleotide (FMN)—The reduced flavine mononucleotide ($FMNH_2$)—The intermediary semiquinone:

The electrons of NADH enter in the chain at the level of the enzyme NADH-Q reductase (NADH dehydrogenase). Two electrons are transferred from the NADH to the FMN, flavine mononucleotide, prosthetic group of this enzyme. There is formation of the reduced form FMN H_2 (Figure 92)

NADH + H^+ + FMN → FMN H_2 + NAD^+

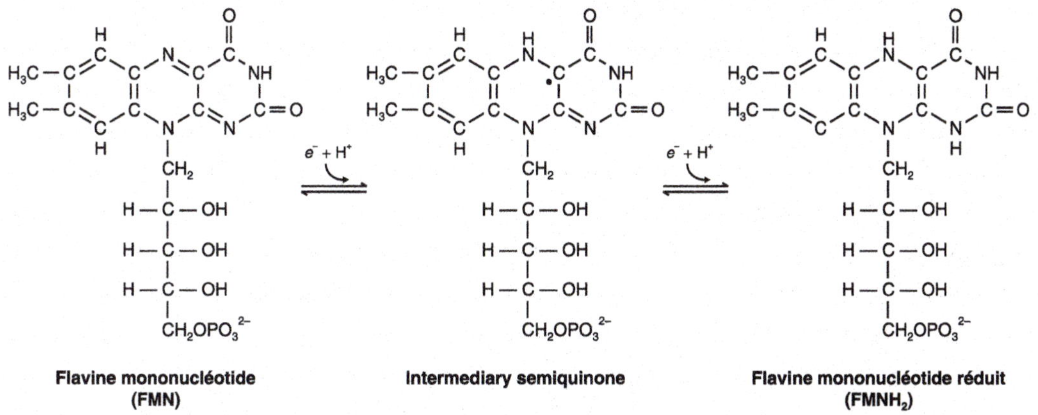

Figure 92. Structure of FMN and $FMNH_2$.

* Iron-sulfur centers. These derivatives constitute a second kind of prosthetic group of NADH deshydrogenase. They are actually simple iron-sulfur proteins. As examples, let us mention that which possesses one iron atom bound to four thiol groups belonging to 4 cysteine rests of the protein. Another contains 2 iron atoms, 2 inorganic sulfur atoms plus 4 cysteine rests. Another one is still more complicated.

* The coenzyme Q or ubiquinone U. Q is a quinone. It possesses a long chain isopren, the number of members of this chain may vary according to the biological species which is considered. Ubiquinone may be reduced by one or two electrons. In the latter case, the obtained derivative is ubiquinol (QH_2) (Figure 93).

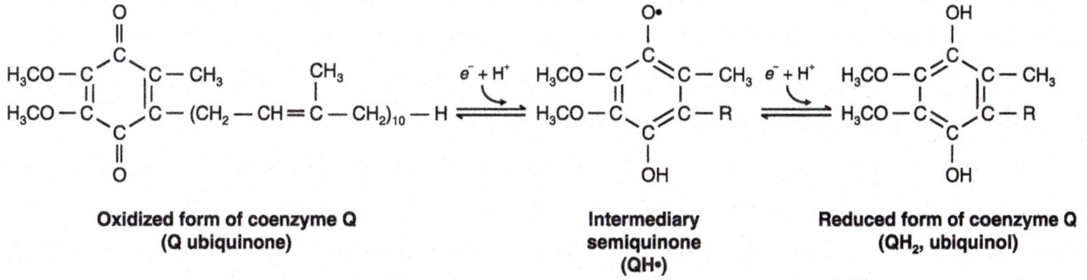

Figure 93. Structures of ubiquinone, the intermediary semiquinone and ubiquinol.

* Derivatives possessing a protoporphyrin ring. For our purpose, these are the cytochromes. These are compounds having a fully conjugated cyclic structure of four pyrrole rings linked together through their 2- and 3-positions by four methine bridges (=CH–).

7) Some comments about the different steps of the respiratory chain

7-1) The electrons of NADH enter into the chain at the level of NADH dehydrogenase. There is a reaction redox between the couples $NAD^+/NADH$ $E'°(NAD^+/NADH) = -0,32V$ and $FMN/FMNH_2 E'°$ ($FAD/FADH_2$) $= -0,22V$. The FMN is the prosthetic group of the NADH deshydrogenase. (A flavin nucleotide is most of the time bound rather tightly to the protein). They do not transfer electrons by diffusing from one enzyme to another. Rather, they provide a means by which they catalyze electron transfer from a reduced substance to an electron

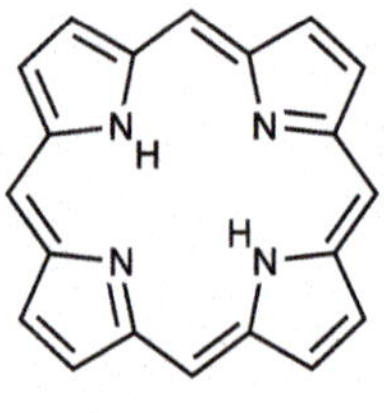

[8]
(94a)

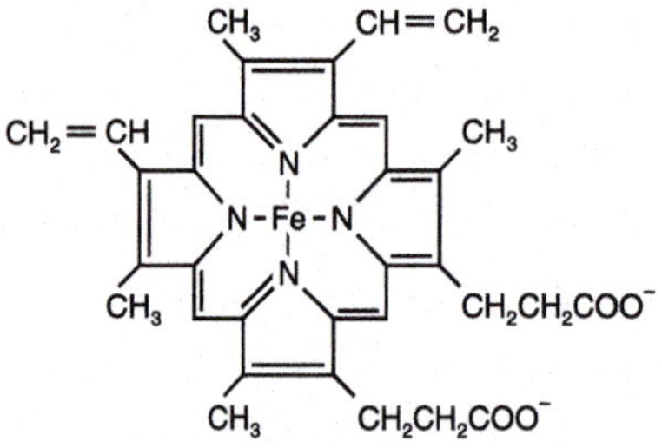

Iron protoporphyrin 1X
(in *b*-type cytochromes)
(94b)

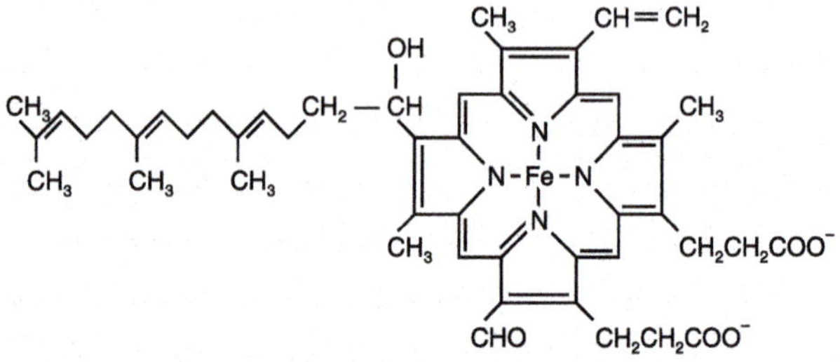

Heme *a*
(in *a*-type cytochromes)
(94c)

Figure 94. Examples of structures of hemes.

acceptor. One important feature of flavoproteins is the variability in the standard reduction potential E'°. Their range values are about –0,40V to +0, 06V. One admits that, in these circumstances, the standard biological redox potential of the couple FMN/FMN H$_2$ allows the following reaction to spontaneously occur:

NADH + H$^+$ + FMN → NAD$^+$ + FMNH$_2$

Concerning the half-reaction defining the couple FMN/FMNH$_2$, it is (see the previous paragraph):

FMN + 2H$^+$ + 2e$^-$ ⇌ FMNH$_2$

- This result is in agreement with the law of thermodynamics. FMN is an oxidant relative to NADH since it has a standard potential of reduction slightly greater than that of the couple NAD$^+$/NADH.

7-2) Then, the electrons are transferred from FMN H$_2$ to a series of aggregates iron-sulfur which constitute the second type of prosthetic group of the NADQ-Q reductase. These aggregates are protein sulfur-iron. Iron atoms in these compounds also participate in redox reactions in which iron "oscillates" between oxidation numbers +2 and +3. One can admit that at the end of this step, the electrons are at a redox potential lower than at the end of the previous step. "The electrons continue to move up to high potentials".

7-3) The electrons in the aggregates Fe-S of the NADH dehydrogenase are then driven to the coenzyme Q also named ubiquinone (see the preceding paragraph). Ubiquinone may be reduced by an electron in the presence of 1 proton or by 2 electrons in the presence of two protons.

(It is interesting to recall that FADH$_2$—the flavin adenine dinucleotide—which is an electron carrier as NAD, is formed during the cycle of citric acid when the succinate ion is oxidised

in fumarate in the presence of the succinate deshydrogenase. The latter is a protein of the internal mitochondrial membrane. The electrons of the formed FADH$_2$ are transferred to the aggregates Fe-S and after to ubiquinone. They enter, through the transfer of electrons into the chain respiratory).

The complex succinate-Q reductase and other enzymes transferring the electrons of FAD H$_2$ to Q are not *protons pumps* (see below); however, the NADH-Q reductase is.

7-4) The second of the three protons that pumps of the respiratory chain is the *cytochrome reductase* also named *ubiquinol-cytochrome c-reductase*. A cytochrome is a protein which transfers electrons. The protein contains an heminic prosthetic group (see the paragraph above). The role of the heminic group is to catalyze the transfer of the electrons of QH$_2$ to the protein c and simultaneously to pump protons from inside the mitochondrial matrice to outside. The protons are pumped through the internal mitochondrial membrane (see the end of this chapter).

7-5) The electrons go from ubiquinol to cytochrome c through the cytochrome reductase. This is the second of the three protons pumps of the respiratory chain. The cytochrome reductase is also-named ubiquinol-cytochrome c-reductase. It contains two kinds of cytochromes, cytochromes b and c1. The reductase also contains a protein Fe-S. The prosthetic group of cytochromes b, c1 and c is the protoporphyrine IX. (The protoporphyrine is one product of the metabolism of the δ-aminolevulinate). The hemes of the cytochromes c and c1 are bound to the protein. It is not the case of those of cytochromes b. The ubiquinol transfers one of its electrons to an aggregate in the reductase. This electron is then sequentially brought to the cytochrome c1 and finally to c. It is transported at a distance from the complex. Following this process, the ubiquinol QH$_2$ is transformed into semi-quinone QH$^\bullet$. The only remaining electron on the semiquinone is transformed according to a reaction of the kind;

$$QH^\bullet + QH^\bullet \rightarrow QH_2 + Q$$

This reaction is a kind of reaction of dismutation.

7-6) The cytochrome oxidase, the third electron pump, catalyzes the transfer of electrons from the reduced cytochrome c to the molecular dioxygen:

$$4 \text{ cyt c} + 4 \text{ H}^+ + O_2 \rightarrow 4 \text{ cyt c} + 2 \text{ H}_2O$$

This is a redox reaction. On the left hand side, the cytochrome c exhibits an oxidation number of +II (Fe^{2+}) whereas on the right it exhibits the state + III (Fe^{3+}). The half redox reactions are:

$$\text{cyt c ox } (+ \text{ III}) + 1 \text{ e}^- \rightleftharpoons \text{ cyt c }_{red(+II)} \qquad E'^\circ = 0,22 \text{ V}$$

$$O_2 + 4e^- + 4 \text{ H}^+ \rightleftharpoons 2 \text{ H}_2O \qquad E'^\circ = 0,82 \text{ V}$$

7-7) The step by step diminution of the electron pressure during the respiratory chain

We present here the successive redox steps of the respiratory chain. In Figure 95, the different steps are located on a scale according to the values of the standard biological potentials of reduction of the corresponding couples.

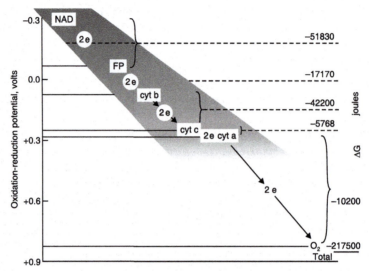

Figure 95. Successive redox steps of the respiratory chain.
(figure reproduced from the book "bioenergetics" by A.L. Lehninger, p. 100, Benjamin Editor, by the courtesy of the Pearson group)

8) The balance sheet of the complete glucose-oxidation

So far, it has not been the question of coupling of electron transport and phosphorylation, that is to say of the conservation of energy as phosphate bond.

Actually, experiments have revealed that both phosphate and ADP are necessary components for obtaining maximum rates of electron transport. *In fact, during the transformation NADH →* O_2*, three molecules of ATP are formed from ADP and phosphate ions.* As a result, the reaction (205) is false. It must be written:

$$NADH + 3 ADP + 3 P + \frac{1}{2} O_2 + H^+ \rightarrow NAD^+ + 3 ATP + H_2O \tag{209}$$

If we sum up all the dehydrogenation steps encountered during the complete respiratory chain of one molecule of glucose up to CO_2 and H_2O, we find 12 steps. The calculation gives that 12 pairs of electrons pass down the whole process of oxidation. We already know that the decline in Gibbs energy accompanying the reaction (see paragraph 3) is $\Delta G'^\circ = -220$ kJ mol^{-1}. As a result, the process of electron transport from NADH to dioxygen accounts for:

$12 \times 220 = 2640$ kJ mol^{-1} per mol of oxidized glucose.

If we recall that the Gibbs energy of combustion of glucose is -2867 kJ mol^{-1}, it appears that almost all the Gibbs energy decrease in the biological oxidation of glucose occurs along the respiratory chain.

9) Coupling oxidation and phosphorylation

The question is now: how are matched oxidation and phosphorylation? As we know, according to the *chimiosmotic hypothesis*, the sequential transfer of electrons of NADH or FADH$_2$ to O_2 and the synthesis of ATP are coupled thanks to a pumping of protons to the outside of mitochondrial matrice. It is due to the occurrence of a pH gradient and of an electrical transmembranar potential. ATP is synthesized when the protons come back into the mitochondrial matrice by passing through an enzymatic complex, the *ATP synthase*. During the first step of the coupling, there is a pumping of protons from the matrice to the outside of the external mitochondrial internal membrane. The proton concentration is higher on its cytosolic face. A transmembranar electrical potential $\Delta\psi$ also appears.

Hence, a protons gradient through the internal mitochondrial membrane is formed during the transfer of the electrons. The transfer of two electrons from NADH through the respiratory chain to molecular dioxygen is highly exergonic ($\Delta G'^\circ = -220$ kJ mol^{-1} in standard conditions). A large part of this energy is used to pump protons out of the matrix. The energy due to the difference in proton concentrations and also due to the separation of charges actually represents the energy temporarily stored which is a part of energy of electron transfer. It is called the *proton-motive force*. Roughly, 200 kJ mol^{-1} of the 220 kJ mol^{-1} are released by oxidation of 1 mol of NADH conserved, thanks to the proton gradient.

When protons flow spontaneously down their gradient, energy is made available to do work. Finally, at the end of the chain, on top of that, there is a remarkable enzyme complex that works by "rotational catalysis". It captures the energy of proton flow in ATP and energy from the regulatory mechanisms that coordinate oxidative phosphorylation with the many catabolic pathways by which fuels are oxidized.

10) Vectorial reaction

The coupling electron transfer/proton gradient introduces a new interesting concept: that is to say that of vectorial reaction. It is somewhat developed in the appendices.

11) Photosynthesis

Photosynthesis is a process which consists in another reaction sequence different from the one in which the flow of electrons is coupled with the synthesis of ATP. This new reaction sequence is coupled itself with light-driven phosphorylation. As it has already been said, there are several points in common between oxidative phosphorylation and photosynthesis.

Photosynthesis in green plants occurs in membranes called *thylakoid membranes* that lie inside chloroplasts (see Chapter 31). As mitochondria (see Chapter 31), chloroplasts possess inner and outer membranes.

Recall that a mitochondria possess two membranar systems, the external and internal ones (see Chapter 31). The structure of the internal membrane is complicated. It is puckered inward in a series of folds called cristae. Therefore, there exist two sorts of compartments. The inner membrane has a much larger area than the outer one. Within the inner compartment, there is a semi-fluid material called the matrix. Mitochondria contain all the enzymes and coenzymes required to carry out the complete oxidation of pyruvate with the complete formation of ATP.

Thylakoid membranes contain the pigment chlorophyll which traps light energy. There are two kinds of chlorophyll, chlorophylls a and b (see Figure 96).

The thylakoid membrane contains several proteins involved in the trapping of light, the transport of electrons, the pumping of protons and other enzymatic reactions. Each of these proteins and protein complexes is oriented in the thylakoid membrane in a specific fashion. Some are located only on one side or on the other **one** of the membrane. Therefore, an asymmetry allowing protons' gradients to occur appears. Here, one finds again the notion of vectorial reaction.

In photosynthesis, the energy of light is trapped by chlorophyll and is used to generate a proton gradient. The latter, in turn, is used to synthesize ATP from ADP and P according to:

$$H^+ + ADP^{3-} + P^{2-} \xrightarrow{\ h\nu\ } ATP^{4-} + H_2O$$

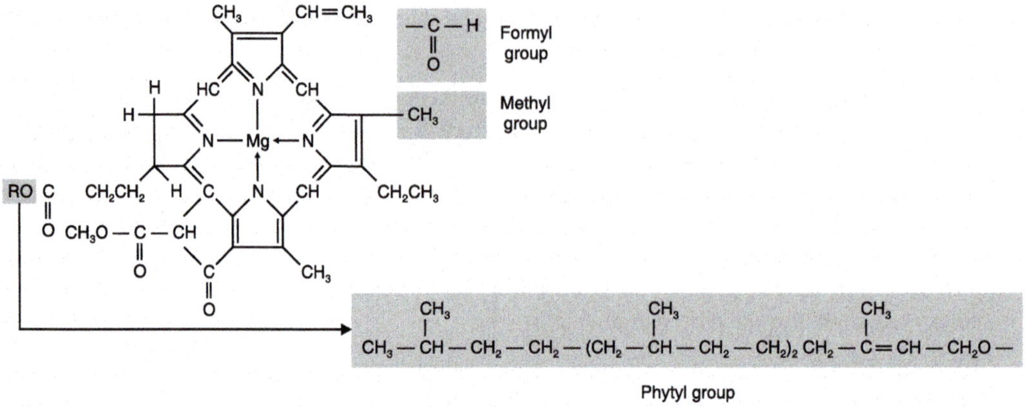

Figure 96. Structures of chlorophylls a and b. In chlorophyll a, the side chain is an ester of phytol. In chlorophyll b, the formyl group replaces the methyl group.

Light energy is also used to split water to form dioxygen and to reduce the oxidized form $NADP^+$ of the electron carrier NADPH:

$$2\ H_2O + 2\ NADP^+ \xrightarrow{h\nu} 2\ H^+ + 2\ NADPH + O_2$$

Notice that this reaction must be coupled with another process because of the redox potential values of the couples $NADP^+/NADPH$ ($E^{\circ'} = -0,32$ V) and $H_2O/O_2,H^+$ ($E^{\circ'} = 0,82$V). This reaction evolving alone, spontaneously, is frankly impossible from the thermodynamic viewpoint.

Once ATP^{4-} and NADPH are formed, they enter in the synthesis of glucose according to the global reaction:

$$6\ CO_2 + 18\ ATP^{4-} + 12\ NADPH + 12\ H_2O \rightarrow C_6H_{12}O_6 + 18\ ADP^{3-} + 18\ P^{2-} + 12\ NADP^+ + 6H^+$$

This global reaction is the resultant of the last two reactions and of the formation of glucose:

$$6CO_2 + 6H_2O \rightarrow C_6H_{12}O_6 + 6O_2$$

qualified for this reason as photosynthetic.

Generation of ATP^{4-} and NADPH is associated with the specialized thylakoid membrane. These membranes contain chlorophylls and enzymes and form closed vesicles which permit the generation of the transmembrane proton gradient used in the synthesis of ATP. Light energy absorbed by the chlorophylls is used to remove electrons from water. These electrons have a very high Gibbs energy content and move through a series of electron carriers located within the thylakoid membrane.

This is why photosynthesis requires the input of energy in the form of light to create a good electron donor at the beginning in the chain (Figure 97).

Light energy absorbed by chlorophylls is used to remove electrons from water. These electrons have a very high Gibbs energy content. They move according to the direction of the respiratory chain through a series of electron carriers located within the thylakoid membrane. At each step, the electrons lose a part of their Gibbs energy. The final acceptor is $NADP^+$ which is reduced to NADPH. The movement of electrons through certain of the carriers is coupled to the pumping of protons across the thylakoid membrane. There is an accumulation of protons within the lumen of the membrane. This results in an accumulation of protons within the lumen of thylakoid (inside

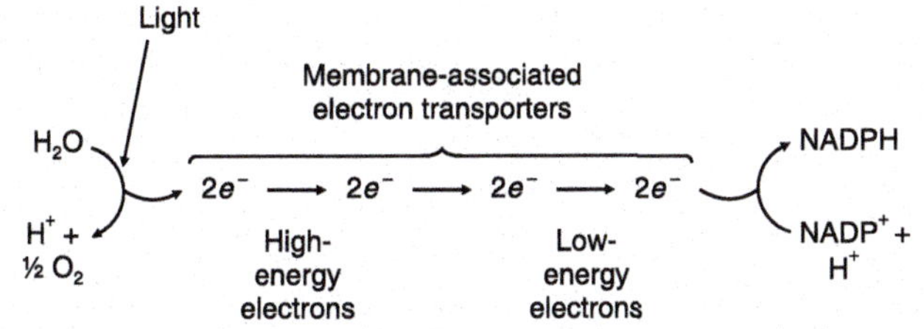

Figure 97. Input of energy in the form of light in the course of photosynthesis.

the vesicle), creating an electrochemical gradient across the thylakoid membrane. As awaited, the proton gradient is the immediate source of energy for ATP synthesis and as in oxidative phosphorylation, movements of protons down their electrochemical gradient are coupled to the synthesis of ATP. This is done in a specialized protein.

The glucose formed in such a manner may be enzymatically converted in other carbon containing components such as cellulose, proteins and lipids. Moreover, some of the newly formed glucose may be oxidized again by plants to CO_2 and H_2O to extract energy, if some need for it is necessary. This is the case at night, when solar energy is not available. During darkness, the carbohydrates, proteins and lipids, which after photosynthesis contain the energy originally derived from sunlight, can then be utilized as foods by cells of the "animal world".

It is chlorophyll which drives the absorbed light energy to *reaction centers*. The light-absorbing pigments of thylakoid membranes are arranged in functional arrays called *photosystems*. All the pigment molecules of a photosystem can absorb photons, but a few chlorophyll associated with the photochemical reaction center can transduce light into chemical energy. The other pigment molecules of a photosystem are called *antenna molecules* or light-harvesting molecules. They absorb light energy and transmit it rapidly and efficiently to the reaction center.

Chapter **37**

The Pentose Phosphates Pathway–Glucogenesis

So far, it was essentially the question of the thermodynamic features of the formation of ATP with glucose as fuel. It was the case of glycolyse, Krebs' cycle, oxidative phosphorylation and of photosynthesis.

Some of the electrons of high reducing potentials (belonging actually to systems possessing strongly negative values of reducing potentials) must be actually conserved for biosynthesis instead of being transferred to dioxygen to form ATP. All these possibilities are respected by the pentose phosphates pathway. The pivotal unity of reduction in cells in this case is NADPH. NADPH is an electron donor (donor of hydride ions) in the reactions of biosynthesis by reduction.

1) An overview of the pentose phosphates pathway

One knows that glucose-6-phosphate has, for major metabolic fate, its glycolytic breakdown to pyruvate followed by oxidization of the latter *via* the citric acid cycle. Finally, it ends by the synthesis of ATP. But glucose-6-phosphate has other catabolic fate. Here, we mention the pentose phosphates pathway.

It consists of two parts. One is an oxidative part, the other being the non-oxidative one. In the oxidative part, NADP$^+$ is the oxidant and is transformed into NADPH. The latter is used to reduce oxidized glutathione GSSG and also does reductive biosynthesis. Another product of the way is ribose-5-phosphate. It is a precursor for nucleotides, coenzymes and nucleic acids (Figure 98).

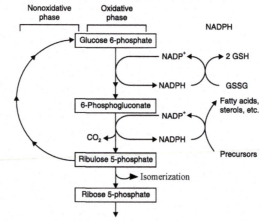

Figure 98. Other catabolic fates of glucose-6-phosphate than its glycolytic breakdown.

There also exists a nonoxidative phase which contributes to the interconversion of sugars possessing three, four, five, six and seven carbons. It allows continued production of NADPH and converting glucose-6-phosphate into CO_2.

2) The pentose-phosphates pathway

2-1) Oxidative phase of the pentose phosphates pathway

In the pentose phosphates pathway, NADPH is formed when glucose-6-phosphate is oxidized to ribulose-5-phosphate in the oxidative part. The consecutive reactions are:

- glucose-6-phosphate + NADP$^+$ → 6-phosphoglucono-δ-lactone + NADPH + H$^+$

Recall that NADPH is the reduced form of the *nicotinamide adenine dinucleotide phosphate* the structure of which is:

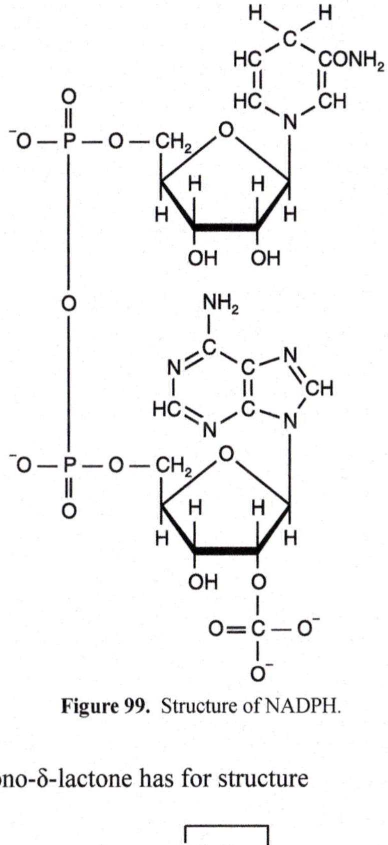

Figure 99. Structure of NADPH.

The 6-phosphoglucono-δ-lactone has for structure

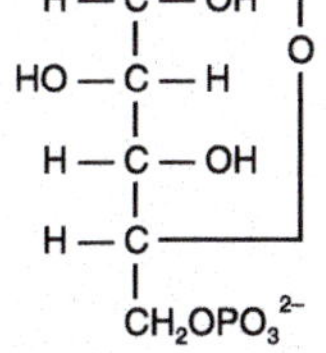

6-Phosphoglucono-δ-lactone

Figure 100. Structure of 6-phosphoglucono-δ-lactone.

The enzyme catalyzing the reaction is the *glucose-6-phosphate dehydrogenase.*

- The lactone is hydrolyzed to the acid-6-phosphogluconate under the action of a specific *lactonase* (Figure 101):

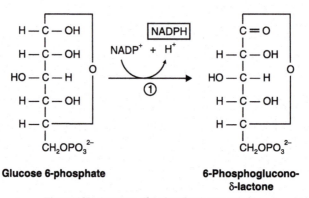

Glucose 6-phosphate   **6-Phosphoglucono-δ-lactone**

Figure 101. Structure of 6-phosphogluconate acid.

- Then, the 6-phosphogluconate acid undergoes oxidation and decarboxylation. The keto-pentose ribulose-5-phosphate is formed under the action of the enzyme *6-phosphogluconate dehydrogenase.* It is interesting to notice that, then, there is formation of a second molecule of NADPH (Figure 102):

6-phosphogluconate dehydrogenase

6-phosphogluconate acid $\longrightarrow$ D-ribulose-5-phosphate

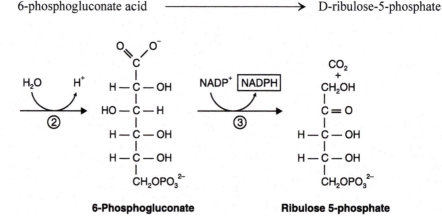

6-Phosphogluconate   **Ribulose 5-phosphate**

Figure 102. Formation of ribulose-5-phosphate.

2-2) Nonoxidative phase of the phosphopentose pathway

At this point, one considers that the oxidative phase of the pentose phosphates pathway is finished and that the nonoxidative one begins. In the non-oxidative phase, the isomerization ribulose-5-phosphate → ribose-5-phosphate occurs and the produced pentose phosphates in the oxidative phase are recycled in glucose-6-phosphate.

- The reaction ribulose-5-phosphate → ribose-5-phosphate evolves through an intermediary enediol as evolve the isomerizations glucose-6-phosphate → fructose-6-phosphate and dihydroyacetone phosphate → glyceraldehyde-3-phosphate.

The isomerization ribulose-5-phosphate ribose-5-phosphate is done through the intermediary of the *phosphopentose isomerase*. The ribose-5-phosphate is a precursor for nucleotide synthesis. These isomerizations ketose-aldose evolve through an intermediary which is an enediol (Figure 103).

$$
\begin{array}{ccc}
H_2C-OH & H-C-OH & O\diagdown{}^H\!/C \\
| & \parallel & | \\
C=O & C-OH & H-C-OH \\
| & | & | \\
H-C-OH \rightleftharpoons & H-C-OH \rightleftharpoons & H-C-OH \\
| & | & | \\
H-C-OH & H-C-OH & H-C-OH \\
| & | & | \\
H_2C-OPO_3^{2-} & H_2C-OPO_3^{2-} & H_2C-OPO_3^{2-}
\end{array}
$$

Ribulose   **Énediol**   **Ribose**
5-phosphate   **intermédiaire**   **5-phosphate**

Figure 103. Isomerization ribulose-5-phosphate → ribose-5-phosphate.

- Recycling pentose phosphates produced in the oxidative phase in glucose-6-phosphate are carried out by several steps.

- Firstly, there is epimerization of ribulose-5-phosphate in xylulose-5-phosphate:

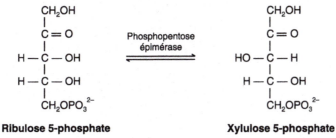

Ribulose 5-phosphate   **Xylulose 5-phosphate**

Figure 104. Epimerization ribulose-5-phosphate → xylulose-5-phosphate.

This transformation is catalyzed by the *ribulose-5-phosphate epimerase*.

* Secondly, a series of rearrangements is carried out under the influence of two specific enzymes: the *transketolase* and the *transaldolase*. (Here the interconversions between sugars of different lengths actually begin).

The enzyme *transketolase* catalyzes the transfer of the two carbon fragment from a ketose donor to an aldose acceptor. Hence, the transferred group by the transketolase is:

$$
\begin{array}{c}
CH_2OH \\
| \\
C=O \\
|
\end{array}
$$

Figure 104'. Group transferred by a transketolase.

For example, the xylulose-5-phosphate reacts with ribose-5-phosphate to give the glyceraldehyde-3-phosphate and the sedoheptulose-7-phosphate under the action of the transketolase (Figure 105):

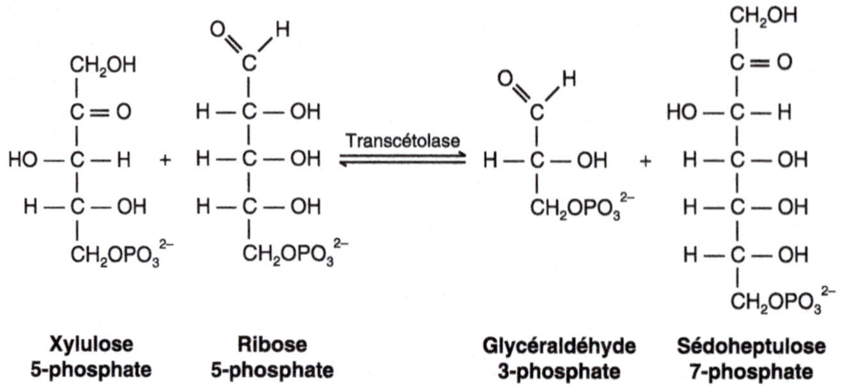

Figure 105. An example of action of transketolase.

Concerning this reaction, an interesting point must be noticed: one ketose is a substrate of the transketolase if, and only if, its hydroxyl group in C3 possesses the configuration of xylulose and not that of ribulose.

The enzyme *transaldolase* catalyzes the transfer of the group (3 carbons) to an aldose:

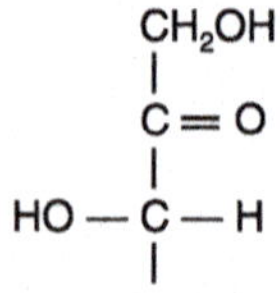

Figure 105'. Group transferred by a transaldolase.

The reaction of sedoheptulose-7-phosphate with glyceraldehyde-3-phosphate gives an example of such a transfer (Figure 106):

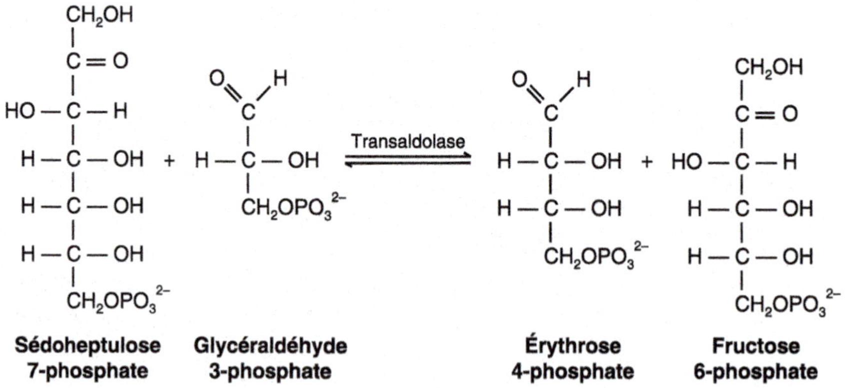

Figure 106. Example of a reaction catalyzed by a transaldolase.

Finally, the fructose-6-phosphate together with glyceraldehyde-3-phosphate are formed through the reaction:

xylulose-5-phosphate + erythrose-4-phosphate $\rightleftharpoons$

fructose-6-phosphate + glyceraldehyde-3-phosphate

2-3) Balance-sheets of the phosphopentose pathway

Concerning the reaction of formation of ribose-5-phosphate from glucose-6-phosphate it evolves through the formation of ribulose-5-phosphate as an intermediary. It is clear that the reaction glucose-6-phosphate $\rightarrow$ ribulose-5-phosphate is a redox one. The glucose-6-phosphate is oxidized by NADP$^+$ which is the oxidized form of the couple NADP$^+$/NADPH. The half-redox reaction is:

$$\text{NADP}^+ + \text{H}^+ + 2e- \rightarrow \text{NADPH} \quad E'^\circ = -0,324 \text{ V}$$

NADP$^+$ is the electron acceptor. The global reaction is:

glucose-6-phosphate + 2 NADP$^+$ + H_2O $\rightarrow$

ribulose-5-phosphate + CO_2 + 2NADPH + 2 H$^+$

Now, concerning the recycling of the hexose-6-phosphates we can write:

3 ribose-5-phosphate $\rightleftharpoons$ 2 fructose-6-phosphate

+ glyceraldehyde-3-phosphate

or

2 xylulose-5-phosphate + ribose-5-phosphate $\rightleftharpoons$

+ 2 fructose-6-phosphate + glyceraldehyde-3-phosphate

3) Neoglucogenesis

Neoglucogenesis is a pathway which converts pyruvate and related three or four-carbon compounds to glucose. Neoglucogenesis is essential since the supplies of glucose from its natural stores are not always sufficient even in physiological conditions, for example, after a vigorous exercise. Neoglucogenesis occurs in all animals, plants, fungi and microorganisms. The reactions are essentially the same in all species and in all tissues.

The important precursors of this process in animals are three-carbon compounds such as pyruvate, lactate, glycerol as well as certain amino-acids. The neoglucogenesis pathway may be summarized by the process:

gluconeogenesis

pyruvate $\xrightarrow{\hspace{3cm}}$ glucose

The non-glucidic precursors enter into this pathway essentially under the form of pyruvate, oxaloacetate and of dihydroxyacetone phosphate. The principal non glucidic precursors are the lactate ions, some amino acids and the glycerol. Lactate ions are formed in squelettic muscles while they are working and when the rate of glycolysis is higher than those of the metabolic cycle of citric acid and of the respiratory chain. Amino acids come from the proteins of the alimentation. The glycerol is a precursor of glucose but animals cannot transform fatty acids in glucose.

As a rule, given the facts that in the glycolysis the glucose is transformed into pyruvate and that during the neoglucogenesis the pyruvate is transformed in glucose, one would imagine that the neoglucogenesis is exactly the inverse of glycolysis. It is not the truth.

It cannot be the truth from the standpoint of pure thermodynamics. The change of Gibbs energy accompanying the global process of glycolysis is:

glucose $\longrightarrow$ pyruvate ions $\Delta G \approx -84$ kJ mol^{-1}

(usual conditions of concentrations)

The most part of the Gibbs energy decline comes from the following three reactional steps which are quasi-irreversible:

hexokinase
glucose + ATP $\longrightarrow$ glucose-6-phosphate + ADP

phosphofructokinase
fructose-6-phosphate + ATP $\longrightarrow$ fructose-1,6-diphosphate + ADP

pyruvate kinase
phosphoenolpyruvate + ADP $\longrightarrow$ pyruvate + ATP

In the neoglucogenesis, these quasi-irreversible reactions are replaced by the following ones:

- the phosphoenolpyruvate formation from the pyruvate through that of oxaloacetate as intermediary. The pyruvate is firstly carboxylated in oxaloacetate at the expense of ATP. The oxaloacetate is then decarboxylated and phosphorylated giving the phosphoenolpyruvate at the expanse of a second energy-rich bond:

pyruvate + CO_2 + ATP + H_2O → oxaloacetate + ADP + P + 2 H$^+$

oxaloacetate + GTP $\rightleftharpoons$ phosphoenolpyruvate + GDP + CO_2

The first reaction is catalyzed by the pyruvate carboxylase and the second by the phosphoenolpyruvate carboxykinase. The sum of these reactions is:

pyruvate + ATP + GTP + H_2O → phosphoenolpyruvate + ADP + GDP + P + 2H$^+$

This formation in two steps of the phosphoenolpyruvate by starting from the pyruvate is possible from the thermodynamic viewpoint because $\Delta G'^\circ$ is +0,84 kJ mol^{-1} whereas the reaction catalyzed by the pyruvate kinase is +31,4 kJ mol^{-1}. Hence, the far more reasonable value +0,84 kJ mol^{-1} results from the addition of a supplementary rich-energy phosphate bond.

- the fructose-6-phosphate formation, starting from fructose-1,6-bisphosphate by hydrolysis of the ester phosphate in C(1). The fructose-1,6-biphosphatase catalyzes this exergonic hydrolysis;

- the glucose formation by the hydrolysis of the glucose-6-phosphate by a reaction catalyzed by the glucose-6-phosphatase:

glucose-6-phosphate + H_2O → glucose + P

The glucose-6-phosphate is transported by a specific proteinic carrier from the cytosol to the reticulum endoplasmic where it is hydrolyzed by the glucose-6-phosphatase, enzyme linked to the membrane. The glucose and phosphate come back to the cytosol. The glucose-6-phosphatase is not present in the brain and in the muscle and, hence, the glucose cannot be formed by these organs.

The following table summarizes the differences in enzymes working in glycolysis and neoglucogenesis:

Table 16. Differences in enzymatic systems of glycolysis and neoglucogenesis processes.

glycolysis	neoglucogenesis
hexokinase	glucose-6-phosphatase
phosphofructokinase	fructose-1,6-bisphophatase
pyruvate kinase	pyruvate carboxylase
	phosphoenolpyruvate carboxykinase

The stoichiometries of the reaction of neoglucogenesis and of the reaction inverse of glycolysis (whole process) are respectively:

$$2 \text{ pyruvate} + 4 \text{ ATP} + 2 \text{ GTP} + 2 \text{ NADH} + 6 \text{ H}_2\text{O} \rightarrow$$

$$\text{glucose} + 4 \text{ ADP} + 2 \text{ GDP} + 6 \text{ P} + 2 \text{ NAD}^+ + 2 \text{ H}^+ \qquad \Delta G'^\circ = -38 \text{ kJ mol}^{-1}$$

and

$$2 \text{ pyruvate} + 2 \text{ ATP} + 2 \text{ NADH} + 2 \text{ H}_2\text{O} \rightarrow$$

$$\text{glucose} + 2 \text{ ADP} + 2 \text{ P} + 2 \text{ NAD}^+ \qquad \Delta G'^\circ = +84 \text{ kJ mol}^{-1}$$

Six energy rich phosphate bounds are used in order to synthesize the glucose when starting from pyruvate in neoglucogenesis whereas only two are formed in glycolysis for the conversion of glucose in pyruvate. The supplementary cost of the neoglucogenesis is, hence, of four energy-rich phosphate bonds per glucose molecule synthesized from pyruvate.

Chapter **38**

The Chemical Work of Biosynthesis

Before studying the metabolisms of the different kinds of fuel molecules encountered in the different metabolic chains, it is useful to recall the biosynthesis of compounds which are transformed into them.

Biosynthesis is an active and dynamic process. It takes place in all types of cells. It involves a chemical work necessary to build the cellular components from small building-blocks which are precursor molecules. Not only does this work involve the formation of characteristic chemical components of cells from simple precursors, it also includes their assembly into what can be qualified as being "suprastructures", such as membranes, mitochondria, nuclei, and ribosomes. The synthesis of suprastructures are in the realm of the supramolecular chemistry. Of course, once a chemical work is involved, chemical thermodynamics are just around the corner! This is the reason why we decided to incorporate chapters devoted to biosynthesis into the book. In this chapter, we begin by considering the biosynthesis of polysaccharides. After that, we deal with the biosynthesis of a kind of lipids, the triacylglycerols and that of amino-acids. We end with some elements devoted to the supramolecular chemistry.

1) Some generalities about biosynthesis

Biosynthesis has not only the mission to build cellular components together with their corresponding suprastructures but it also has it also aims at multiplying because they have no control over their environment and self-multiplying is a means for them to survive.

The principal steps of cellular biosynthesis are:

simple $\rightarrow$ building $\rightarrow$ major biochemical $\rightarrow$ Supramolecular $\rightarrow$ cell

    precursors   blocks   molecules   structures

The rate of growth of cells varies greatly. As an example, some bacterial cells can make over 1000 molecules of cell-proteins per second from their component amino-acids. This is equivalent to the creation of about 500 peptide bonds between its amino-acids, which, furthermore, must be linked in a determined order! In plants and animals, cells grow much more slowly than in the bacteria.

Another aspect of biosynthesis is the fact that some cells which do not grow in mass may be, however, cells in which biosynthetic work takes place. In these cells, all their components (lipids, proteins, polysaccharides, etc.) are built up and broken down continuously in such a way that the rate of their synthesis equals that of their breakdown. We know that the system is in a steady state (see Chapter 24).

2) Thermodynamic aspects of biosynthesis

Each chemical reaction goes to completion with a definite heat of reaction in well-definite reactional conditions (see Chapter 7). It is quantitatively related to the number of reacting molecules. This fundamental property has led to the notion of bond energies which exhibit some constancy for a given bond in analogous conditions. Of course, this property is essentially statistical but it may be very useful. Table 17 mentions heats of combustion of some cellular fuels.

Table 17. Heats of combustion of some cellular fuels. In A.L. Lehninger, "Bioenergetics", Ed. W.A. Benjamin, Inc, 1965, New York.

Fuel	Molecular weight	ΔH J.mol^{-1}
Carbohydrate — D-glucose	180	−2813140
lactic acid	90	−1362680
Lipids — palmitic acid	256	−9948400
tripalmitin	809	−31391,800
Amino acids — glycine	75	−978120

Table 18 mentions typical enthalpy changes of some chemical reactions.

Table 18. Enthalpy changes of some chemical reactions. In A.L. Lehninger "Bioenergetics", W.A. Benjamin, INC, New York, 1965 "Bioenergetics", W.A. Benjamin, INC, New York, 1965.

Enthalpy Changes of Some Representative Chemical Reactions

Type	ΔH cal/mole	J.mol^{-1}
Oxidation		
glucose + 6 O_2 → 6 CO_2 + 6 H_2O	−673,000	−2813140
Hydrolysis		
sucrose + H_2O → glucose + fructose	−4,800	−20064
glucose 6-phosphate + H_2O → glucose + H_3PO_4	−3,000	−12540
Neutralization		
NaOH + HCl → NaCl + H_2O	−13,800	−57684
Ionization		
CH_3COOH + H_2O → CH_3COO^- + H_3O^+	+1,150	+4807
$^+NH_3CH_2COOO^-$ + H_2O → $NH_2CH_2COO^-$ + H_3O^+	+10,806	+45169

We have already seen the possibilities of calculations offered by this property which is a direct consequence of the first principle (Chapters 7 and 8).

Other interesting thermodynamic aspects for our purpose are related to the second principle. There are two important aspects which must retain attention in the thermodynamics of the cellular biosynthesis.

It is the fact that the formation of a large macromolecule from many small molecules (precursors) is a process which is accompanied by a large decrease in entropy. It is, indeed, clear that a system composed by several molecules of precursors is characterized by more disorder than the same system whose same small molecules are agglomerated in only one. They are, for example, the cases of one solution containing a large molecule of glycogen and of another containing one molecule of protein once they are formed compared to solutions, respectively containing molecules of glucose or amino-acids. The case of the protein is all the more striking because an excess order is obligatorily present once the protein is formed compared with the solution containing the molecule of glycogen. The molecules of amino-acids are not, indeed, incorporated into the chain of a protein at random whereas it is the case of glucose molecules in the chains of glycogen. For the second aspect and in the same order of ideas, the fact that all the reactions take place in dilute aqueous solutions must not be forgotten. This condition of dilution is not in favor of the formation of the chemical linkages of the building-blocks for the same entropic reason as above.

Living cells use the chemical energy of ATP to perform the chemical work of biosynthesizing cellular components from precursor molecules. They use the common intermediate principle. We have seen that this principle makes possible the conservation of oxidation-reduction energy as the phosphate bond energy of ATP. Recall, for example, the formation of sucrose from glucose and fructose (Chapter 33). Glucose-1-phosphate is formed by the enzymatic transfer of a phosphate group from ATP to glucose. The bond between glucose and phosphate has about the same Gibbs energy of hydrolysis as the glucosidic bond which links fructose and glucose in sucrose. Once formed, glucose-1-phosphate reacts enzymatically with fructose to produce sucrose. The latter is readily formed. The overall reaction is downhill. Its $\Delta G'$ is frankly negative ($\Delta G' = -6270$ J mol^{-1}):

ATP + glucose $\rightarrow$ ADP + glucose-1-phosphate

glucose-1-phosphate + fructose $\rightarrow$ sucrose + phosphate

The overall reaction is:

ATP + Glucose + fructose $\rightarrow$ sucrose + ADP + phosphate

Hence, the chemical energy of ATP is used to cause the coupled synthesis of sucrose through the common intermediate glucose-1-phosphate. The same principle is used in all other biosynthetic reactions in which building blocks are linked in condensation reactions.

It is important to notice that the presence of common intermediate is an essential condition because the transfer of Gibbs energy cannot be done as it is the case with heat, that is to say by the direct transfer of heat itself. It can only be done through the transfer of a chemical group bringing a certain value of Gibbs energy.

3) Biosynthetic reactions resulting from a loss of a pyrophosphate rest

Many biosynthetic reactions for which ATP provides the driving force do not proceed by the loss of a single terminal phosphate rest but, rather, by the loss of the two terminal phosphate groups of ATP under the form of one piece, that is to say under the form of pyrophosphate rest.

After the loss of pyrophosphate, ATP "remains" as AMP. Both following equations stress the differences between the two processes:

"orthophosphate cleavage"

$$A - B - P \sim P \sim P \quad \rightarrow \quad A - B - P \sim P \quad + \quad P$$
$$\qquad \text{ATP} \qquad\qquad\qquad \text{ADP} \qquad\qquad \text{phosphate}$$

"pyrophosphate cleavage"

$$A - B - P \sim P \sim P \quad \rightarrow \quad A - B - P \quad + \quad P \sim P$$
$$\qquad \text{ATP} \qquad\qquad\qquad \text{AMP} \qquad\qquad \text{pyrophosphate}$$

In these equations, the symbol ~ means a "high energy" bond and A-B is the molecule support. The standard Gibbs energy changes are about the same for the two kinds of hydrolysis, since:

$$ATP^{4-} + H_2O \rightarrow ADP^{3-} + P^{2-} + H^+ \qquad \Delta G^{\circ\prime} \approx -30,5 \text{ kJ mol}^{-1}$$

$$ATP^{4-} + H_2O \rightarrow AMP^{2-} + P \sim P^{3-} + H^+ \qquad \Delta G^{\circ\prime} \approx -30,5 \text{ kJ mol}^{-1}$$

$$ATP^{4-} + 2 H_2O \rightarrow AMP^{2-} + 2 P^{2-} + 2H^+ \qquad \Delta G^{\circ\prime} = -61,0 \text{ kJ mol}^{-1}$$

Pyrophosphate cannot be used by the cell for the direct phosphorylation of ADP during glycolysis or oxidative phosphorylation. It must be first hydrolyzed to orthophosphate. This is done enzymatically by *pyrophosphatase*:

$$P \sim P^{4-} + H_2O \rightarrow 2HPO_4^{2-}$$

The enzymatic hydrolysis of pyrophosphate is accompanied by a large negative Gibbs energy change, pyrophosphate being a "high energy" phosphate compound. Hence, after pyrophosphate cleavage and after hydrolysis of the liberated pyrophosphate, there is hydrolysis of two high-energy phosphate bonds of ATP. As a result of this latter process, there is a stronger thermodynamic pull in favor of such coupled reactions than with only a phosphate cleavage.

4) Channelling of ATP energy via other triphosphates

Nearly all cells contain many phosphate derivatives other than ATP, ADP and AMP. Their structures and functions are very similar to those of ATP. They participate in the channeling and transfer of the phosphate bond energy. They belong to two series of compounds: those derivating from ribonucleoside-5'-triphosphates and those deriving from deoxyribonucleoside-5'-triphosphates.

Ribonucleoside-5'-triphosphates are identical to ATP except for the fact that the adenine ring of ATP is replaced by the purine guanine or by the pyrimidines uracil or cytosine. The structures of these derivatives are given in Figures 107 and 108.

The structures of some deoxyribonucleoside-5'-triphosphates are given in Figure 108. In this series, the ribose of ATP is replaced by the 2-deoxyribose.

ATP is the mainline vehicle of transfer of bond energy whereas all the other nucleoside-5'-triphosphates together with the deoxynucleoside-5'-triphosphates are derivatives, the functioning of which is to channel ATP energy into *different* biosynthetic pathways. Hence, for example, ATP, GTP, UTP and CTP are involved in the biosynthetic work of RNA whereas dATP, dGTP, dTTP and dCTP are involved in that of DNA and so forth.

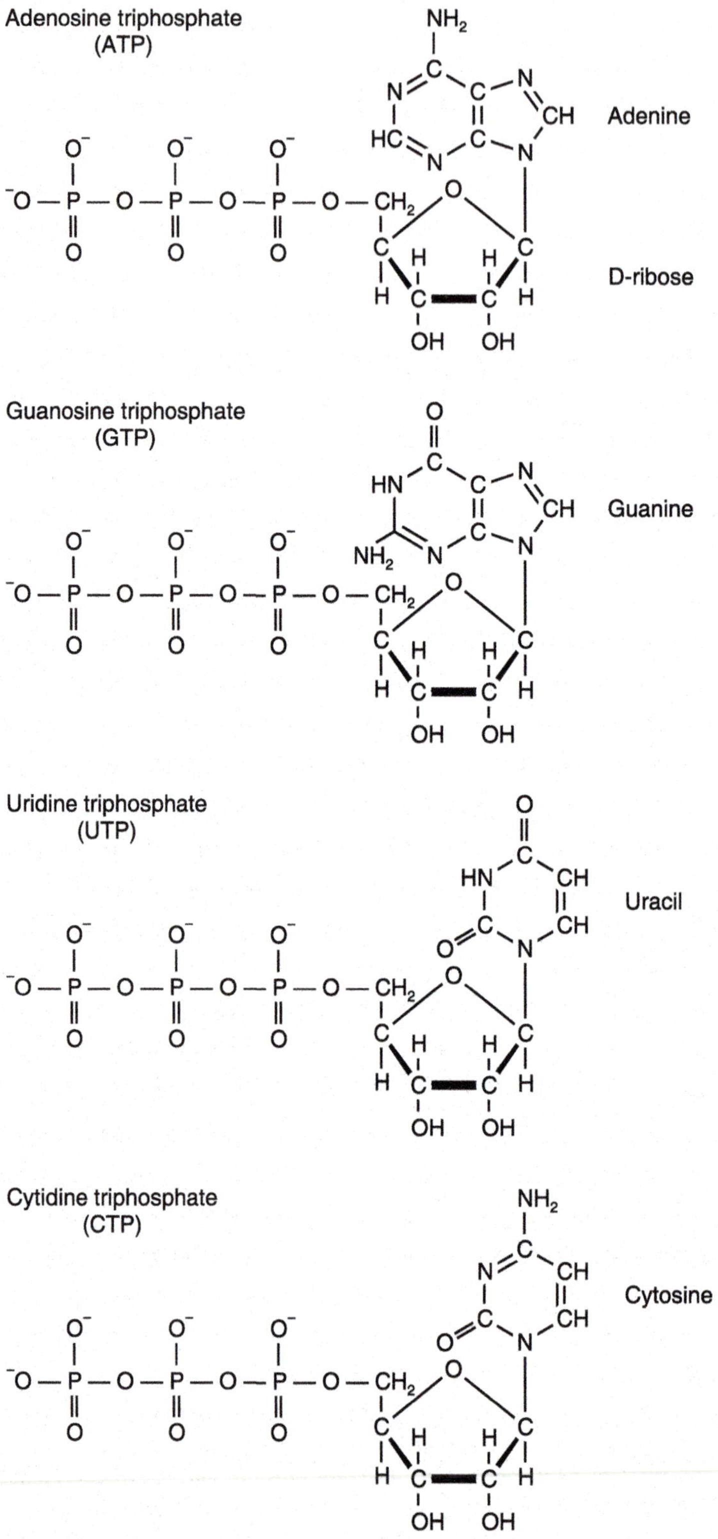

Figure 107. Structures of some ribonucleoside-5'-triphosphates.

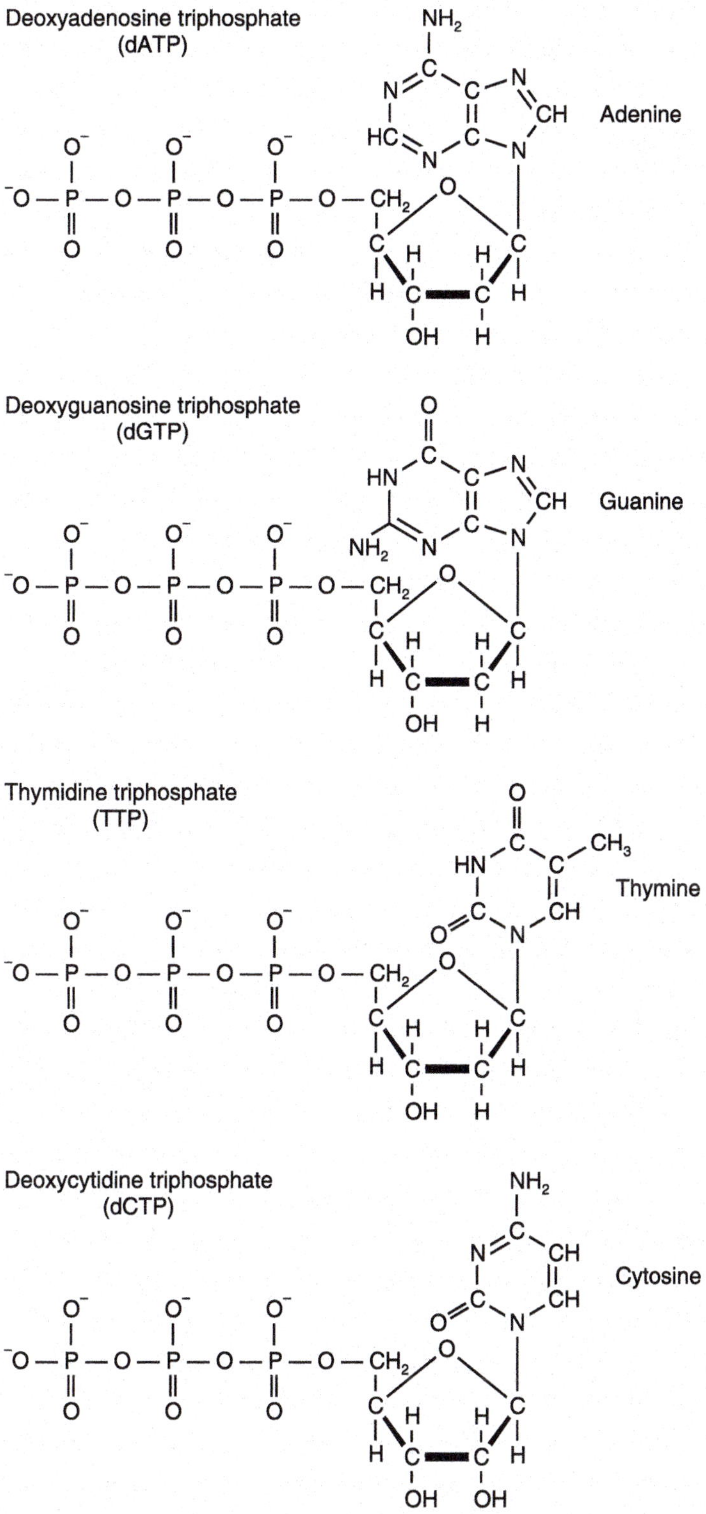

Figure 108. Structures of some deoxyribonucleoside-5'-triphosphates. The symbol of such a derivative is dATP (deoxyadenosine triphosphate), for example.

The channelling is possible because the terminal phosphate group can be enzymatically transferred to the 5'-diphosphates of the other nucleosides by the action of enzymes called *nucleoside diphosphokinases*. Hence, the following reactions are catalyzed in this manner:

ATP	+	GDP	→	ADP	+	GTP
		guanosine diphosphate				guanosine triphosphate

ATP	+	UDP	→	ADP	+	UTP
		uridine diphosphate				uridine triphosphate

ATP	+	CDP	→	ADP	+	CTP
		cytidine diphosphate				cytidine triphosphate

ATP	+	dADP	→	ADP	+	dATP
		deoyadenosine diphosphate				deoxyadenosine triphosphate

ATP	+	dGDP	→	ADP	+	dGTP
		deoxyguanosine diphosphate				deoxyguanosine triphosphate, etc.

GTP, UTP, CTP and dATP all have about the same Gibbs energy of the hydrolysis of the terminal phosphate group as ATP: as a result, the equilibrium constant of these reactions is about 1,0. From the study of these reactions, it appears that the ATP/ADP couple is necessary to phosphorylate GDP, UDP, CDP and, hence, to fill each channel with the high-energy phosphate group.

5) Biosynthesis of polysaccharides

Polysaccharides are comprised of long chains of simple sugar molecules bond by glycosidic linkages. They may have weights of 10 millions and may be equal to proteins in size. We mention:

– amylose which is the major component of starch. It is essentially a storage form of glucose in plant cells. The glucose molecules are essentially joined by 1-4-glycosidic linkages. It contains no other building block than α-D-glucose (Figure 109 and appendix I-5);

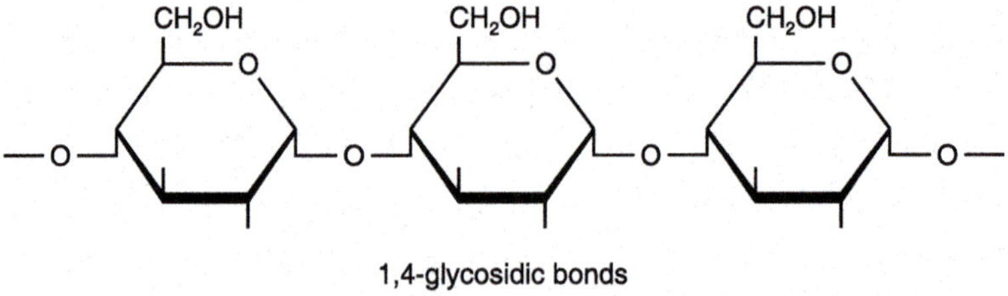

1,4-glycosidic bonds

Figure 109. Structure of amylose.

– The glycogen is the polysaccharide counterpart of amylose, but in animals. Glycogen has the same structure as amylose but its chains are more branched than those of amylose;

– cellulose which is an insoluble fibrous compound. It is composed of lengthy chains of β-glucopyranoses.

Glycogen is enzymatically synthesized from glucose by a repetitive process according to which a glucose molecule is attached to the end of a glycogen chain in building. Each repetitive step is the sum of six sequential reactions. They are:

1)   glucose + ATP → glucose-6-phosphate + ADP

2)   glucose-6-phosphate → glucose-1-phosphate

3)   glucose-1-phosphate + UTP → UDP-glucose + pyrophosphate

The structure of uridine diphosphate glucose is given just below

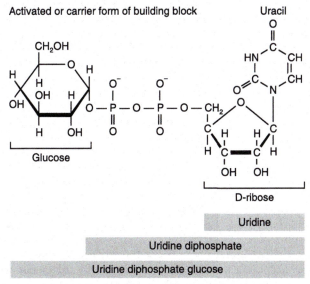

Figure 109'. Structure of uridine diphosphate glucose.

4)   UDP-glucose + glycogen $_n$ → Glycogen $_{n+1}$ + UDP

5)   ATP + UDP → ADP + UTP

6)   pyrophosphate + H_2O → 2 phosphate

The overall reaction is:

glucose + 2 ATP + glycogen$_n$ → Glycogen$_{n+1}$ + 2 ADP + 2 P

It can be noticed that glucose must be converted into a derivative of UDP just before the reaction forming the glycoside linkage occurs. No other nucleoside triphosphate can replace UTP in this reaction, except in the biosynthesis of cellulose in which guanosine diphosphate serves as the specific carrier. A second point is that two molecules of ATP are split to ADP and phosphate for each glycosidic linkage formed, one in the phosphorylation of glucose and the second in the transformation UDP → UTP. The Gibbs energy ΔG' for hydrolysis of two moles of ATP to ADP and P is 2 × 29260 = –58620 J mol^{-1} whereas the ΔG°' for the synthesis of a glycosidic linkage is about + 20900 J mol^{-1}. The net Gibbs energy is:

–58620 + 20900 = –37720 J mol^{-1}

This result is the reason why the reaction goes towards the expansion of the chain.

6) Biosynthesis of lipids

Lipids constitute a group of major elements of the cell structure. Their biosynthesis is complex because most of them contain more than one kind of chemical bond. Lipids are very important elements for at least three physiological parts that they play:

- they are important components of biological membranes,
- some of their derivatives play the part of hormones,
- *they are molecules of fuel.* It is essentially this part that will retain our attention.

Here, we are specially interested in the neutral lipids or triglyceraldehydes or triacylglycerols because of their quality of fuels. (We do not mention the case of phosphatidyl choline or lecithin which is a phospholipid. Phospholipids are present largely in cell membranes).

Triglycerides have glycerol and three long-chain fatty acids as building-blocks which are esterified to the glycerol. An example of triacylglycerol is given just below (Figure 110):

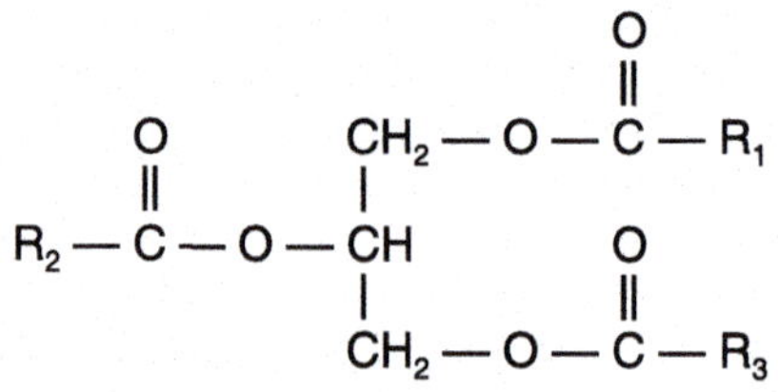

Triacylglycérol

Figure 110. Structure of a triglyceride.

Fatty acids change according to their chain-length and by the extent of their insaturation, should an insaturation happens. As examples of fatty acids, let us mention laurate (C12), palmitate (C16), stearate (C18) for the ions and the bases of saturated ones, palmitoleate base of the palmitoleic acid $CH_3(CH_2)_5CH=CH(CH_2)_7COOH$ (cis derivative) and oleate (oleic acid $CH_3(CH_2)_7CH=CH(CH_2)_7COOH$ - cis derivative). Triglycerides are extremely concentrated forms of stored energy. (Recall that in mammals, the sites in which triacylglycerols accumulate themselves the most, are adipocytes).

Here, we only regard the synthesis of fatty acids.

1) The synthesis of fatty acids begins by the carboxylation of acetyl CoA to give a malonyl CoA (Figure 111). This is an irreversible reaction. It is the essential step of the synthesis of malonylCoA

Acetyl CoA   **Malonyl CoA**

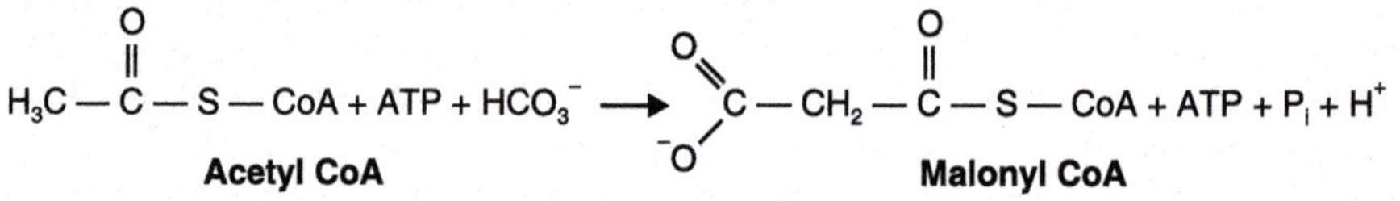

Figure 111. Carboxylation of acetyl CoA.

The synthesis of malonyl CoA is catalyzed by the *acetyl CoA carboxylase* which contains the biotine as a prosthetic group. The acetyl CoA is carboxylated in two steps. In the first one, an intermediary carboxybiotine is formed at the expense of one molecule of ATP:

biotine-enzyme + ATP + HCO_3^- ⇌ CO_2-biotine-enzyme + ADP + P

In the second step, the rest CO_2, activated in this intermediary, is transferred to acetyl CoA. Malonyl CoA is formed:

CO_2-biotine-enzyme + acetyl CoA → malonyl CoA + biotine-enzyme

2) and 3)   The second and third steps consist in the reactions of acetyl CoA with one acyl carrier protein (ACP) and of malonyl CoA with ACP according to the reactions:

acetyl CoA + ACP $\rightleftharpoons$ → acetyl-ACP + CoA

malonyl CoA + ACP $\rightleftharpoons$ → malonyl-ACP + CoA

The corresponding enzymes are the *acetyltransacylase* and the *malonyltransacylase*. This description is that of the synthesis of fatty acids of *E. coli*. The intermediaries of synthesis of the latter ones are linked to an *acyl carrier protein (ACP)*.

4)   Then the acetyl-ACP and the malonyl-ACP react together to form the acetoacetyl-ACP:

acetyl-ACP + malonyl-ACP → acetoacetyl-ACP + ACP + CO_2

The reaction is catalyzed by the *acyl-malonyl-ACP condensating enzyme*. This reaction is a kind of rearrangement as it would be named in organic chemistry. There is, indeed, a transfer of an acetyl rest from a thioester linked to a carrier protein to another acetyl rest coming from the decarboxylation of the rest malonyl.

5)   Formation of D-3-hydroxybutyryl-ACP by reduction with NADPH

The enzyme is the *β-ketoacyl-ACP-reductase*. It must be noticed that, in this reaction, it is the epimer D which is formed. It is not the epimer L. This reaction differs from the corresponding one occurring in the degradation of fatty acids in which it is the isomer L which is formed. It must also be noticed that the reductant is NADPH whereas it is NAD^+ which is oxidant in the β-oxydation (see the following chapter). Figure 112 represents these reactions:

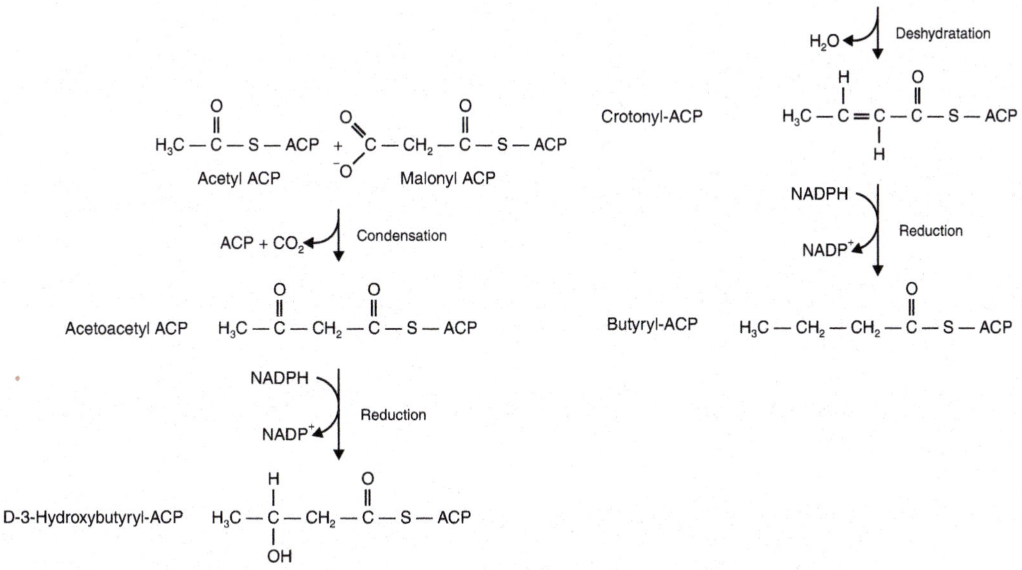

Figure 112. Successive steps in the synthesis of fatty acids *(in Escherichia coli)*.

6) Then the D-3-hydroxybutyryl-ACP is dehydrated and forms a crotonyl-ACP: the trans-$\Delta 2$-enoyl-ACP. The enzyme is the *3-hydroxyacyl-ACP-deshydratase*:

7) Finally, there is reduction by NADPH of the crotonyl product of the preceding step. The butyryl-ACP is formed. The enzyme is the *enoyl-ACP-reductase*.

The sequence of reactions 1 to 7 constitutes the first part of a synthesis of fatty acids, the end of which being the formation of butyryl-ACP.

The second part begins with the condensation of butyryl-ACP with malonyl-ACP and so forth as before. The whole process continues until C_{16}-acyl-ACP is formed. This derivative is not a substrate for the enzyme of condensation. It is hydrolyzed in palmitate and in ACP and the synthesis is blocked at this point.

It is evident that all these reactions show that all the intermediates in the synthesis of fatty acids are linked to one acyl carrier protein (ACP).

We shall also see that fatty acids are synthesized and degradated according to different ways in accordance with the fact that they are concerned by their synthesis or by their degradation (see Chapter 39).

From the pure energetic viewpoint, the following interesting question calls for an answer. In the reaction of condensation, one unit of 4 carbons is formed from one unit of two carbons and from another of three carbons while one mole of CO_2 is liberated. Why the reactants are not two units of two carbons (in the occurrence of two molecules of acetyl-ACP)? The answer is: it is because the equilibrium of the reaction 2 acetyl-ACP $\rightarrow$ acetoacetyl-ACP is far from being in favor of the right-term. Conversely, the equilibrium of the reaction between 1 acetyl-ACP + 1 malonyl-ACP with one molecule of CO_2 liberated is in favor of the right side. This is because there is a displacement towards the right due to the decarboxylation subsequent to the condensation of the formed malonyl compound. The decrease in Gibbs energy becomes spontaneous.

The stoichiometry of the synthesis of fatty acids can be calculated. For example, that of the synthesis of the palmitate is:

acetyl CoA + 7 malonyl CoA + 14 NADPH + 14 H$^+$ $\rightarrow$

$$\text{palmitate} + 7CO_2 + 14NADP^+ + 8CoA + 6H_2O$$

The equation of the synthesis of malonyl CoA is:

7 acetyl CoA + 7CO$_2$ + 7ATP $\rightarrow$ 7 malonyl CoA + 7 ADP + 7P

The global stoichiometry for the synthesis of palmitate is:

8 acetyl CoA + 7ATP + 14 NADPH + 14H$^+$ $\rightarrow$

$$\text{palmitate} + 14 NADP^+ + 8 CoA + 6H_2O + 7ADP + 7P$$

7) Biosynthesis of amino-acids

  – Molecular dinitrogen N $\equiv$ N represents about 80% of the earth's atmosphere. It is unavailable to most living organisms until it is reduced. However, nitrogen enters into the biosynthesis of numerous nitrogenous biological molecules such as amino-acids, purines, pyrimidines, nucleosides, nucleotides, proteins, etc. It can enter only when it is reduced, for example under the form of ammonium ion NH_4^+ (oxidation number of nitrogen–III) by some bacteria and blue-green algae. This possibility is called "nitrogen fixation". The triple bond, whose energy is 940,5 kJ mol^{-1}, is very resistant to any chemical attack. Besides, one knows that the synthesis of ammonia (Haber) from dihydrogen and dinitrogen involves hard conditions;

– Nitrogen is fixed through a vast cycle. In the first step, atmospheric nitrogen is fixed by reduction in NH_3 or NH_4^+ by soil bacteria, the best known being *rhizobium*. After that, nearly all formed ammoniac is oxidized in the nitrite ion NO_2^- (oxidation number: + III) and even in the subsequent level of oxidization, the nitrate ion NO_3^- (oxidation number + V). The process is called nitrification;

– Then, nitrates are transformed into ammonia in higher plants;

– The synthesis of amino-acids is done from ammonia by all organisms;

– The conversion of nitrates to N_2 is carried out by denitrifying soil bacteria. There is, then, an aerobic oxidization of ammonia to nitrogen. In this case, nitrite ions play the part of an oxidant.

This brief summary calls for the following comments:

– The fixation of N_2 as NH_3 is carried out enzymatically with the aid of the *nitrogenate complex*. This system is constituted of two kinds of proteic components: one reductase of strong reducing potential, and a nitrogenase which reduces N_2 in NH_4^+. Each component is a protein iron-sulfur. The nitrogenase also contains a molybdenum atom. The reduction of N_2 in NH_4^+ requires the occurrence of ATP and of a powerful reductant. The reduction reaction is:

$$N_2 + 6e^- + 12\ ATP + 12\ H_2O \rightarrow 2\ NH_4^+ + 12\ ADP + 12\ P + 4H^+$$

This reaction is equilibrated if we consider that the working pH is such that the liberated phosphate ion is the dihydrogenophosphate one $H_2PO_4^-$ and if we admit that ATP and ADP are under the same state of ionization. This is justified (Chapter 32).

– Reduced nitrogen under the form NH_4^+ is thought as forming amino-acids through entry points which are the amino-acids *glutamate* and *glutamine*. Both play a central role in the catabolism of ammonia and amino groups (see the next chapter).

– Without going into the details of the transformation, it must be known that all amino acids are derived from intermediates in glycolysis, the citric acid cycle and the pentose phosphate pathway. The entries are made through the entry points glutamate and glutamine. Humans are incapable of synthesizing half of the twenty common amino acids and the essential amino acids must be provided in the diet. They are: histidine, isoleucine, leucine, lysine, methionine, phenylalanine, threonine, tryptophan and valine. Organisms vary greatly in their ability to synthesize the 20 common amino acids. Amino acids are grouped by their metabolic precursor. One retained the following results:

* from α-ketoglutarate as precursor following are formed: glutamate• glutamine• proline• arginine•;

* from pyruvate: alanine• valine•, leucine•, isoleucine•;

* from phosphoenolpyruvate and eryrhrose-4-phosphate: tryptophan•, phenylalanine•, tyrosine•;

* from oxaloacetate: aspartate• asparagine• methionine•, threonine•, lysine•;

* from ribose-5-phosphate; histidine•.

Of course, amino acids grouped in the same family exhibit a structural relationship.

8) Super structures–supramolecular chemistry

To finish with this chapter it is the "*lieu et place*" to mention some points which are in the realm of *supramolecular chemistry.*

Up to now, we can say that we have essentially considered the building of molecular components of cells in terms of covalent bonds, that is to say we have only considered the bonding of molecular blocks in terms of covalent bonds. There subsist other aspects of cell assembly also involving the consideration of energy. One of them is the fact that living cells are equipped with superstructures such as membrane systems, mitochondria, nuclei, ribosomes and so forth. Each of the intracellular structures has a very complex fine structure of its own. Now, it remains to try tackling the molecular organization of such functional units between them in one cell. In this brief account, we only consider the corresponding general thermodynamic aspects.

Some authors have defined the supramolecular chemistry as the chemistry beyond the molecule. It investigates molecular systems in which the components are held together reversibly by intermolecular forces and not by covalent bonds. This sentence explains what we have written just above: *we have only considered the bonding of molecular blocks in terms of covalent bonds.* The forces at the disposal of the supramolecular chemist are already known. They are—electrostatic ones, hydrogen bonding, π–π stacking interactions, van der Waals forces, and hydrophobic forces (see appendix I-2).

The principles of chemical thermodynamics apply to the supramolecular chemistry. Hence:

– the equilibrium constants K are defined. They are expressed in terms of dissociation or association constants. The latter are also called *binding constants.*

– the equilibrium constants are related to the corresponding standard Gibbs energies $\Delta G°$.

– the change of Gibbs energy of a process with the temperature is related to its entropy change by the relation:

$$d\Delta G/dT = -\Delta S$$

and:

$$d \ln K/dT = \Delta H/RT^2$$

By calorimetic measurements, it is possible to know if the process of formation, for example, is of enthalpimetric or entropic origin.

In brief, much of the physical chemistry of the supramolecular structures looks like that of complexes.

Subsequently there is still a lot to explore in vast domain of the subcellular units of biological cells.

Chapter 39

Lipids and Amino-Acids as Fuel

At this point, we have seen the extraction of energy from glucose. It was through glycolysis, Krebs' cycle and oxidative phosphorylation.

Fatty acids and amino acids can also, through different biochemical pathways, be fuels. In this chapter, we justify this assertion.

1) Fatty acids as fuel

Firstly, it is interesting to notice that triacylglycerols are molecules in which **the** energy from metabolic origin is stocked. This is due to the facts that these derivatives are highly reduced and that they are quasi-anhydrous. By way of comparison, there is a consensus which says that the chemical energy values per gram of fats, proteins and carbohydrates are as follows:

fats: 39 kJ/g;   proteins: 13 kJ/g;   carbohydrates: 16 kJ/g

The yield of complete oxidation of a fatty acid is about 37,6 kJ/g whereas it is about 16,7 kJ/g for glucoids and proteins. One gram of fat stocks about six times the energy content of 1 g of hydrated glycogen. A man of 70 kg possesses energetic reserves of 418000 kJ in its triacylglycerols, 104500 kJ in its proteins, 2508 kJ in its glycogen and 167,2 kJ in its glucose.

In mammalians, triacylglycerols are located essentially in the cytoplasm of adipocytes. One can say that adipocytes are specialized in the synthesis and in the "stockage" of triacylglycerols and in their "mobilisation" as molecules of fuel which are brought to other "tissues" by blood.

To provide living cells with energy, there is firstly the hydrolysis of the triacylglycerols by enzymes called *lipases*:

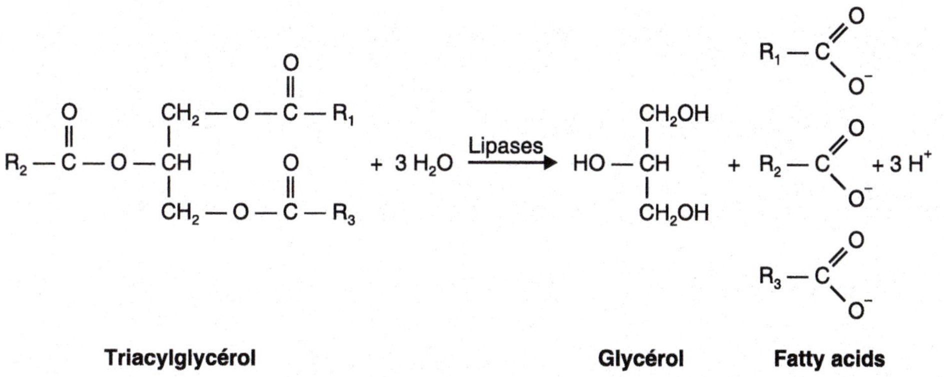

Triacylglycérol   **Glycérol**   **Fatty acids**

Figure 113. Hydrolyse of triacylglycerols.

The activity of lipases of adipocytes is regulated by some hormones: adrenaline, noradrenaline, glucagon, ACTH, etc.

– The *glycerol* formed by the lipolysis is phosphorylated and oxidised in dihydroxyacetone-phosphate which is itself isomerized in glyceraldehyde 3-phosphate. This compound is also found in glycolysis and in neoglucogenesis. Hence, glycerol can be transformed in pyruvate and in glucose. This is done in the liver.

– Concerning now the *fatty acids* liberated by lipolysis, it has been found that they are degraded by oxidation taking place at the carbon β:

β   α

$$RCH_2CH_2COOH$$

Fatty acids are actually oxidised in mitochondria and they are activated before entering into the matrice of the latter ones. Under the action of ATP, there is formation of a thioester bond between the carboxyl rest and the thiol –SH group of CoA. The reaction takes place in the external mitochondrial membrane where it is catalyzed by acyl CoA synthetase.

$$RCOO- + ATP + HS\text{-}CoA \rightleftharpoons RCOS\text{-}CoA + AMP + PP \qquad (210)$$

Actually, the reaction is realized in two steps. Firstly, the acid reacts with ATP by forming one acyl adenylate. The linkage is realized with expulsion of one molecule of pyrophosphate P-P. After, the rest thiol of CoA attacks the acyl adenylate and forms acyl CoA and AMP:

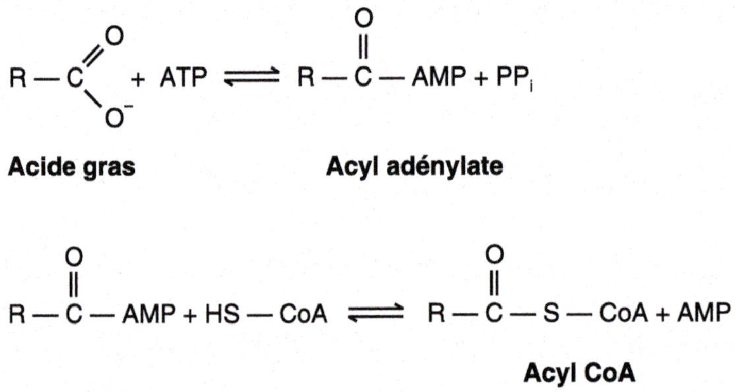

$$R - C \overset{O}{\underset{O^-}{\big\backslash}} + ATP \rightleftharpoons R - \overset{O}{\overset{\|}{C}} - AMP + PP_i$$

Acide gras   **Acyl adénylate**

$$R - \overset{O}{\overset{\|}{C}} - AMP + HS - CoA \rightleftharpoons R - \overset{O}{\overset{\|}{C}} - S - CoA + AMP$$

Acyl CoA

Figure 114. Decomposition of the reaction of the fatty acid with acyl CoA.

This is another example of a coupled reaction. These reactions are easily reversible. The equilibrium constant of reaction (207) is of the order of 1. An energy-rich bond is broken down whereas an energy-rich one is formed. It is the bond thioester of acyl CoA. Actually, there are two energy-rich bonds which are formed instead of one only since the liberated-molecule of pyrophosphate is quickly hydrolyzed by a phosphatase:

$$RCOO^- + ATP + HS\text{-}CoA + H_2O \rightarrow RCOS\text{-}CoA + AMP + 2\,P + 2H^+$$

This is why the reaction is irreversible.

Fatty acids are activated in the external mitochondrial membrane whereas they are oxidized in the mitochondrial matrice. A zwitterion, named carnitine:

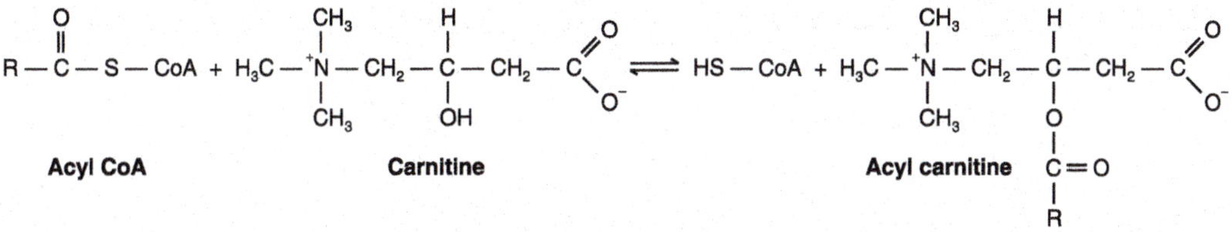

$$R-\overset{\overset{\text{O}}{\|}}{C}-S-CoA + H_3C-\overset{\overset{CH_3}{|}}{\underset{\underset{CH_3}{|}}{N^+}}-CH_2-\overset{\overset{H}{|}}{\underset{\underset{OH}{|}}{C}}-CH_2-C\overset{\diagup O}{\diagdown O^-} \rightleftharpoons HS-CoA + H_3C-\overset{\overset{CH_3}{|}}{\underset{\underset{CH_3}{|}}{N^+}}-CH_2-\overset{\overset{H}{|}}{\underset{\underset{O}{|}}{C}}-CH_2-C\overset{\diagup O}{\diagdown O^-}$$

Acyl CoA   Carnitine   Acyl carnitine $\overset{|}{\underset{\underset{R}{|}}{C}}=O$

Figure 115. Metabolic energy production.

transports the activated fatty acids through the internal mitochondrial membrane. The acyl carnitine which is formed is transported with the help of a *translocase*.

Concerning, now, the recurrent sequence of degradation, we can say that it evolves in four steps: oxidization by FAD, hydratation, oxidation by NAD+ and thiolysis by CoA. After this sequence, the acyl chain is shortened from two carbon atoms. The sequence is (Figure 116):

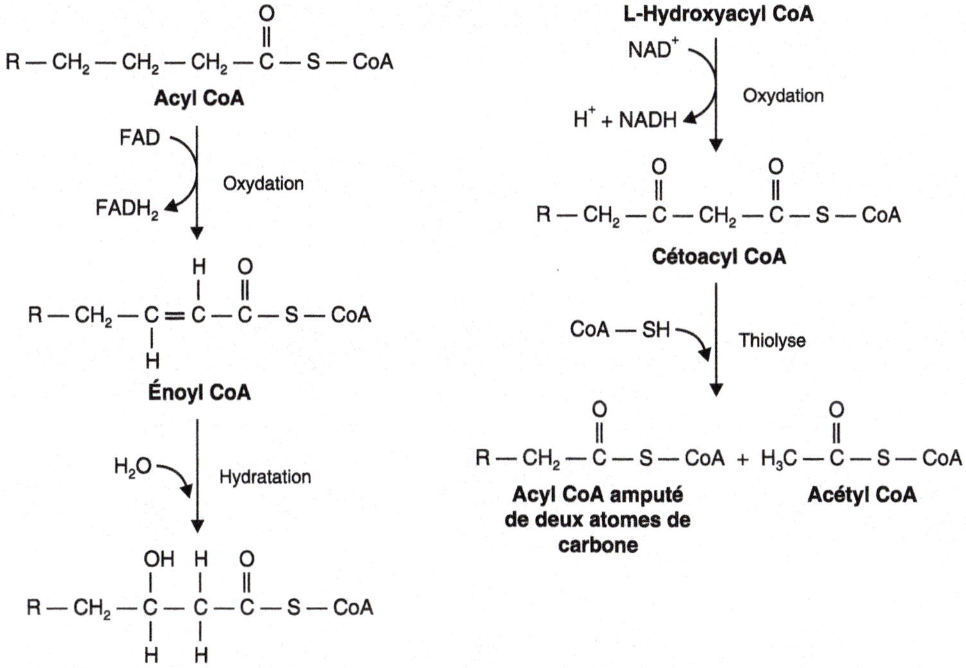

$$R-CH_2-CH_2-CH_2-\overset{\overset{\text{O}}{\|}}{C}-S-CoA$$
Acyl CoA

FAD ↘   Oxydation   ↙ FADH₂

$$R-CH_2-\overset{\overset{H}{|}}{C}=\overset{\overset{H}{|}}{C}-\overset{\overset{\text{O}}{\|}}{C}-S-CoA$$
Énoyl CoA

H₂O ↘ Hydratation

$$R-CH_2-\overset{\overset{OH}{|}}{\underset{\underset{H}{|}}{C}}-\overset{\overset{H}{|}}{\underset{\underset{H}{|}}{C}}-\overset{\overset{\text{O}}{\|}}{C}-S-CoA$$

L-Hydroxyacyl CoA

NAD⁺ ↘   Oxydation   H⁺ + NADH ↙

$$R-CH_2-\overset{\overset{\text{O}}{\|}}{C}-CH_2-\overset{\overset{\text{O}}{\|}}{C}-S-CoA$$
Cétoacyl CoA

CoA — SH ↘ Thiolyse

$$R-CH_2-\overset{\overset{\text{O}}{\|}}{C}-S-CoA + H_3C-\overset{\overset{\text{O}}{\|}}{C}-S-CoA$$
Acyl CoA amputé   **Acétyl CoA**
de deux atomes de carbone

Figure 116. Steps of oxidation of fatty acids.

- Oxidation by FAD. It is the oxidization of the acyl CoA

  There is formation of the derivative called the enoyl CoA. It is the trans-Δ^2-enoyl CoA. This is actually a dehydrogenation under the action of an *acyl CoA dehydrogenase*. The symbol Δ shows there is a double bond formed and the superscript indicates its location. Notice that the configuration of the double bond is *trans*.

- the following step is the hydratation of the double bond located between the carbons C2 and C3. The enzyme is the *enoyl CoA hydratase*. The hydratation is stereospecific. The isomer L is formed alone. It is the L-hydroxyacyl CoA.

- the third step is a new step of oxidation. The hydroxyl group in C3 of the L hydroxy derivative is oxidized by NAD⁺ in a keto derivative with formation of NADH. A ketoacyl CoA is formed.

The reaction is catalyzed by the *L-3-hydroxyacyl CoA deshydrogenase* which is absolutely specific of the preceding L isomer.

– the final step is the cleavage of the 3-ketoacyl CoA by the thiol group of a second molecule of CoA. The cleavage is catalyzed by the *β-ketothiolase*. The reaction is:

3-ketoacyl CoA + HS-CoA $\rightleftharpoons$ acetyl CoA + acyl CoA

   n carbons   (n–2) carbons

The total yield in ATP of the full oxidization of the palmitate ion can be calculated.

Recall that the palmitic acid is the saturated fatty acid in C16. In each sequence of the four steps, 1 acyl CoA is liberated from two carbons while 1 molecule of $FADH_2$, 1 molecule of NADH and 1 of acetyl CoA are formed:

C_n acyl CoA + FAD + NAD^+ + H_2O + CoA $\rightarrow$

$$C_{n-2} \text{acyl CoA} + FADH_2 + NADH + \text{acetyl CoA} + H^+$$

The degradation of the palmitoyl CoA involves 7 cycles of reactions. In the seventh, the ketoacyl CoA in C4 is cut by thiolysis in two molecules of acetyl CoA. The stoichiometry of the palmitoyl CoA is hence:

palmitoyl CoA + 7 FAD + 7 NAD^+ + 7 CoA + 7 H_2O $\rightarrow$

$$8 \text{ acetyl CoA} + 7 FADH_2 + 7NADH + 7 H^+$$

3 ATP are formed when each of these NADH is oxidized by the respiratory chain whereas 2 ADP are formed for each $FADH_2$ because their electrons enter into the chain at the level of ubiquinol. Now, recall that the oxidisation of acetyl CoA by the citric acid cycle provides 12 ATP. The number of formed ATP during the oxidization of palmitoyl CoA is hence 14 starting from $7FADH_2$, 21 from 7NADH and 96 starting from 8 molecules of acetyl CoA. All that gives 131 molecules. Two rich-energy phosphate bonds have been consumed for the activation of palmitate during which 1 ATP is cut in AMP and 2 P. The net yield of the oxidation of the palmitate is hence 129 ATP.

One estimates that the efficiency of the conservation of energy during the oxidization of fatty acids in standard conditions is about 40%. This value is identical to those found in glycolysis, in the Krebs' cycle and in the oxidative phosphorylation.

2) Amino-acids as fuel

Amino-acids, in excess relatively to those necessary for the synthesis of proteins and other biomolecules, cannot be stocked on the contrary to fatty acids and glucose and can no longer be excreted. The excess of amino-acids is used as fuel. In the metabolism, the rest amino acid is removed from the carbon bone and the latter becomes an important metabolic intermediary. Most α-amino acids rests of amino in excess are transformed in urea whereas their carbon bones are transformed in acetyl CoA, in acetoacetyl CoA, in pyruvate ions and in intermediaries of the citric acid cycle. As a consequence, fatty acids, ketonic derivatives and glucose can be formed from amino-acids.

Some of these points are "reconsidered" now briefly.

– The α-amino rests of several amino acids are transferred to α-ketoglutarate and form molecules of glutamate. Reactions are catalyzed by *transaminases* according to the scheme (Figure 117):

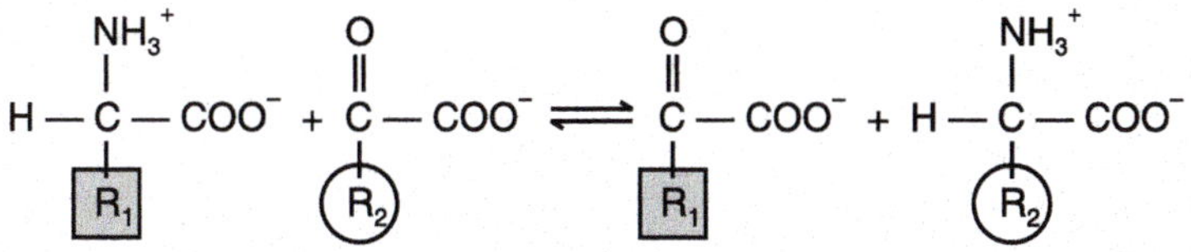

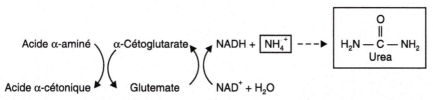

Figure 117. Reactions catalyzed by transaminases.

They are the cases, for example, of aspartate and alanine. Then, the enzymes are, respectively, the *aspartateaminotransferase* and the *alanineaminotransferase*. The reactions are:

aspartate + α-ketoglutarate   ⇌   oxaloacetate + glutamate

alanine + α-ketoglutarate   ⇌   pyruvate + glutamate

Other schemes of desamination can exist. It is the case for serine and threonine for which there is a direct desamination under the action of *serine deshydratase* and *threonine deshydratase*.

– Most of α-amino groups of amino acids in excess are transformed in urea. In the most part of the vertebra, the formation of the ammonium ion is the intermediary step. The ammonium ion is formed from the glutamate by oxidative desamination according to Figure 118:

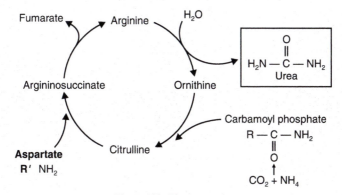

Figure 118. Transformation of ammonium ion in urea.

The reaction is catalyzed by the *glutamate dehydrogenase*, enzyme which can work with NAD^+ or $NADP^+$. In the vertebrates, urea is synthesized by the urea cycle:

Fumarate — Arginine H_2O

Argininosuccinate   Ornithine

$H_2N - C - NH_2$
Urea

Aspartate
R' NH_2 Citrulline

Carbamoyl phosphate
$R - C - NH_2$
$CO_2 + NH_4$

Figure 119. The urea cycle.

Briefly, one of the nitrogen atoms of urea comes from the amino acid *aspartate*. The other nitrogen atom and the carbon atom come from the ion NH_4^+ and from CO_2. The immediate precursor of urea is arginine which is hydrolyzed in urea and ornithine by *arginase* (Figure 120):

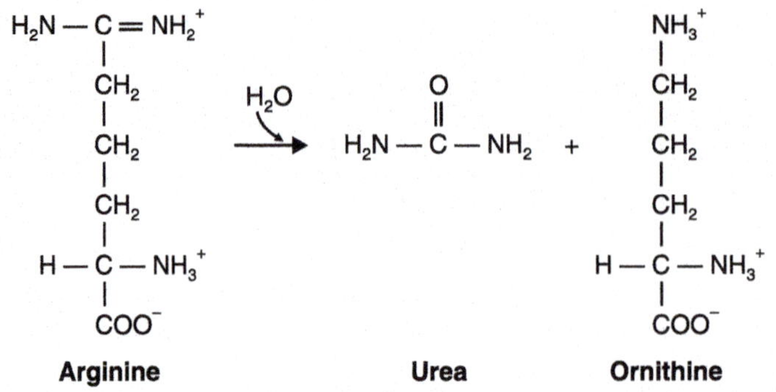

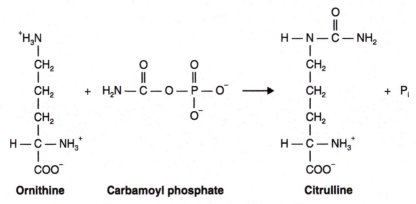

Figure 120. Transformation of arginine into ornithine.

In the cycle, arginine is formed from ornithine. During this transformation, a carbamoyl group is transferred to ornithine. Citrulline is formed. The donor of carbamoyl is the carbamoyl phosphate (Figure 121):

Figure 121. Transformation of ornithine citrulline.

There is then the condensation of citrulline and aspartate under the catalyze of *arginino synthetase* (Figure 122). This reaction is possible because of the cleavage of ATP in AMP and pyrophosphate and by the subsequent hydrolysis of pyrophosphate.

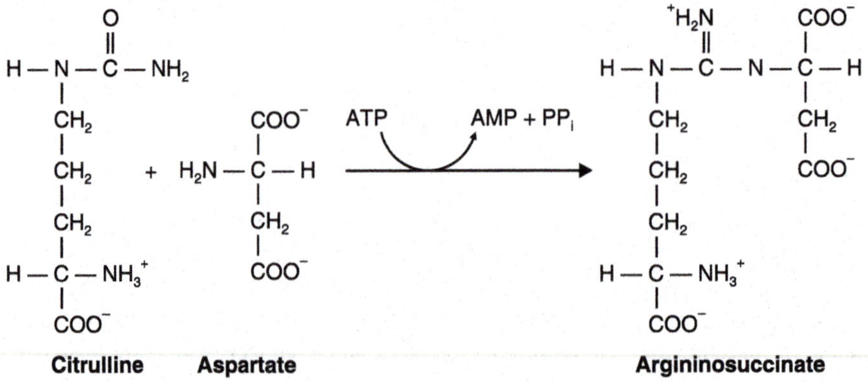

Figure 122. Transformation of citrulline argininosuccinate.

Finally, the *argininosuccinase* cleaves the argininosuccinate into arginine and fumarate (Figure 123).

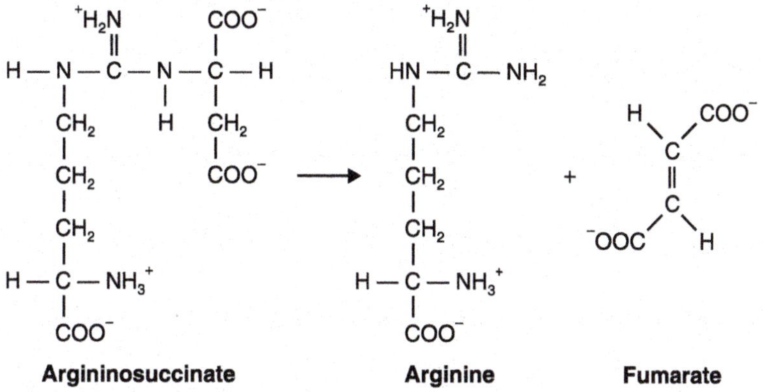

$$\begin{array}{ccc}
{}^{+}H_2N & COO^- & {}^{+}H_2N \\
\| & | & \| \\
H-N-C-N-C-H & & HN-C-NH_2 \\
| & | & | & | \\
CH_2 & H & CH_2 & CH_2 \\
| & | & | \\
CH_2 & COO^- & CH_2 \\
| & | \\
CH_2 & CH_2 \\
| & | \\
H-C-NH_3{}^{+} & H-C-NH_3{}^{+} \\
| & | \\
COO^- & COO^-
\end{array}$$

Argininosuccinate   **Arginine**   **Fumarate**

Figure 123. Cleavage argininosuccinate/arginine + fumarate.

The carbamoyl phosphate is synthesized starting from $NH_4{}^{+}$, CO_2, ATP and H_2O (Figure 124)

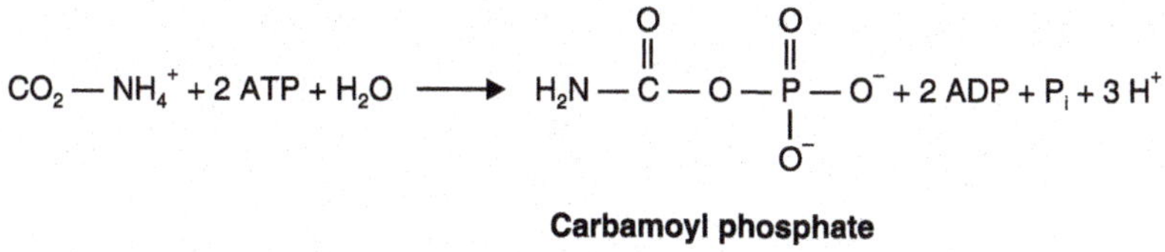

$$CO_2 - NH_4{}^{+} + 2\ ATP + H_2O \longrightarrow H_2N-C-O-P-O^- + 2\ ADP + P_i + 3\ H^+$$

Carbamoyl phosphate

Figure 124. Biosynthesis of carbamoyl phosphate.

The stoichiometry of the reaction of synthesis of urea is:

$CO_2 + NH_4{}^{+} + 3\ ATP + aspartate + 2\ H_2O \rightarrow urea + 2ADP + 2P + AMP + PP + fumarate$

– The cycles of urea and of citric acid are linked together.

The pyrophosphate is quickly hydrolyzed and 4 rich-energy bonds ($\sim$ P) are consummated.

The synthesis of fumarate by the urea cycle is important because it links the cycles of urea and citric acid. The different steps and the crossing of both cycles are summarized in Figure 125:

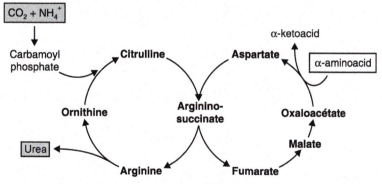

Figure 125. Cycles of urea and of citric acid.

The fumarate is hydrated in malate which is itself oxidized in oxaloacetate. One knows the different pathways in which the oxaloacetate (transamination in aspartate, conversion in glucose-neoglucogenesis, condensation with acetyl CoA, conversion in pyruvate) participates. It is interesting to notice that the formation of NH_4^+, its incorporation in the carbamoyl phosphate and the citrulline synthesis are carried out in the mitochondrial matrice. The three other reactions of the urea cycle are carried out in the cytosol.

Chapter 40

Active Transport and Electrical Work

There are three types of work done by living organisms: the chemical work, the work of transport and concentration (also named osmotic work) and the mechanic work. So far, the chemical work, which was essentially in connection with catabolic and anabolic pathways of cellular metabolism, has been largely dealt with in this book. The present chapter is devoted to the osmotic and mechanic works. We begin by considering a kind of transports through the biological membranes, that is to say the crossing across them under active transport and more precisely by considering what is named osmotic work. We shall give some examples of such transports and conditions under which they are operating. We shall also consider the case where an active transport results in a bioelectric phenomena such as an *action potential*.

Since the osmotic work essentially concerns the passing of solutes across biological membranes, it is judicious to begin by briefly recalling the structure of the latter ones.

1) Structure and properties of cell membranes

All the membranes of living cells are similar in their gross chemical composition, structure and properties. Hence, it can be said that they all contain about 60% protein and 40% lipids. Most of the latter are under the form of phospholipids. They possess high electric resistance and low surface tension. It is found that they all have about the same thickness and the same type of organization. Their organization is such that each membrane possesses (see Figure 126):

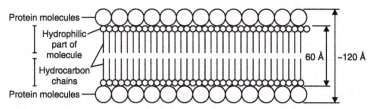

Figure 126. Structure of biological membranes.
(figure reproduced from the book "bioenergetics" by A.L. Lehninger, p. 160, Benjamin Editor, by the courtesy of the Pearson group)

– two monolayers of phospholipid molecules, in which the hydrophobic hydrocarbon chains of the lipids face each other;

– each double layer is coated with a single layer of protein molecules.

Most membranes allow neutral uncharged molecules to pass through them by simple diffusion. Not surprisingly, the rate of penetration of uncharged molecules is directly proportional to their solubility in non polar solvents or in a fat. Curiously, however, water passes rather easily through them because, probably, the membranes are hydrated. Another atypical behavior is that of glucose which passes through membranes at a higher rate than it would be expected from its very low solubility in hydrocarbons. In general, ions do not pass through membranes readily and large protein molecules do not pass through cell membranes.

Solutes do not pass through membranes *via* pores. They pass by dissolving themselves in one side of the membrane. The driving force for the passage of the solute is due to the phenomenon of diffusion.

2) Solute transports across membranes

 – Some nonpolar compounds can dissolve in the lipid bilayer of the membranes. They can cross membranes unassisted.

 – For any polar compound, a membrane protein is essential. In some cases, it simply facilitates the transport transmembrane down its concentration gradient. But the transport can occur against its concentration gradient. Then, it requires energy. Of course, the polar derivative may be an ion.

 – Crossing membranes can also evolve *via* ion channels formed by proteins or *via* ionophores which are small molecules which mask the charge of ions.

(The notion of gradient is approached in the mathematical appendix II-3).

In the present case, it can be grasped as considering a simple derivative with the aid of the following simple reasoning. Consider the plan normal to the lining of the membrane at the abscisse x_0. The profile of concentration of the solute in the plan is given by the curve $C_A C_B$. This curve passes by the point of coordinates $x_0 C_0$ (Figure 127).

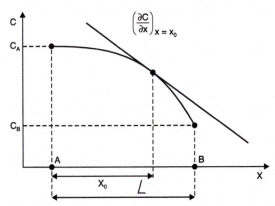

Figure 127. Gradient of concentration at the interface membrane/surroundings.

The gradient of concentration is the slope of the curve $C(x)$ at the absisse x_0 of the membrane, that is to say $(dC/dx)_{x0}$.

3) The osmotic work

According to what is preceding, one can distinguish passive and active compounds. The first ones are those which can dissolve in the lipid bilayer and which, more generally, can cross the membrane unassisted.

However, all cells are capable of accumulating some substances coming from the surroundings so that their concentration inside the cell may far exceed their external one. The converse is also true. They may secrete substances in the surroundings so that their external concentrations may exceed the internal ones. For example, cells may accumulate ions potassium K^+ and glucose molecules. They may also secrete sodium ions. Another important example is provided by the accumulation of a solute in a given zone from another one where its chemical potential is lower. All cells, hence, carry out an important and fundamental activity for the work of concentrating molecules; this process requires a large input of metabolic energy. These transfers are not spontaneously possible from the thermodynamic standpoint but they are realizable under the conditions of *active transports* which we shall specify. According to most authors, active transports are possible thanks to the so-called *osmotic work.* It remains to explain why. We already have introduced the notion of osmotic pressure (see Chapter 19).

The occurrence of osmotic pressure is easily explained by the notion of chemical potential. Recall that the chemical potential of a substance is a quantity which quantifies its tendency to leave its current thermodynamic state by every sort of process, physical, chemical or biochemical one (Chapter 17). Recall also that a chemical potential μ of a substance is given by the expression:

$$\mu = \mu° + RT \ln a$$

where $\mu°$ is its standard potential, a its activity, R the perfect gas constant and T the absolute temperature of the medium. $\mu°$ is a constant for given solute, solvent, and temperature of the medium. In some conditions, the numerical value of the activity may be equal to its concentration. It is the case for sufficiently dilute solutions. It must also be recalled that a chemical potential has the physical meaning of a molar Gibbs energy. Usually, but not obligatorily, it is moreover a partial molar Gibbs energy. Let us suppose that in a solution, the chemical potential of the solute be μ_B at the point B and μ_A at the point A and that $\mu_B > \mu_A$, that is to say for example $C_B = 10^{-4}$ mol l^{-1} and $C_A = 10^{-6}$ mol l^{-1}. We can write:

$$\mu_A = \mu° + RT \ln C_A < \mu_B = \mu° + RT \ln C_B$$

* *Consider the transfer A → B*

$$\Delta G = \mu_B - \mu_A$$

$$\Delta G = RT \ln 10^{-4}/10^{-6}$$

$$\Delta G = 11416 \, J \, mol^{-1}$$

The Gibbs energy change of the process is positive. It cannot spontaneously evolve in this direction. Attention must be paid to the fact that this numerical value is the minimal one which must be delivered to the system in order to counterbalance it, since it is calculated in the conditions of reversibility.

* *Now, consider the opposite process B → A*

$$\Delta G = RT \ln 10^{-6}/10^{-4}$$

$$\Delta G = -11416 \, J \, mol^{-1}$$

The Gibbs energy change of the process is negative. It spontaneously evolves in the studied direction.

These considerations show that these active transports are not truly due to the occurrence of osmotic pressure even if, basically, the deep cause of these phenomena is the difference of chemical potentials of solutes in different locations of the system.

This means that the process of dilution is a spontaneous one, that of concentration is not. Nevertheless, it remains feasible, provided energy is brought to the system. Roughly speaking, these results explain themselves by the fact that the concentration of the solute in a zone decreases the entropy or the randomness of the system. It is the inverse for the dilution. Hence, active transports can only evolve with the aid of an input of metabolic energy, such as that furnished by glycolysis, respiration or ATP.

Another example of such a type of active transport is afforded by the red blood cells. Chemical analysis shows that the ionic composition of the internal aqueous phase of the latter is different from that of the blood plasma. The intracellular compartment is rich in ions K^+ but contains little Na^+. It is the inverse for the extracellular plasma blood. It might be thought that this result is due to the fact both ions might possess inability to pass through the membrane. It is not the reason. Researches with radioactive Na^+ and K^+ show that K^+ is actively "pumped" in the cell, whereas Na^+ is actively "pumped" outside. It is demonstrated that the maintenance of the characteristics of Na^+ and K^+ concentrations inside the red blood cell is the result of an energy dependent process.

It is important to notice that transport mechanisms of cells are specific for given solutes. For example, some cells have a pump specific for amino-acids whereas they do not operate with glucose. Other cells have a pump of opposite behavior and so forth.

It is also important to notice that such a kind of active transport can maintain the internal solute and ion composition of cells remarkably, constant even when the external medium fluctuates widely in composition. Some yeast cells can live and grow while keeping normal their cellular behavior when the pH of the culture medium varies from pH = 3 to 10. *Therefore, the pumping mechanisms (even if their functioning is actually not as that of a pump) must be based on the presence of sensible devices which can determine the concentration of a specific solute in the internal and external media and can adjust their activity on them automatically.*

The general behavior we have described in this paragraph is that of active transports, named *homocellular active transport* mechanisms. In brief, they appear to have three main functions. They maintain a constant pH and ionic composition for a normal behavior of all the enzymes in the cell. They also maintain an adequate internal concentration of fuel such as glucose or amino acids. Finally, they contribute to rid the cell of waste products and toxic substances.

Some other active transports are also distinguished.

4) Transcellular active transport

Now, we briefly consider the notion of *transcellular active transport*. Contrary to the homocellular transport mechanism, transcellular active transport takes place across a whole cell or a whole layer of cells.

In this process, the "pumps" work at different rates on the opposite sides of cells. "Pumps" may be of different kinds. This type of active transport is seen only in multicellular organisms such as plants or higher animals. The transport is between two aqueous compartments. An example is provided by the secretion of hydrochloric acid into the gastric juice by epithelial cells of the gastric mucosa. Gastric juice is the most acid of the body fluids. Its pH value is about 1. This result is striking because gastric juice is formed from blood plasma, the pH of which is about 7. Hence, the characteristic composition of both compartments must be maintained. This is done by "pumps" of different activities and specificities. They can also work according to adapted directions (see appendix I-7).

5) Intracellular active transport

We know that some of the internal organelles of cells are capable of accumulating or secreting solutes. Each of these organelles is surrounded by a membrane and the solutes are pumped across it, located between the internal fluid compartment and the "ground substance" of the cell. We have already encountered such behaviors with mitochondria and chloroplasts. For example, isolated mitochondria can accumulate some cations such as Ca^{2+}, Mn^{2+}, Mg^{2+}, and some anions.

6) Action potentials

We have already noticed that ions, in particular ions Na^+ and K^+, are transported across cell membranes thanks to the conversion of the chemical energy of ATP. It is an experimental fact that there exists a membrane electric potential across a cell surface when a gradient of Na^+ and K^+ is established by action of one ATP-driven pump. In excitable tissues (nerves and muscles), the potential difference maintained across the cell membrane in the absence of stimulation is called the *resting potential* and the cell is said to be in the *resting state*. The inside of the cell is negative with respect to the outside. The magnitude of this potential difference depends on the ratio of the concentrations of the ions on each side. K^+ ions are ten to twenty times more concentrated near the inner surface of the membrane and Na^+ are much more concentrated outside. Because of this electrical configuration, which is a steady state (resulting from active pumping and back diffusion across the membrane), the potential difference is usually of about 50 to 70 mV.

When an impulse passes down a neurone, a movement of negative charges along the axon is observed. (An axon is a single fiber that conducts the nerve impulse away from the cell body. In humans, axons may be a meter or more in length). It appears that negative charges (electrons) are propelled along the outer surface (Figure 128).

When the nerve cell is excited by reception of an impulse from the next cell, or by electrical stimulation, it is found that a "wave" travels along the axon at a high rate. The "wave" consists in an abrupt change in the potential difference and its rapid return to the initial state. This change in potential is called the *action potential* (Figure 129).

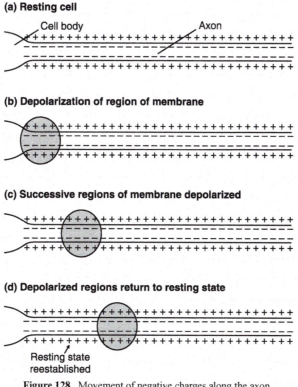

Figure 128. Movement of negative charges along the axon.

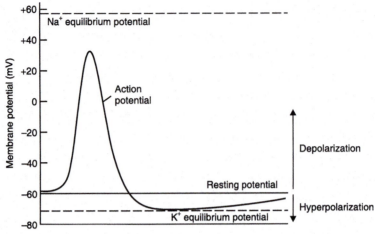

Figure 129. The action potential.

The time scale is measured in ms and the unit of electrical conductance is the siemens. The resting potential is about –60 mV. The action potential results successively from a rapid depolarization period followed by a rapid hyperpolarization.

From the theoretical standpoint, the energetic work of displacement of an ion depends no longer only on its profile of concentrations but also from the membrane potential. It depends on the *electrochemical potential* ΔG_{total} defined by:

$$\Delta G_{total} = RT \ln C_2/C_1 + Z\, F \Delta \psi$$

$\Delta \psi$ is the electric membrane potential, F is the faraday and Z the charge on the ion. We find in the above relation the term diffusive gradient $RT \ln C_2/C_1$ which has its origin in the definition of the chemical potential $Z\, F \Delta \psi$ is the electric gradient. Notice that the membrane potential across a cell surface membrane is not given by the Nernst equation. A better one is the following one. It is for the case in which the responsible ions are Na^+, K^+ and Cl^-:

$$E = RT/F \ln [P_K K_0 + P_{Na} Na_0 + P_{Cl} Cl_i]/[P_K K_i + P_{Na} Na_i + P_{Cl} Cl_0]$$

where P_K, P_{Na} and P_{Cl} are the *plasma membranes*, and K, Na and Cl are the concentrations (activities) of ions K^+, Na^+ and Cl^-. Indices o and i mean outside and inside. Plasma membranes are inserted in order to take account of the permeability of ions. P is a measure of the permeability of an ion across a membrane of unit area (1 cm^2) driven by a 1-M difference in concentration.

7) Contraction and motion

The question now is to know how the energy of fermentation, respiration, and sunlight is conserved when a mechanical work is performed. The concerned mechanical works are those carried out by contractile and motile systems of cells.

In the intact organism, muscles are supplied with fuels and oxygen by the blood. It is well-known that muscles use more dioxygen when they are active. But, we also know that dioxygen is not an absolute requirement for muscular contraction. Muscles can also contract under fully anaerobic circumstances. In this case, where does the energy come from? It comes from glycogen, the amount of which decreases during exercises in these conditions. There is simultaneously an increase in lactic acid.

Furthermore, the contractile system of muscle can be uncoupled from respiration and glycolysis and can perform mechanical work without utilization of glucose and cellular foodstuffs. When this was discovered, a problem of explanation of the phenomenon was pointed out.

Actually, one now knows that important chemical changes take place during contraction in the latter conditions. It is not at the level of consumption of some fuel. It is at the level of high-energy phosphate compounds of muscle. The product particularly concerned is the phosphocreatine, which is a derivative of the creatine (Figure 130). Formula of both compounds are:

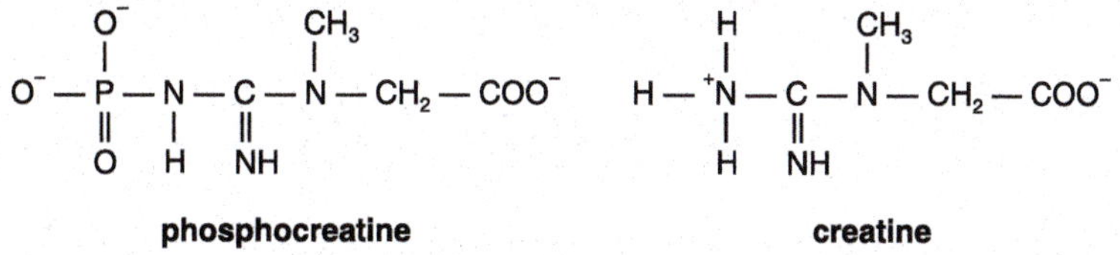

$$O^- - \overset{\overset{\displaystyle O^-}{|}}{\underset{\underset{\displaystyle O}{||}}{P}} - \overset{}{\underset{\underset{\displaystyle H}{|}}{N}} - \overset{\overset{\displaystyle CH_3}{|}}{\underset{\underset{\displaystyle NH}{||}}{C}} - N - CH_2 - COO^- \qquad H - \overset{\overset{\displaystyle H}{|}}{\underset{\underset{\displaystyle H}{|}}{{}^+N}} - \overset{\overset{\displaystyle CH_3}{|}}{\underset{\underset{\displaystyle NH}{||}}{C}} - N - CH_2 - COO^-$$

phosphocreatine **creatine**

Figure 130. Structures of phosphocreatine and creatine.

Phosphocreatine, present in muscles and nervous cells, disappears quickly during contraction in completely anaerobic conditions, including in the case where 3-phosphoglyceraldehyde is completely inhibited by the poison iodoacetate ICH_2COO^-. (By action of the latter, no conversion of glycogen to lactic acid occurs).

Phosphocreatine disappears with formation of free creatine and inorganic phosphate. The reaction is coupled with that of formation of ATP from ADP according to:

phosphocreatine + ADP $\rightleftharpoons$ creatine + ATP

The reaction is catalyzed by the enzyme *creatine phosphokinase*. The above reaction is reversible but the equilibrium point is located far on the right. In other words, the reaction is strongly displaced towards the right. This is not astonishing. To be convinced, it is sufficient to consider the table giving the Gibbs energy of hydrolysis of phosphate compounds (see Chapter 32):

phosphocreatine + H_2O $\rightarrow$ creatine + phosphate $\qquad \Delta G'^\circ = -43890$ J mol^{-1}

ATP + H_2O $\rightarrow$ ADP + phosphate $\qquad \Delta G'^\circ = -29260$ J mol^{-1}

Chapter 41

The Molecular Basis of the Informational System–The Replication of DNA–The Trancription to mRNA– Protein Biosynthesis

Here, we begin by very briefly recalling the biosynthesis of informational macromolecules DNA and *messenger RNA* and, as a result, the building of proteins.

Nucleic acids (DNA and RNA—see later) are molecules adapted for the storage and transcription of biological information and, in some way, the formation of proteins "realizes" the biological information. We finish the chapter by some comments about the biological information.

1) Structure of desoxyribonucleic acid

As we know, proteins are formed by condensation of amino acids. The listing of the 20 common amino acids of proteins is given in the appendix. A formal example of peptide (in the occurrence a dipeptide) is given in Figure 131:

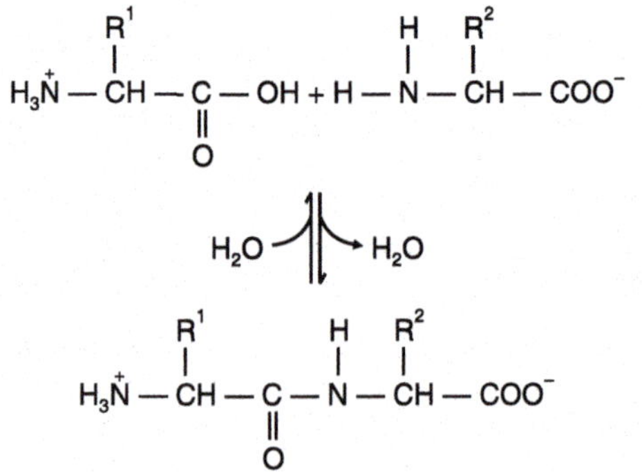

Figure 131. General structure of a dipeptide.

(Notice the location of the acido-basic sites and their charges). Both amino acids are linked by a peptide bond. Desoxyribonucleic acid, or DNA, consists of two chains that form a double helix (Figure 132).

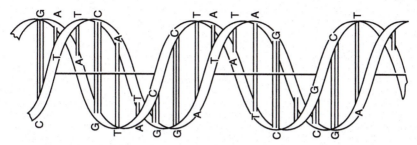

Figure 132. Schematic representation of the DNA double helix.

Each chain may be considered as a polymer of nucleosides. (Recall that nucleosides are compounds consisting of a purine or pyrimidine base covalently linked to a pentose.) The nucleosides, indeed, are linked by phosphodiester bonds which form the backbone structure of DNA (Figure 133).

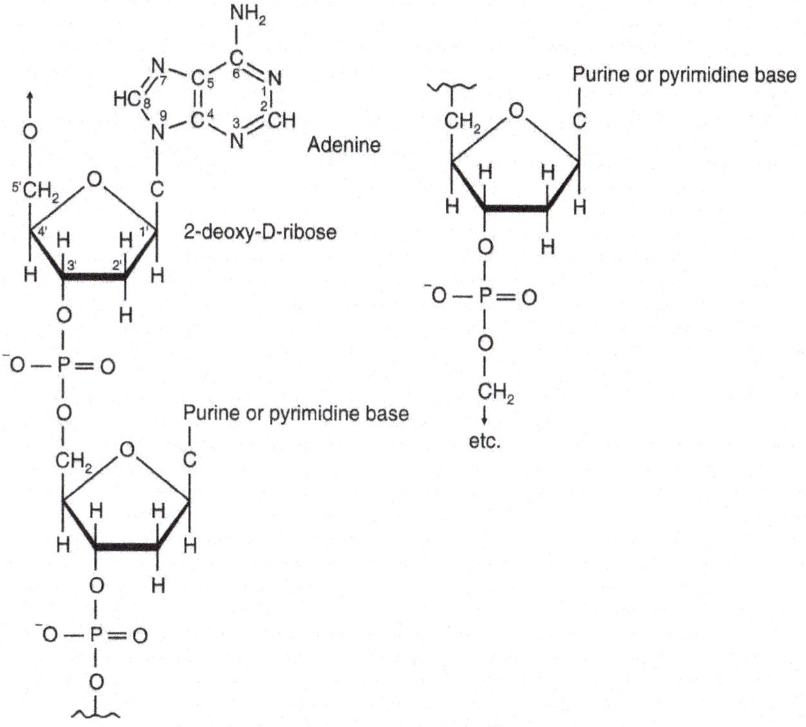

Figure 133. Backbone structure of DNA.

Each nucleoside contains a 2'-deoxyribose molecule and a base, either adenine A or thymine T or cytosine C or guanine G (Figure 134).

2-deoxyribose is a derivative of the sugar ribose (Figure 135)

The phosphodiester linkage is through the 5' and 3' of two rests 2'deoxyribose. DNA is an extremely long chain, the links of which are located at four different recurring subunits, the mononucleotides. (Recall that a nucleotide is a nucleoside phosphorylated at one of its pentose

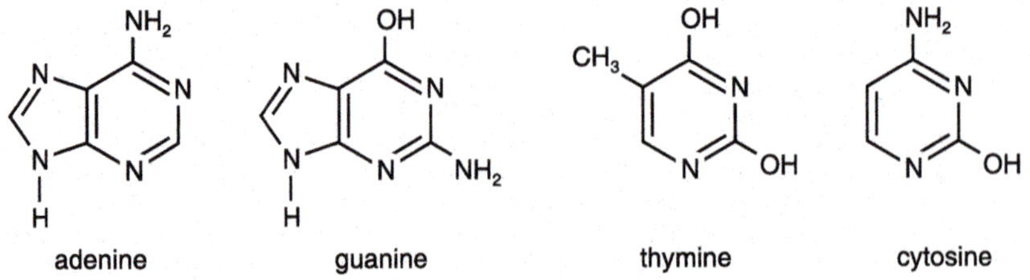

Figure 134 I, II, III. Structures of adenine, thymine, cytosine and guanine.

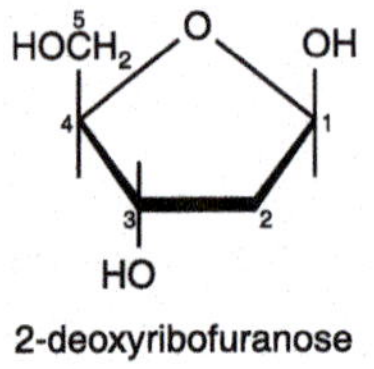

2-deoxyribofuranose

Figure 135. Structure of the 2-deoxyribofuranose.

hydroxyl groups). Each mononucleotide unit contains either a purine or a pyrimidine base, one molecule of 2-deoxy-D-ribose and one molecule of phosphoric acid.

The chains of the double-helix are arranged in an antiparallel fashion and form a right-handed helix. The bases are paired through hydrogen bonds. The base-pairs encountered are (Figure 136):

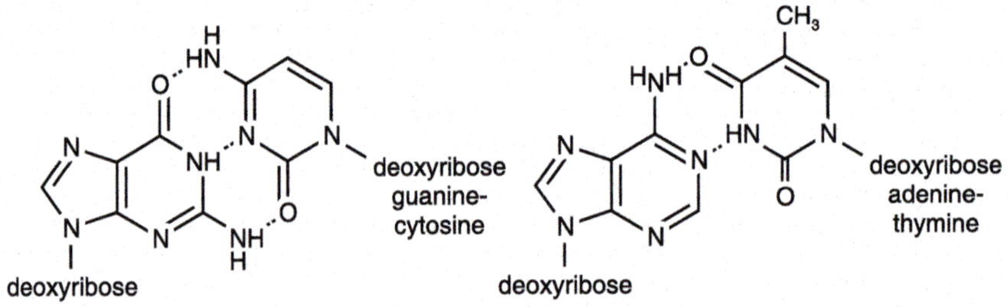

Figure 136. Hydrogen-bonding between DNA strands involving the base-pairing of guanine and cytosine on one hand and, on the other, of adenine and thymine.

Table 19 mentions the thermodynamic parameters for base pairing in deuterochloroform. We notice that the bonds are weak as it was awaited for H-bonds. They also tend to form spontaneously, at least in deuterochloroform. When cells divide, each daughter cell receives one of the complementary strands of the parent DNA and then synthesizes a complementary strand to provide the daughter cell with a complete double-stranded DNA. The process is called *replication*.

Table 19. Thermodynamic parameters for base pairing in deuterochloroform; (U: uracile). According to G.G. Hammes, "Thermodynamics and kinetics for the biological sciences": see general bibliography.

base-pair	$\Delta G°$(kJ mol^{-1})	$\Delta H°$(kJ mol^{-1})	$\Delta S°$(J mol^{-1} K^{-1})
A-A	−2,80	−16,72	−47,65
U-U	−4, 47	−17,97	−45,98
A-U	−11,37	−25,92	−49,32
C-C	−8,23	−26,33	−62,7
G-G	−17,14 to −22,57	−35,53 to −41,8	−62,7
G-C	−22,57 to −28,42	−41,80 to −48,07	−62,7

2) RNA

The information contained in DNA must first be transcribed to a chemical messenger. The latter is a ribonucleic acid *named messenger RNA* (mRNA). Messenger RNA has a chemical structure very similar to that of DNA. However, it has one single strand and contains four different types of mononucleotides which possess the sugar D-ribose instead of the 2-deoxyribose. The four characteristic bases of mRNA are adenine, guanine, cytosine and uracile. mRNA contains uracil instead of the thymine found in DNA (Figure 137).

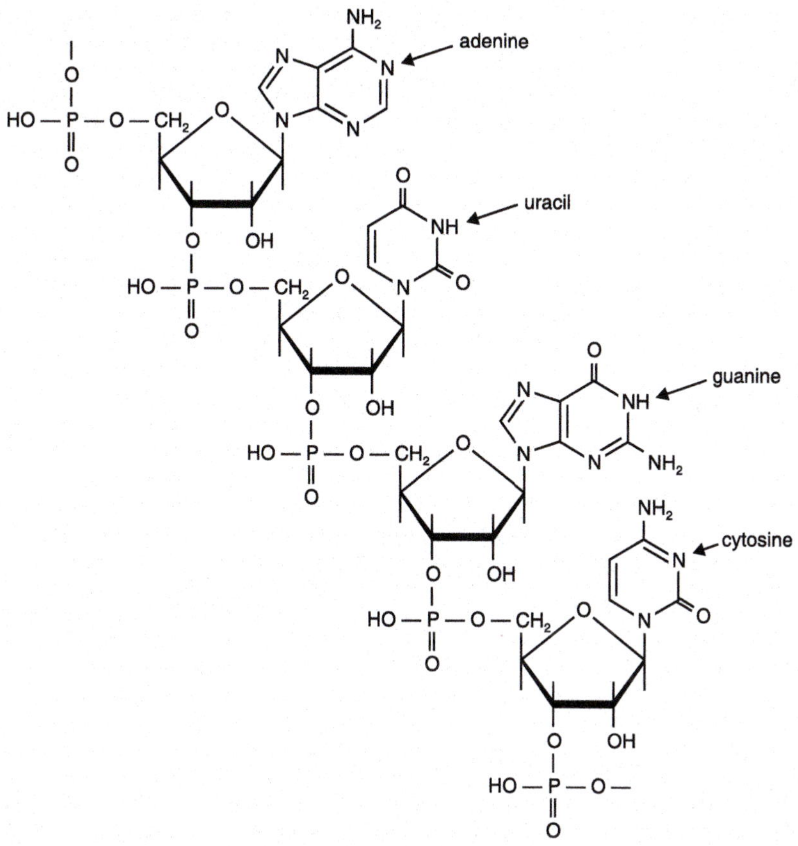

Figure 137. Structure of a strand of RNA.

Actually, it is a transcription of the DNA molecule. It is synthesized enzymatically in such a way that the DNA is the template for the sequence of the bases in the messenger RNA.

The complete mRNA diffuses into the cytoplasm from the nucleus and attaches to the ribosomes and the protein synthesis occurs on the surface of these ones.

After the encoding, there is formation of the peptide bond between the amino acid and its predetermined neighbor. After many repetitions of the process, the protein being built is formed.

3) Encoding

The messenger RNA molecule bears the code for directing the specific sequence of amino acids which are to be inserted into the peptide chain of the protein being built. *The principle of encoding is that a sequence of three consecutive mononucleotide units in the mRNA molecule codes a single, specified amino acid. The process in the ribosome consists in "reading out" the consecutive nucleotide triplets, selecting the activated amino acids which correspond to each consecutive triplet and, finally, in forming the peptide bond.*

4) The replication of DNA

The synthesis of a new strand of DNA which, structurally complementary to the single-stranded DNA, takes place in the daughter cells during or after cell division is called *replication* (of DNA). The replication is catalyzed by a single enzyme molecule called the *DNA polymerase*. It can build such a chain of DNA only when a single strand form of DNA is present to provide the template, otherwise it is inactive. The reaction of biosynthesis evolves only in the presence of the 5'-triphosphates of the four deoxyribonucleosides dATP, dGTP, dTTP and dCTP (see Chapter 38) and also of ions Mg^{2+}. The enzyme causes the sequential formation of new deoxy monophosphates by splitting out the terminal two phosphate groups from the precursor triphosphate in the form of pyrophosphates, as follows:

n dATP			d AMP$_n$		
n dGTP		DNA	d GMP$_n$		
	+ DNA	$\longrightarrow$		----	DNA + 4n P–P
nTTP		polymerase	TMP$_n$		
n dCTP			d CMP$_n$		
	template		formed double-stranded DNA		pyrophosphate

From the energetic standpoint, we can notice that for each mononucleotide subunit added to the template, one molecule of pyrophosphate is formed. The latter is hydrolyzed into two molecules of phosphate by *pyrophosphatase*. This reaction exhibits a large decrease in Gibbs energy ($\Delta G'^\circ = -29260$ J mol^{-1}). Since the Gibbs energy of the reaction of formation of the phosphate diester linkage is about -27170 J mol^{-1}, there remains a considerable tendency towards the formation of the double strand.

5) The transcription to mRNA

Recall that the transcription is the enzymatic process whereby the genetic information contained in one strand of DNA is used to specify a complementary sequence of bases to an mRNA chain. It proceeds through an enzymatic process which is analogous to that taking place in the enzymatic replication of DNA chains. The specific enzyme, the *RNA polymerase*, present in the nucleus, catalyzes the reaction. It is the assembly of mRNA from the four ribonucleoside 5'-triphosphates, that is to say: ATP, GTP, UTP and CTP (see Chapter 38). In this reaction, DNA is required as the template. The reaction is:

n ATP			AMP$_n$		
n GTP		RNA	GMP$_n$		
	+ DNA	$\longrightarrow$		----	DNA + 4n P–P
n UTP		polymerase	UMP$_n$		
n CTP			CMP$_n$		
	template		formed DNA-mRNA hybrid		pyrophosphate

At each step, a nucleoside triphosphate is selected according to its fit with a base in the template DNA in the complementary way evoked.

6) Protein biosynthesis

The protein biosynthesis is by far the most elaborate biosynthetic mechanism known. It is the reason why it seems interesting to us to mention very briefly its steps before finishing this book by considering the biological information. The biosynthesis is in several steps.

– The first step is the activation of the twenty different amino acids A-A at the expense of ATP. The reactions are (Figure 138):

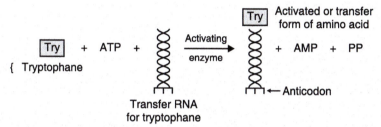

Figure 138. Schematic representation of an amino-acid activation. Example of one amino-acid (tryptophane).

Twenty different activation enzymes are required, each specific for one of the twenty amino-acids. Through the activation reaction, the amino-acid is esterified to form a high-energy bond with a specific amino acid carrier molecule. The amino-acid carriers are molecules of ribonucleic acid. The latter is not the same as the mRNA. This type of RNA is known as soluble RNA:sRNA or transfer RNA:tRNA. It is a relatively small molecule (molecular weight about 20 000 whereas mRNA of the order of 10^6). There is at least one specific sRNA molecule for each amino-acid. Hence, for each amino-acid, there is a specific activating enzyme and at least one specific sRNA. The amino-acid becomes linked to both. It is activated. The activated amino-acids are now ready to be assembled. Attaching the right amino-acid to the right tRNA is critical. This reaction takes place in the cytosol and not in the ribosome. For example, let us choose the alanine for amino-acid (Figure 139):

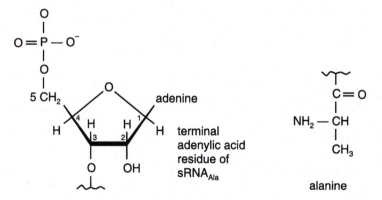

Figure 139. Structure of alanine linked to the terminal adenylic acid, residue of $sRNA_{ala}$.

The reaction of activation and the activated amino-acid structures are, respectively (Figure 140):

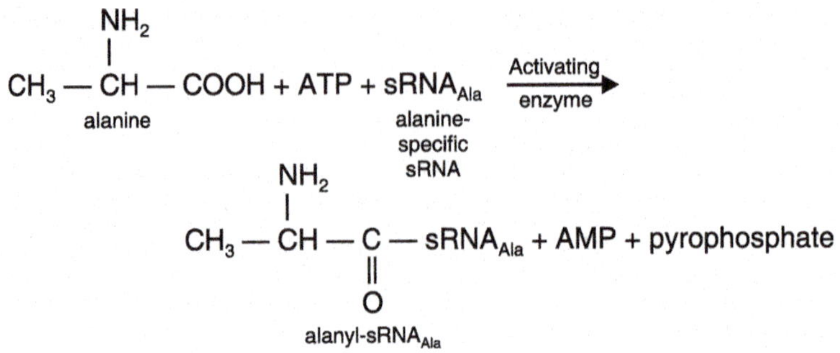

$$CH_3 - \underset{\substack{| \\ \text{alanine}}}{\overset{\substack{NH_2 \\ |}}{CH}} - COOH + ATP + sRNA_{Ala} \xrightarrow{\substack{\text{Activating} \\ \text{enzyme}}}$$

alanine-
specific
sRNA

$$CH_3 - \underset{\substack{| \\ O}}{\overset{\substack{NH_2 \\ |}}{CH}} - \underset{\substack{\| \\ O}}{C} - sRNA_{Ala} + AMP + \text{pyrophosphate}$$

alanyl-sRNA_{Ala}

Figure 140. The activating reaction of alanine.

– During the preceding process, the messenger RNA molecules are attached firmly to the ribosomes. One mRNA molecule or the portion of it which is attached to the surface of the ribosome comprises the template for the sequential assembly of the peptide chain from amino-acid and binds to the initiating aminoacyl-tRNA. The base sequence of three consecutive mononucleotide residues in the mRNA chain may code a single amino-acid. Such a coding triplet is called a *codon*. For example, the codons for alanine and leucine are CUG and UAU, respectively. The amino acids "recognize" their codons on the mRNA template not directly but through a sequence of recognition nucleotides in the specific sRNA molecules to which they are attached. The recognition site is the *anticodon*. The anticodon is believed to be a complementary triplet of bases in the sRNA molecule which can fit the codon on the mRNA uniquely. The complete amino acids RNA molecule thus attaches to the ribosome by some form of very specific bonding between the anticodon of the sRNA and the codon of the mRNA. When the amino acid is thus fixed in position, an enzyme causes the formation of the peptide bond (Figure 141).

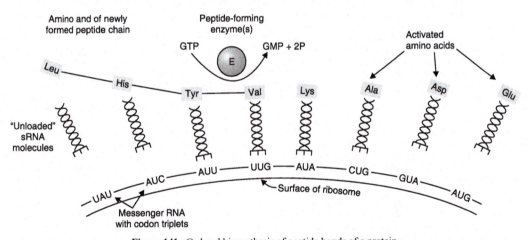

Figure 141. Ordered biosynthesis of peptide bonds of a protein.
(figure reproduced from the book "bioenergetics" by A.L. Lehninger, p. 213, Benjamin Editor, by the courtesy of the Pearson group)

From the energetic standpoint, ATP is transformed into pyrophosphate which, in turn, is enzymically hydrolyzed into two moles of phosphate. Two high-energy bonds of ATP are consumed to create the chemical bond of the amino-acid with the transfer RNA. It is important to notice that the amino-acid is activated through its carboxylic rest which becomes linked to the 2' or 3'-hydroxyl group of the ribose. This linkage is of high-energy (hydrolysis Gibbs energy about -27170 J mol^{-1}).

A total of three high-energy phosphate bonds of ATP permits to create each peptide bond. Each peptide bond has a Gibbs energy of formation of 23000 joules. Clearly, the input of 88000 joules (by ATP) is sufficient to provide a large pull.

- In the next step, another specific amino acid-sRNA molecule is attached to its specific codon and is "locked" into place by the codon-anticodon fit and the process repeats. The nascent polypeptide is lengthened by covalent attachment of successive amino-acid, each carried to the ribosome and correctly positioned by its tRNA which "base-pairs" to its corresponding codon in the mRNA.
- Termination and ribosome recycling.
- Folding and posttranslational processing.

The protein biosynthesis is by far the most elaborate biosynthetic mechanism known. It is the reason why it seems interesting to us to mention very briefly its steps before finishing this book by considering the biological information. It is carried out under the influence of a genetic flux of information.

Genes determine the kinds of proteins which are built by cells. However, the DNA is not the direct matrice for the synthesis of proteins. Actually, the templates for the synthesis of proteins are some molecules of RNA.

A kind of RNA molecules, called messenger RNA (mRNA) gather intermediaries bringing information during the synthesis of proteins. Other molecules of RNA such as transfer RNA (tRNA) and also the ribosomal RNA (rRNA) also participate to the synthesis of proteins. All the forms of the cellular RNA are synthesized by RNA *polymerases* which take their instructions in the matrice of DNA. This phenomenon is called *transcription*. It is followed by that of *traduction* which is the synthesis of proteins according to the instructions given by the templates of mRNA. Hence, the flux of genetic information (into a normal cell) evolves as follows:

DNA $\xrightarrow{\text{transcription}}$ RNA $\xrightarrow{\text{traduction}}$ protein

The genetic code, which has just been precisely involved, is the relation between the arrangement of the bases of DNA (or of that which is its "transcript") and the amino acids of a protein. A sequence of three bases, named *codon*, determine one amino acid. The codons of mRNA are sequentially read by molecules of tRNA. A molecule of tRNA brings a specific amino acid under an activated form up to the synthesis site. The carboxylic acid group is esterified by the 2' and 3'rests of a ribose unit located at the end of the chain of tRNA. An aminoacyl-tRNA is built according to a reaction specifically catalyzed by an *activation enzyme*. The recognition site of the matrix on the tRNA is a sequence of three bases called *anticodon*. The Figures 145, 143 and 142 schematically represent the linkage between an amino acid and a tRNA and the linkage site of the amino acid and the anticodon.

Up to the stage of the synthesis of proteins we have just described, it is not a finished one we have in our hands but only a long peptide chain. It must be folded into a characteristic three-dimensional conformation. The biological function of a protein molecule is vitally dependent on its specific three dimensional folded conformation. Recall that proteins fall into two major classes depending on their three dimensional structure. They are the fibrous proteins which have all their peptide chains in an extended conformation located on one axis and the globular ones. Globular proteins are nearly spherical in shape. The long peptide chains are folded inside them. The study of protein folding is a major field of research.

The synthesis of proteins are carried out on the ribosomes which are complex assemblies of tRNA and several proteins. The newly built proteins contain signals which allow them to be directed towards purposes.

Chapter **42**

Biological Information

In brief, in this chapter, we are concerned by the handling of cellular information. DNA is the master informational molecule of the cell. The DNA of each species is specific for that species and directs its faithful reproduction. Its four mononucleotides are elements of the coding system. Living organisms possess an extraordinary property, namely information, in their organization. The new science of information theory says that information, whether in an encyclopedia or a living cell, is actually a form of energy.

In this respect, we shall now consider the biosynthesis of the nucleic acids and the proteins. In doing so, we come face to face with a new aspect or quality of molecular components of the cell, namely the information. Nucleic acids are molecules adapted for the storage and transcription of biological information and the proteins are the molecules for its expression. The biosynthesis of nucleic acids and proteins is rather difficult to understand because their building block molecules must be inserted into the structure of these long chain molecules in an exact specific order or sequence and the entire biological function of the nucleic acids and proteins is dependent on the exactness of this sequence.

The theoretical relationships between information and entropy tell us that assembling the cell structures from a collection of molecules is a process that must proceed with a very large decrease in internal entropy.

1) Information theory

The information theory is a theory of signal. It is due to Cl. Shannon (1948). By definition, an information points out one or several events among a finite number of possible events.

For example, if we search for a file among other ones and if one tells you that the file is red, we have received one information. On the practical standpoint, it reduces the time to find it. An important point is that the information is not of the same quality. For example, in the preceding case, if among 800 files there are 50 red ones, one sets up, by definition, that the quantity of information I is given by the relation:

$I = \log (800/50)$

If instead of 50 red files, we have 200 red files, the information I' would be:

$I' = \log (800/200)$

It would have been more difficult to find the file. The second information is of less quality than the first one.

2) A particular interesting example of information of high quality

It is that obtained from each answer to binary questions, questions which on one hand are only answerable by yes or no and which, on the other, permits to gain more information from each answer. To illustrate this point, let us suppose that we have sixteen equal boxes and a coin which is in one of these boxes (Figure 142). We have to find where it is.

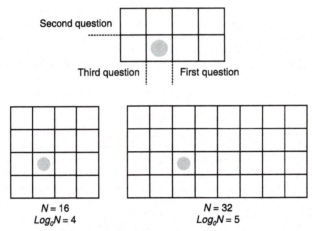

$N = 16$
$Log_0N = 4$

$N = 32$
$Log_0N = 5$

Figure 142. Different information received during the followed strategy.
(figure reproduced from the book "entropy demystified" by Arieh Ben-Naim, p. 49 revised edition, copyright 2008, by courtesy of World Scientific edition)

To acquire this information, one can ask only binary questions. There are many strategies. Here, we exemplify that which gives the best quality of information. The first question may be: is the coin present in the first two horizontal lines? The answer is no. That is, it is in the two following ones. We have already got a supplementary information. The second worthwhile question may be: is the coin in the third line? The answer is for example no. We have still got a new information and so forth. We can notice that, very often, this strategy is quicker than another one which would consist of directly asking the questions of the kind: is the coin present in the third rank and in the fourth column?

This reasoning is due to A. Ben-Naim.*

3) Some theoretical points of the information theory

From the general standpoint, one can say that:

I = log (N/n)

The analogy with Boltzmann's formula relative to the entropy S in the microcanonical ensemble (see statistical thermodynamics):

S = k log W

is troublesome. W is the number of possible repartitions of the particles in the isolated system and k is a constant. Actually, the pivotal formula of Shannon is the following one:

$H = -\Sigma_i P_i \log_2 P_i$

---

* A. Ben-Naim "Entropy demystified", World Scientific Publishing Co, Singapore, 2008).

H is the quantity of the circulating information. P_i is the emission probability of the message. This relation is identical to those giving the entropy in the cases of the canonical and grand-canonical ensembles (see statistical thermodynamics). The logarithm of base 2 $\log_2$ is introduced into the basic quantitative unit of international content called the binary digit or *bit*. The amount of information in a message is expressed in terms of the probability of a sequence of binary choices or bits.

It is interesting to notice that an interpretation of entropy is that of missing information. For these authors (Shannon-Ben-Naim), it is a better understanding of entropy than is its meaning of "disorder".

The amount of information in a message is expressed in terms of probability of a sequence of binary choices or bits. If the amount of information in a message is 4, this means that four correct binary choices (with a probability of 1) would have been made to get the knowledge of the hidden impossibilities. The approximate information content of protein molecules and DNA molecules can be calculated.

Suppose we have protein molecules containing 1000 amino acids' residues of sixteen different kinds arranged in an absolutely specific sequence of order. (In other words, only sixteen amino acids can be present). The probability to choose the right amino acid is only one out of sixteen. To specify each amino acid in the chain of sixteen amino acids, hence, requires about four bits of information. So there are 1000 sets of 4 binary choices in such a *protein molecule*.

By such approaches, it is calculated that a single bacterial cell having a diameter of only 2 μm and weighing 6×10^{-13}g contains 10^{12} bits of information!!! This is an enormeously large number. Another calculation shows that the information in one volume of Encyclopedia Britannica would contain? 10^6 bits!!!!

It is clear that living cells do possess immense amounts of information.

4) Entropy and information (following)—an interesting thought experiment: The Maxwell's demon experiment

This experiment still brings relations between the thermodynamic entropy and the information. Let a gas be allowed to escape from one chamber through a narrow orifice into another one which is empty (Figure 143). The gas molecules diffuse evenly throughout both containers as it is expected from the second law. Let us suppose that both flasks are of equal sizes and that a demon sits at their common orifice. When a fast or hot molecule comes along, it lets it through to the other container. Contrarily, when a cold molecule comes, the demon closes the hole and the cold molecule must stay behind. Such a process would decrease the entropy (or the randomness of the system) without changing its total energy. It is in flagrant contradistinction with the second law. *Indeed, since the system has evolved, the system of both flasks (which is an isolated one) might have its entropy enhanced.* For years, there seemed to be no reasonable explanation until an author (Szilard) pointed out that, in this experiment, the demon requires the use of information to be successful in his process to select the hot molecules. *This virtual experience obviously set up a direct numerical correspondence between the amount of information in a system and a lack of entropy.*

It has been deduced that about 10^{23} bits of information are required to reduce the entropy of a system by 4,18J $mol^{-1}K^{-1}$. Thus one joule seems to be equivalent to an enormous amount of information.

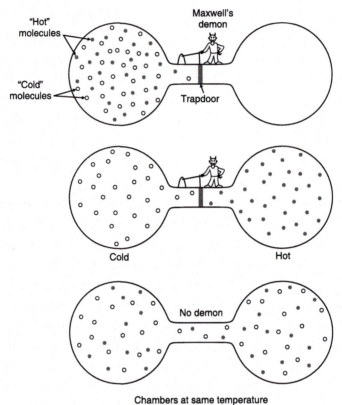

Figure 143. Maxwell's demon experiment.
(figure reproduced from the book "bioenergetics" by A.L. Lehninger, p. 226, Benjamin Editor, by the courtesy of the Pearson group)

The figures above, relative to the informational content of living cells, are very very high. This is the reason why they are acknowledged with great difficulty. It has been proposed that there is some underlying simplicity in cellular development and growth according to A.L. Lehninger (1965).

Appendices

I) Physico-Chemical and Biochemical Appendices

I-1) Calculations of the molality and of the molarity of a solute from its molar fraction

Calculating the molality and the molarity of a solution from its molar fraction is not trivial. Such calculations involve the solution's density. They emphasize the fact that in the molarity, it is the solution volume that is considered, whereas in the molality, it is the mass of the pure solvent. Let us suppose that the solution contains n_0 solvent moles, n_A n_B moles of solutes A and B. Let us consider solute A.

By definition:

$$x_A = n_A/\Sigma n_I \qquad \Sigma n_I = n_0 + n_A + n_B + \ldots..$$

and

$$C_A = n_A/V$$

where V is the solution volume. We want to find a relationship between C_A and x_A. The solution mass $\Sigma n_I M_I$ (grams) is:

$$\Sigma n_I M_I = n_0 M_0 + n_A M_A + n_B M_B + \ldots..$$

and so forth, where M_A, M_B are the molar masses (g/mol) of the solvent and of the solutes A, B and so forth. The solution volume V is:

$$V = \Sigma n_I M_I/\rho \, . \, 1000$$

where ρ is the volume mass of the solution (g/cm³). The factor 1000 permits us to express the volume in liters. We deduce immediately from the first three relations of this appendix:

$$C_A = (1000\rho/\Sigma n_I M_I)n_A$$

$$C_A = (1000\rho/\Sigma n_I/\Sigma n_I M_I)x_A$$

From a strict mathematical standpoint, C_A and x_A are not in a linear relationship since Σn_I and $\Sigma n_I M_I$ do change with x_A. However, the linear relationship appears when the solution is sufficiently diluted. In this case, indeed,

$$\Sigma n_I \approx n_0$$

and

$$\Sigma n_I M_I \approx n_0 M_0$$

Thereby, we have:

$$C_A = (1000\, \rho/M_0)x_A$$

where ρ is the volumic mass of the pure solvent since the solution is diluted. In particular, for water at 25°C:

$$\rho \approx 1$$

$$C_A = (1000/M_0)\, x_A \quad \text{(room-temperature water)}$$

Then, by definition:

$$m_A = 1000.n_A/n_0 M_0$$

The factor 1000 is introduced since M_0 is expressed in grams while m_A is in mol/kg. By introducing the first relation of this appendix into the latter, we find:

$$m_A = (\Sigma n_I.1000/n_0 M_0)x_A$$

Again, m_A and x_A are not in a linear relationship. However, in diluted solutions:

$$\Sigma n_I \approx n_0$$

$$m_A = (1000/M_0)x_A$$

The 5th and the 9th relations of this appendix permit the calculation of C_A and m_A from x_A. The relationship between C_A and m_A is obtained after eliminating x_A in these relations. We find

$$m_A/C_A = \Sigma n_I M_I/\rho N_0 M_0$$

The latter relation clearly shows that in diluted aqueous solution,

$$\Sigma n_I M_I \approx n_0 M_0$$

$$m_A \approx C_A$$

since $\rho \rightarrow 1$. In brief, it is only in sufficiently diluted solutions that numerical values of the molarity and the molality of a solute are equal and, thus, in these conditions, the molarity and the molality are proportional to their molar fraction.

I-2) Weak bonds

The strongest forces that hold the atoms of a molecule together are covalent bonds. Usually, their values range from 210 to 840 kJ mol^{-1}. However, not all the bonds responsible for maintaining the structures of large biomolecules are covalent. The forces that stabilize the three-dimensional architecture of large molecules are much weaker. Their energy is of the order of 4 to 20 kJ mol^{-1}. In this appendix, we briefly consider the hydrogen bond, the van der Waals interactions and the hydrophobic bond.

• The hydrogen bond

The nature of hydrogen bonding can be illustrated in the first place by water. The boiling-point of water is much higher than that of hydrogen sulphide. This suggests that water molecules are bound to each other in the liquid state. The bond between water molecules is relatively weak compared to the bond between the atoms in the water molecule itself. Two water molecules can associate. There is an attractive force between the proton bound to an oxygen atom and the unshared electrons of the oxygen atom of another water molecule. No other element can replace hydrogen. The kinds of hydrogen-atom bonding are those involving two oxygen atoms, two nitrogen atoms or one nitrogen or one oxygen atom. Sulfur atoms are sometimes incriminated. The energy of a hydrogen bond is about 21 kJ mol^{-1}. Hydrogen bonding may be intermolecular. This is the case in water. It is also the case in the mutually bonded chains of desoxyribose nucleic acid (see Chapter 41). Hydrogen bonding may also be intramolecular.

Hydrogen bonding is important in proteins. The carbonyle C = O of one amide group forms a hydrogen bond with the N–H of another (Figure I-1);

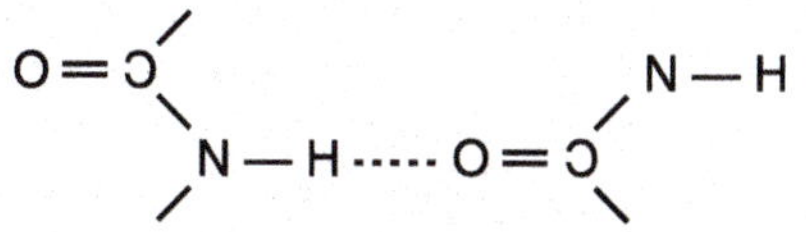

Figure I-1. Hydrogen bonding.

• van der Waals forces

Frequently, one encompasses three distinct kinds of weak interactions into the heading van der Waals forces. They are Keesom, Debye and London forces.

– Keesom forces are interaction forces between two permanent dipoles. They are due to electrostatic forces, the positive pole of one molecule attracting the negative pole of another;

– Debye forces are due to the interactions between a permanent dipole and another which is induced by a polar molecule which creates an electric field all around it;

– London forces are also named dispersion forces. In the cases of neutral atoms or non polar molecules, there exists no permanent dipole but there exist transient ones, owing to the fact that electrons rotate around the nucleus. Hence, the instantaneous moment of an atom creates an induced moment in another and reciprocally. The energy of the system constituted by both atoms is, thus, decreased. London forces are always the strongest. They are of the order of 15 kJ mol^{-1}.

Van der Waals interactions occur among all types of molecules, both polar and non-polar. For example, they are responsible for the cohesion among the molecules of nonpolar liquids and solids. The van der Waals between two large molecules are appreciable if they have complementary shapes.

• Hydrophobic interactions

They result from the tendency of molecules to avoid water. They are called hydrophobic molecules in water, hydrophobic molecules are surrounded by water molecules which more or less solvate them. These water molecules form a network stabilized by hydrogen bonds. When two water molecules approach mutually, they tend to bind. The single resultant molecule has less need of water molecules to solvate itself than the two previously separated. This is the hydrophobic interaction. It is thermodynamically favored by the increased disorder due to the liberated water molecules during the binding. This is an entropic effect. As a conclusion, we can say that hydrophobic interactions are not at all due to formation of bonds.

Hydrophobic interactions among lipids and between lipids and proteins are the most important determinants of the structures of biological membranes. They also stabilize the three-dimensional structures of proteins by their intervention at the level of the non-polar parts of the amino acids.

I-3) Steady state—Rate determining state

- **Steady state**

The steady state treatment is of great importance in chemical kinetics. It permits the analysis of composite mechanisms since they are often endowed with mathematical difficulties that make impossible to obtain an explicit solution of the rate expressions for them. (Composite reactions involve more than one elementary reaction).

Let's consider, for example, the mechanism:

$$A + B \rightleftharpoons X \tag{1}$$

$$X \rightarrow Z \tag{2}$$

The rate equations that apply to these two chemical equations are:

$$d[A]/dt = k_1[A][B] - k_{-1}[X] \quad \text{with} \quad -d[A]/dt = -d[B]/dt$$

$$d[X]/dt = k_1[A][B] - k_{-1}[X] - k_2[X]$$

$$d[Z]/dt = k_2[X]$$

It is impossible to find an explicit solution $[Z] = f(t)$ of the system. Let us apply the steady state principle. It consists in saying that the concentration $[X]$ is practically constant, i.e.,

$$d[X]/dt = 0$$

or:

$$k_1[A][B] - k_{-1}[X] - k_2[X] = 0$$

As a result:

$$[X] = k_1[A][B]/(k_{-1} + k_2) \tag{3}$$

$$d[Z]/dt = k_2 k_1[A][B]/(k_{-1} + k_2) \tag{4}$$

- Rate determining state

When, globally, a chemical reaction consists in successive elementary reactions and when one of them imposes its proper rate, it is called the "rate determining step".

The preceding example can give rise to two hypothesis of rate determining steps.

- First hypothesis: the intermediate X is converted very rapidly into Z, that is to say:

$$k_2 \gg k_{-1}$$

Neglecting k_{-1} in the denominator of (4), only the constant k_1 remains:

$d[Z]/dt = k_1[A][B]$

The initial step is the rate determining state.

– Second hypothesis: the rate constant for the second reaction $X \rightarrow Z$ is very small, i.e.:

$k_2 \ll k_{-1}$

Neglecting k_2 in the denominator of (4) gives:

$d[Z]/dt = (k_2 k_1 / k_{-1}) [A][B]$

Reaction (2), therefore, becomes the rate determining step.

I-4) Some recalls concerning the optical activity and chirality

In this appendix, we recall some elements of the part of chemistry usually called "stereochemistry". It is devoted to optical chemistry and chirality.

The treatment of the subject seems to us justified by the fact that most of the *natural* molecules exhibit one (at least), somewhat amazing, characteristic related to the chirality. For example, natural amino-acids, whose chaining constitutes the primary structure of proteins and enzymes, are all of the series L (see under).

The examples taken in this appendix are extracted from the realm of organic chemistry. However, the concept of chirality and of optical activity is a general one and also applies to all the domains of the chemistry, biochemistry included, and perhaps overall!

4-1) A preliminary: configurations and conformations

A configuration of a molecule is an arrangement in space of the atoms or groups of atoms constituting it. Configurations can be experimentally isolated since they are sufficiently energetically stable. In order to change a configuration, some chemical bonds must be broken. Optical isomers have different configurations, and Z and E isomers too.

A conformation of a molecule is one of the multiple momentaneous spatial arrangements of the atoms (or groups of atoms) of one molecule. Conformations differ from each other by rotations around one or several bonds of the molecule. A particularly simple example is that of the ethane molecule. Its multiple conformations correspond notably to the different angles which can exist between the two methyl groups which can rotate more or less around the central C-C bond. Whereas the configurations can be isolated, the conformations can not. The energy barriers between the different conformations are too weak. This is the reason why they transform into each other very easily. There is no need of breakdown of bonds for a change of conformation. A point which markedly shows the difference between a conformation and a configuration is that for a configuration, there may exist several conformations.

4-2) Optical activity and chirality in brief

Any material that rotates the plane of polarized light is said to be *optically active*. If a pure compound is optically active, its molecule is non-superimposable on its mirror image. If it is superimposable on its mirror image, it does not rotate the plane of polarized light. It is *optically inactive*. The property of non-superimposability of an object on its mirror image is called *chirality*. According to the fact that a molecule is non-superimposable on its mirror image or its converse, it is said as being *chiral* or *achiral*.

A category of compounds exhibiting the phenomenon of optical activity is that containing species possessing an asymmetric carbon. Asymmetric carbons are connected to four different groups according to the disposal of a tetraedre. If there is only one such atom, the molecule must be optically active. There are then two isomers called enantiomers (or enantiomorphs). They rotate the plane of polarized light in opposite directions, but in the same amount. The isomer which rotates the plane counterclockwise is called the levo isomer, the other the dextro isomer. The former is designated (–) isomer, the latter (+) isomer. Each isomer is the mirror image of the other.

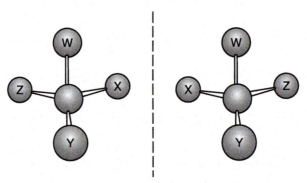

Figure I-2. Two enantiomers.

The amount of rotation α (the observed rotation) for a given enantiomer depends on several parameters. When it is in solution, it is given by the relation:

$[\alpha] = \alpha/l\ c$

l is the length of the measurement cell length, c the concentration of the species, and $[\alpha]$ is the specific rotation of the compound.

4-3) Molecules displaying optical activity

Some tests may be used to deceal optical activity prior that of superimposability. The tests consist in the research of some elements of symmetry present or not in the studied molecule. They are:

–   a plane of symmetry: compounds possessing such a plane are always optically inactive;

–   a center of symmetry: compounds possessing such an element are inactive;

–   an alternating axis of symmetry of order n also has inactivity for consequence. (An alternating center of symmetry is such that when an object is rotated by 360°/n about the axis and then reflection is effected across a plane at right angles to the axis, a new object is obtained that is indistinguishable from the original one).

An axis of symmetry (not alternating) is not a criterion of optical activity or inactivity.

There exist different categories of chiral compounds. We confine ourselves to only continue the study of the most important category, that which is constituted by the derivatives possessing one asymmetric carbon atom, at least. It is easy to verify that it does not possess any symmetry element cited previously.

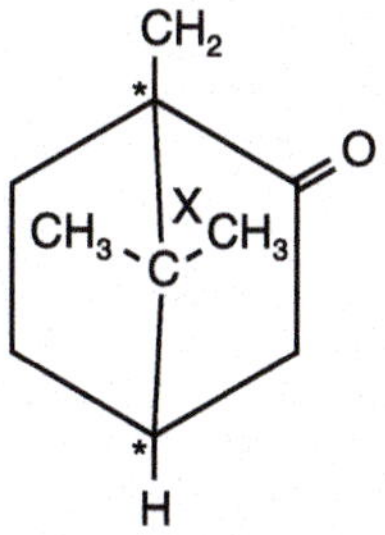

Figure I-3. Structure of camphor.

In principle, for n asymmetric carbons C^*, there exist 2^n optical isomers called enantiomers. This is not an absolute rule. When $n = 1$, it is always true. When $n \geq 2$, there can exist exceptions. This is the case of camphor for example which does possess three asymmetric carbons.

Camphor would exhibit 8 optical isomers. Actually, there exist only two enantiomorph camphors. The reason is that some configurations are not possible for steric strain reasons. Another example is provided by tartaric acid. The explanation of this exception is given in the following paragraph.

It is interesting to notice that α-deuterobutanol is optically active despite the very slight difference of structure of two substituents (here, the presence of a deuterium atom in

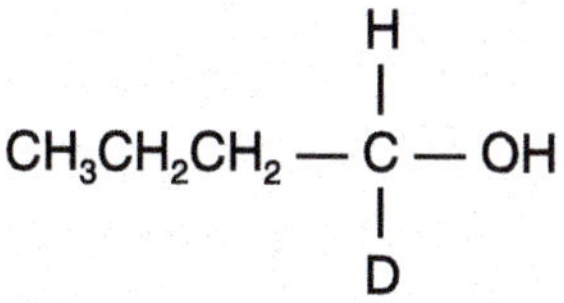

Figure I-4. Structure of α-deuterobutanol.

place of an hydrogen atom). Hence, this property does not preclude the occurrence of optical activity and it proves the generality of the symmetry criterion (Figure I-4):

4-4) Configurations of asymmetric carbons

Before discussing the problem of the absolute configuration of an asymmetric carbon, it is necessary to recall Fischer's convention and, after, that of Cahn, Ingold and Prelog.

4-5) Fischer's convention

– compounds possessing one asymmetric carbon

Fischer's convention is a conventional representation of a molecule possessing an asymmetric carbon. The atoms or groups of atoms fixed on a tetrahedric center are projected on the paper plane so that the atoms (or groups of atoms) appearing above or under the central atom (on the projection) are actually behind the central atom and so that those appearing on the left and on the right of the central atom are actually in front of the paper plane. The principal chain is vertically drawn with its smallest length directed towards the upper part of the paper. The Figure I-5 gives the Fisher's representation of glyceraldehyde.

By convention, the glyceraldehyde having the hydroxyl group on the left is said to belong to the series L (it is the glyceraldehyde levogyre) whereas the aldehyde having the

$$CH_2OH - \overset{*}{C}HOH - CHO$$

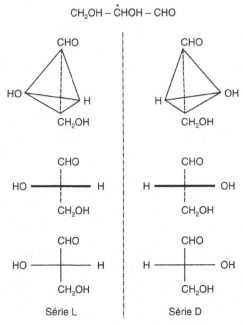

Figure I-5. Fischer's representation of glyceraldehyde.

hydroxyl group on the right is said to belong to the series D (glyceraldehyde dextrogyre). In this example, the hydroxyl group is called the group of "average dimensions".

– compounds possessing several asymmetric carbons—Nomenclature threo-erythro

The nomenclature threo-erythro we now briefly investigate is obsolete but it can be still encountered sometimes in literature, especially in that devoted to the chemistry of sugars. It is closely related to Fischer's representation. Threo-erythro nomenclature applies to systems containing two neighbouring asymmetric carbons with configurations similar to those of the sugars named threose and erythrose. The structures of erythrose and threose are given in Fischer's representations (Figure I-6). They are four carbons sugars. In all these sugars, the chains constituted by the carbon atoms are represented by the vertical line. The bond between carbons 2 and 3 is in the plane of the paper whereas those between carbons 1 and 2 and 3–4 are in the plane normal to the paper, the trace of which is precisely the line 2–3, the carbons 1 and 4 pointing behind the paper (Figure I-6).

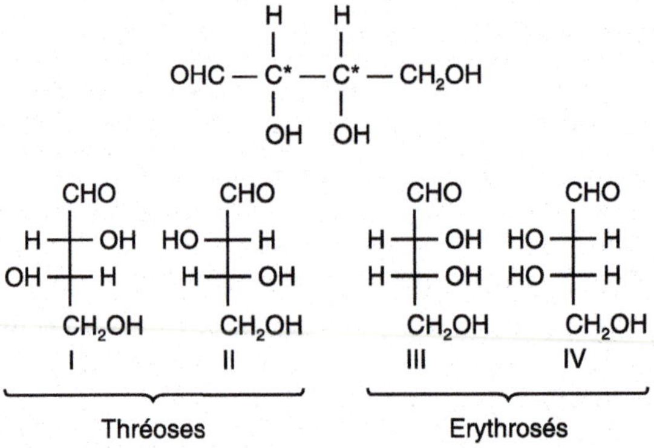

$$OHC - \overset{\displaystyle H}{\underset{\displaystyle OH}{C^*}} - \overset{\displaystyle H}{\underset{\displaystyle OH}{C^*}} - CH_2OH$$

	CHO		CHO			CHO		CHO	
H	OH	HO	H		H	OH	HO	H	
OH	H	H	OH		H	OH	HO	H	
	CH₂OH		CH₂OH			CH₂OH		CH₂OH	
	I		II			III		IV	

Thréoses   Erythrosés

Figure I-6. Configurations of threoses and of erythroses.

There exist two enantiomers of erythrose. In Fischer's representation, they have both groups of average dimensions (hydroxyl groups) on the same side of the vertical line. They are mirror images. In the same configuration, other molecules with different groups of average dimensions would be named "erythro" D or L According to the fact that the first asymmetric carbon next to the lower carbon of the chain brings its group of average dimension on the right or on the left of the principal chain, the compound is said to be of series D or L. The case is similar for threose. There are two enantiomers and the groups of average dimensions are on each side of the vertical line. Both threose are of the series "threo" D or L. According to Fischer, the aldehyde having the hydroxyl group on the left of the carbon chaîn (vertical line) is said to belong to the series L whereas the aldehyde having the hydroxyl group located on the right is said to belong to the series D.

Therefore, when a molecule has two chiral centers, there exist two couples of enantiomers called diastereoisomers which are not mirror images (Figure I-7). They exhibit the threo-erythro isomerism:

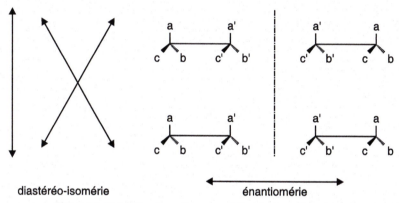

diastéréo-isomérie   énantiomérie

Figure I-7. Examples of enantiomeric and diastereoisomeric couples.

It may arrive that compounds having two asymmetric carbons have fewer isomers than four. It is the case of mesotartaric acid. This is due to the occurrence of a supplementary plane of symmetry. The three isomers of tartaric acid are represented in Figure I-8. The mixture in equal parts of both enantiomorphs threo and erythro constitutes the racemic mixture.

It is easy to verify that isomers B and C are threo derivatives and that they are enantiomers. They are optically active. Derivatives A and B on one hand and A and C on the other are diastereoisomers. The derivative A is optically inactive because of the symmetric plane, the trace of which is perpendicular to the vertical line and passes by its middle. It is called the isomer *meso*.

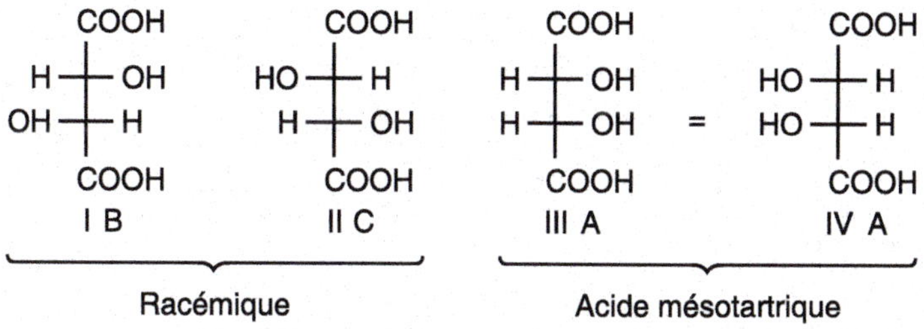

Racémique   Acide mésotartrique

Figure I-8. The three stereoisomers of tartaric acid.

4-6) Configuration of an asymmetric carbon according to Cahn, Ingold and Prelog

A more general system of designation of the configuration of an asymmetric carbon is known under the name of the sequential rule of Cahn, Ingold and Prelog. The principle of this nomenclature is the following: The four (different) substituents of the carbon are placed according to an order of priority based on very well specific rules. Suppose a, b, c, d are the four substituents of an asymmetric carbon and that the priority rules give the order:

a > b > c > d

Once the order is determined, the molecule is held so that the lowest group is pointed away from the observator. Then, if the other groups, in the order listed, are oriented clockwise, the molecule is designated R and if they are counterclockwise, it is designated S (Figure I-9). For example in the glyceraldehyde, the four substituents must be arranged in the order, OH, CHO, CH_2OH, H. According to the rules, the (+) enantiomer is R.

The fundamental rule on which the priority is given is that the substituents are listed in order of decreasing atomic number of the atom directly joined to the carbon. When two or more of the atoms connected to the asymmetric carbon are the same, the atomic number of the second atom of the substituent determines the order, and so forth.

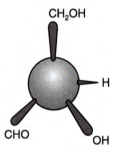

Figure I-9. Configuration according to Cahn, Ingold and Prelo.

4-7) Absolute configuration

The need to determine the absolute configuration of an enantiomer took its origin when chemists were faced with the following experimental evidence:

the fact that a molecule belongs to the series D or L does not imply that it is obligatory (respectively dextrogyre or levogyre). The character dextrogyre or levogyre can be qualified as being unpredictable. An example (among plenty others) is the case of glyceric acid which is in the series D and is levogyre:

CH_2OH-CHOH-COOH
glyceric acid D (–)

Let us consider, as an example, the case of glyceric aldehydes (Figure I-10).

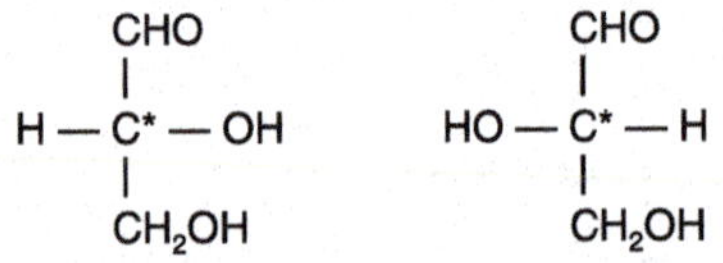

$$
\begin{array}{cc}
\text{CHO} & \text{CHO} \\
| & | \\
\text{H} - \text{C*} - \text{OH} & \text{HO} - \text{C*} - \text{H} \\
| & | \\
\text{CH}_2\text{OH} & \text{CH}_2\text{OH}
\end{array}
$$

D(+) glycéraldéhyde   L(–) glycéraldéhyde

Figure I-10. R and S glyceric aldehydes.

Even if the existence of two enantiomers had been known since a long time, the following problem has arisen: to which configuration (a or b) could we attribute the rotatory angles (+) or (−) and how was that possible? At the beginning chemists arbitrarily decided that the D glyceraldehyde of Fischer was the dextrogyre isomer. Once this decision is taken, the absolute configurations of plenty other asymmetric carbons, *relative to that of the (+) glyceraldehyde,* have been determined with the aid of one-to-one chemical reactions.

But, more recently (1951), it became possible to find without any ambiguity the absolute configuration of the sodium and rubidium tartaric acid double salt by using a particular X-ray technique. The (+) tartrate anion was found to have the R, R configuration. Then the (+) tartaric acid has been correlated with other chiral compounds. *Hence the (arbitrary) attribution of the dextrogyre rotation to the R configuration (or equivalently) to the D glyceraldehyde was accurate. There was one chance out of two that it was the case!*

4-8) Racemates

Mixtures of equal amounts of enantiomers are optically inactive since the equal and opposite rotations cancel. Such mixtures are called *racemates* (the name of racemic mixtures is ambiguous).

4-9) Physico-chemical properties of the different isomers

Concerning this question, there exists a rule which can be qualified as being an *"iron rule."* It is: *enantiomers have identical properties in a symmetrical environment, but their properties may differ in an unsymmetrical environment.* As consequences:

– enantiomers may react at different rates if an optically active catalyst is present,

– they may have different solubilities in optically active solvents,

– they may have different indexes of refraction or absorption spectra, when examined with circularly polarized light.

The properties of racemates are not always the same as those of the individual enantiomers. The properties in the gaseous and liquid states or in solution are usually the same since such mixtures are nearly ideal. This is not the case in the solid state. Some properties such as melting points, solubilities, and heats of fusion are often different from those of the corresponding enantiomers.

There is a difference of reactivity between the couples threo-erythro. It results from the difference of interatomic distances between the substituents. From a general standpoint, diastereoisomers are actually different compounds.

This is such a truth that a racemate is often resolved through the temporary formation of diastereoisomers!

4-10) Molecules with at least three centers of asymmetry

Here, we only consider the case of hexoses, sugars of general formula $C_6H_{12}O_6$. They are aldoses $CH_2OH-(CHOH)_4-CHO$ which possess four asymmetric carbons and ketoses of formula $CH_2OH-(CHOH)_3 CO-CH_2OH$. Aldoses possess four asymmetric carbons and, as it is awaited, exhibit 2^4 optical isomers. Ketoses have only three asymmetric carbons and exhibit 2^3 optical isomers.

I-5) Optical activity and carbohydrates

5-1) Filiation of oses

By way of examples of the preceding appendix, we give the following filiation (Figure I-11).

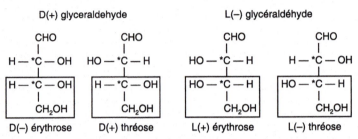

Figure I-11. Some tetroses, their filiation and optical properties.

We see that starting from glyceraldehyde, the introduction of a new secondary alcohol function leads to the sugar with a four carbons chain possessing two asymmetric carbons. Hence, it leads to 2^2 active forms. Two come from the D glyceraldehyde. Hence, they will belong to the series D. Two come from the L glyceraldehyde. They belong to the series L. These active sugars are both erythroses and both threoses.

The principal observations which can be drawn from these figures are:

– the qualification D or L only concerns the absolute configuration of the carbon which is the nearest from that which brings the function primary alcohol. When one speaks of D-erythrose and D-Threose, that means that their carbon 3 has the same configuration as the asymmetric carbon of the D-glyceraldehyde, that is to say, it is R;

– both sugars of the same series D(–)erythrose and D(+) threose on one hand and L(+) erythrose and L(–) threose on the other are diastereoisomers. Their physical and chemical properties, in each pair, are different. They are frankly different compounds;

– the filiation in the series D and L have nothing to do with the character dextrogyre(+) or levogyre (–) of the molecule.

It is very interesting to notice that the great majority of natural sugars are of the series D. It is a puzzling fact.

Let us recall the following correspondences:

D (–) erythrose	optical isomers	L(+) erythrose
diastereoisomers ↓		↓ diastereoisomers
D (+) threose	optical isomers	L (–) threose

We confine ourselves to giving the structures of some other carbohydrates;

– Among the pentoses, let us mention:

the D (–) ribose, which enters into the structure of nucleic acids;

– Among the hexoses, the D (–) glucose, the D (–) fructose (levulose), the D (+) galactose and the D (–) mannose.

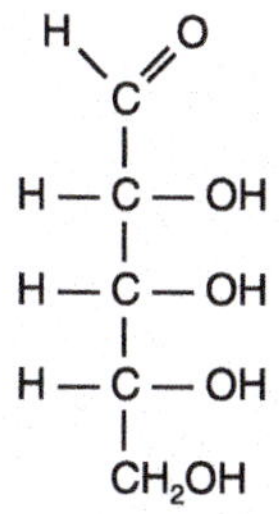

H
C=O
|
H — C — OH
|
H — C — OH
|
H — C — OH
|
CH₂OH

Figure I-12. Structure of D (–) ribose.

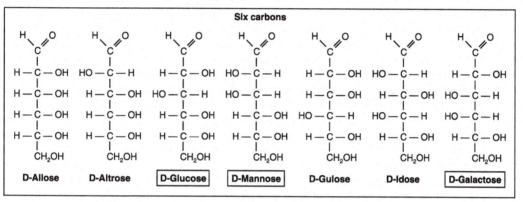

Figure I-13. Formula of some hexoses.

We give a simplified writing of some hexoses where horizontal little lines represent hydroxyl groups (Figure I-14):

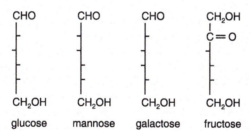

Figure I-14. Simplified representations of some hexoses.

5-2) Cyclic structure of oses

Different experimental results are in favor of cyclic structures for some oses, at least in some conditions. For example, glucose exhibits most of the aldehydic characters. Hence, it is reducing. It forms an oxime and a cyanohydrin. However, on the contrary to other "normal" aldehydes, it does not self-oxidize. It becomes truly subject to oxidation when it is only in alkaline medium.

These anomalies are explained by the fact that glucose is under some conditions under a cyclic structure. The latter is intra-molecular. Its occurrence is due to the formation of a hemiacetal by the carbonyl group of the aldehyde, with a formation of an etheroxide between the remaining hydroxyl of the hemiacetal and one of the hydroxyl rests of the sugar (see the schemes below, Figure I-15):

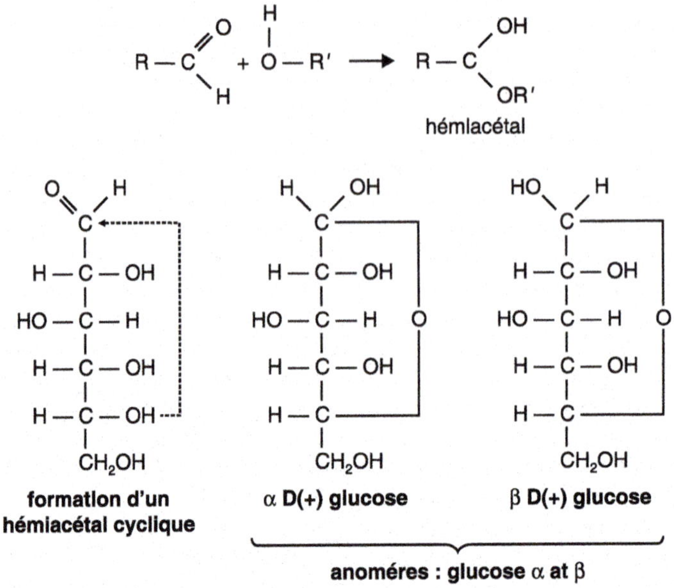

Figure I-15. Hemiketal formation (case of glucose).

We represent some heterocyclic structures of oses in Figures I-16, I-17 and I-18, I-19 represents the glucose and I-20 that of saccharose.

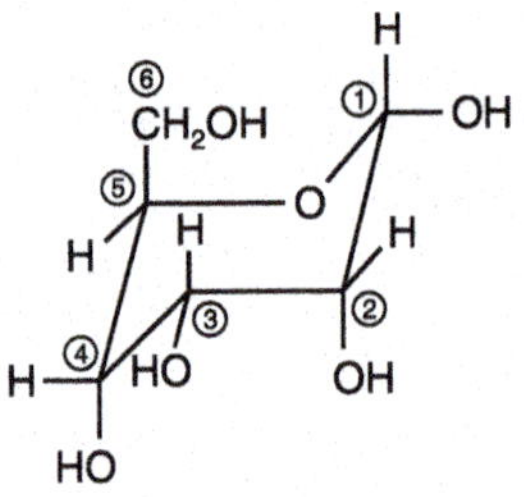

Figure I-16. Cyclic structure of glucose (glucopyranose).

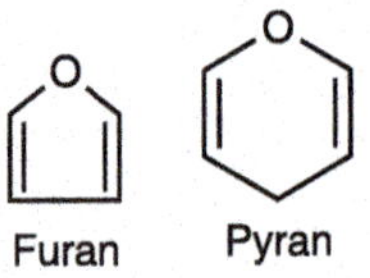

Furan   Pyran

Figure I-17. General representation of pyran and furan.

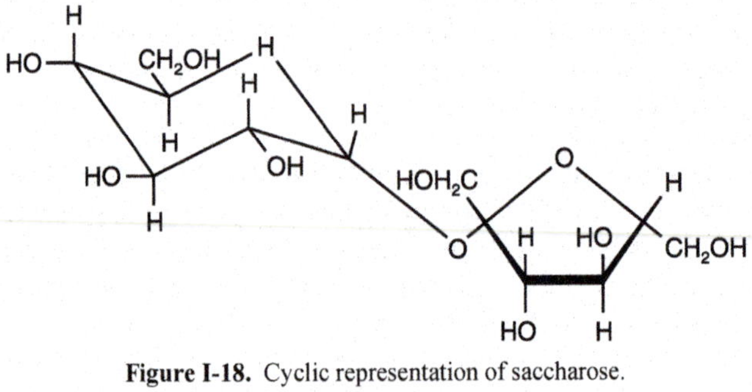

Figure I-18. Cyclic representation of saccharose.

The closing of the ose molecule by formation of the hemiketal can lead to two structures called *anomers*. A new asymmetric center is created in place of the carbon 1 (that of the carbonyl group) by the hemiacetal formation. Therefore, two stereoisomeric forms of D-glucose are formed. They are α-D-glucose and β-D-glucose (see Figure 1-19).

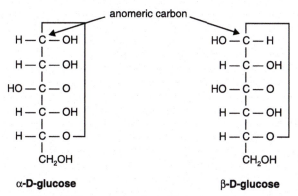

α-D-glucose   **β-D-glucose**

Figure I-19. Structures of α and β anomers of glucose.

Finally, a hexopyranose can exhibit both conformations chair and boat (Figure I-20).

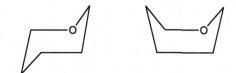

Figure I-20. Conformations chair and boat of a hexopyranose.

5-3) Case of amino-acids

Although α-amino acids are not, of course, carbohydrates, very frequently, they manifest the phenomenon of optical isomerism. We know it is due to the fact that their carbon α brings a carboxylic acid rest together with an amino function. Except the case of the glycocolle (glycine), their carbon α is asymmetric. They also exhibit the very puzzling property that the natural ones are amino-acids of the series L.

The configuration of the asymmetric carbons of amino-acids has been related to those of glyceraldehydes by working on the natural amino-acid serine by judicious chemical and biochemical reactions.

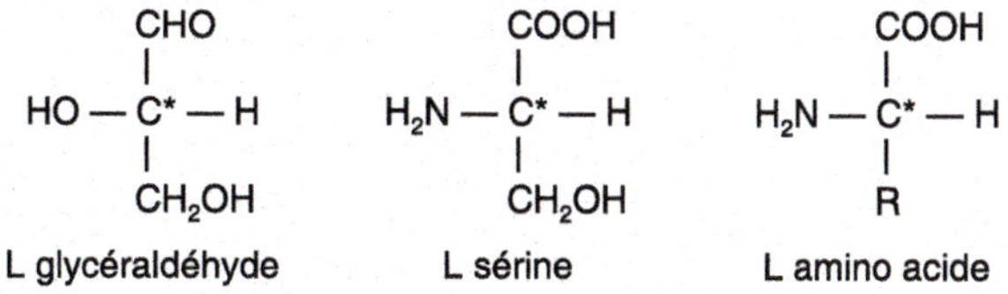

$$
\begin{array}{ccc}
\text{CHO} & \text{COOH} & \text{COOH} \\
| & | & | \\
\text{HO} - \text{C*} - \text{H} & \text{H}_2\text{N} - \text{C*} - \text{H} & \text{H}_2\text{N} - \text{C*} - \text{H} \\
| & | & | \\
\text{CH}_2\text{OH} & \text{CH}_2\text{OH} & \text{R}
\end{array}
$$

L glycéraldéhyde   L sérine   L amino acide

I-6) Determination of the different Gibbs energies involved during the hydrolysis of ATP when several equilibria simultaneously occur

Recall that the studied reaction is:

$$ATP + H_2O \rightleftharpoons ADP + P$$

with:

$$K_\Sigma = [ADP][P]/[ATP] \quad \text{and} \quad \Delta G_\Sigma^\circ = -RT\ln K_\Sigma \tag{1}$$

Recall also that in the above reaction, ATP, ADP and P are mixtures of several different species in different proportions according to the pH values. The species to consider in the neighborhood of pH = 7 are mentioned in the following Table.

Table Species which must be taken into account in the course of the hydrolysis of ATP near pH $\approx$ 7.

$$[ATP] = [HATP^{3-}] + [ATP^{4-}]$$

$$[ADP] = [HADP^{2-}] + [ADP^{3-}] \tag{2}$$

$$[P] = [H_2PO_4^-] + [HPO_4^{2-}]$$

The choice of the retained species is based on the examination of the Figure (63) (Chapter 32).

The goal is to obtain the "constants" K_Σ and ΔG_Σ°. (K_Σ and ΔG_Σ° are not thermodynamic constants. They are only constants for given values of pH and $[Mg^{2+}]_{tot}$).

The determination is carried out in two steps. The first consists of the determination of constants K_Σ and ΔG_Σ° and the values of different other constants for a given value of pH and $[Mg^{2+}]_{tot}$. The second step is identical but is successively carried out with other values of pH and $[Mg^{2+}]_{tot}$.

Let us make the choice to particularly study the hydrolysis reaction:

$$ATP^{4-} + H_2O \rightarrow ADP^{3-} + HPO_4^{2-} + H^+$$

the equilibrium constant of which is K. It is defined *sensu stricto* by the expression:

$$K = [ADP^{3-}][HPO_4^{2-}][H^+]/[ATP^{4-}] \tag{3}$$

The value of K at 298 K is 0,6 (It is determined during the course of this determination). K is a true thermodynamic constant.

– 1st step: It consists first in expressing the concentrations of all the species of expression (1) as a function of those present in (3). This is done easily by introducing the acid dissociation constants K_{a1}, K_{a2} and K_{a3} of the acids $HATP^{3-}$, $HADP^{2-}$ and $H_2PO_4^-$. The corresponding values are respectively $1,12 \ 10^{-7}$; $1,32 \ 10^{-7}$; $1,66 \ 10^{-7}$. (The latter ones also can be determined in the course of the global determination). Substituting these values in expression (1) gives:

$$K_\Sigma = (K/[H^+]) \cdot (1 + [H^+]/K_{a2})(1 + [H^+]/K_{a3})/(1 + [H^+])/k_{a1}) \tag{4}$$

In general, the experimental data are the pH of the medium and the remaining (after reaction) total concentrations [ATP], [ADP], [P]. They are often experimentally accessible. In these conditions, K_Σ is accessible through relation (1). An arbitrary but judicious choice of values of K, K_{a1}; K_{a2}, K_{a3} permits the *calculation*, with the aid of Equation (4), of the value of K_Σ which must be the closest possible to the experimental one. The values of the constants which lead to the closest approach are adopted as being the accurate ones. Mathematical techniques are very often indispensable for the finding of the closest approach. It may be a non-linear less squares technique.

– 2nd step: The second step is practiced when the complexation constants with metallic ions such as Mg^{2+} are searched for. In this case, the Equation (4) permitting the calculation of K_Σ is completed by terms taking into account the formation constants of the different complexes (see the Chapter 31). The successive operations are the same as before, except the fact that the entire operation must be carried out for each value of complex formation constant tried in order to find the best one.

The description of this strategy is an adaptation of that described by G.M. Barrow (see general bibliography) which, in turn, was formerly described by R.A. Alberty J. Biol. Chem. (1969), 244, 3290.

I-7) The vectorial action of enzymes

The problem is to know the exact details of how any one of the many known cellular pumps function.

The current hypothesis is that a directional transport of a solute is brought about by an enzyme located in a membrane.

We have seen that all enzymes have an active site at which the catalyzed reaction occurs. When an enzyme acts on its substrate, the enzyme first combines with it to form an enzyme-substrate complex. The complex undergoes attack by another group on the enzyme molecule or perhaps by an H^+ or OH^-. As a consequence, there is a cleavage of the substrate and its discharge from the active site to the surrounding medium. The process is repeated over and over. The enzyme-substrate complex is very specific. The result is that the substrate molecule is always oriented in a specific direction relative to the long axis of the enzyme molecule. The active-site of most enzymes are asymmetric as is the ADP-ase. However, enzyme-catalyzed reactions in solutions show no evidence of asymmetry or directionality. This is because, in solution, all the enzyme molecules in a solution are randomly oriented with respect to each other. The conclusion is the same for the specific direction of the substrate molecule.

Now, let us suppose that the asymmetric enzyme (for example) and the ATP-ase molecules are all bound perpendicularly to the plane of a membrane and that they are, hence, parallel. The ATP molecules, already in the active sites, are also parallel. Let us also suppose that the catalyzed reaction is the attack by the ion hydroxide of the last phosphoryl group. OH^- ions can only attack from the opposite side of the membrane and the formed ADP can only depart into the left part.

One can deduce easily that there is formation of numerous ATP molecules, which are in parallel and in the same direction. This is an example of the vectorial action.

I-8) Gibbs energies values of processes involving some compounds of biochemical interest according to "Lehninger Principles of biochemistry" (general bibliography)

Investigated Reaction	$\Delta G'^\circ$ (kJ mol^{-1}) (biochemical standard states)
acetic anhydride + $H_2O \rightarrow$ 2 CH3COO$^-$	−91,1
ATP + $H_2O \rightarrow$ ADP + P	−30.5
ATP + $H_2O \rightarrow$ AMP + PP	−45.6
PP + $H_2O \rightarrow$ 2P	−19.2
UDP-glucose + $H_2O \rightarrow$ glucose 1-phosphate	−43.0
glucose 6-phosphate + $H_2O \rightarrow$ glucose + P	−13.8
glutamine + $H_2O \rightarrow$ glutamate + NH_4^+	−14.2

maltose + H_2O → 2 glucose	−15.5
lactose + H_2O → glucose + galactose	−15.9
glucose 1-phosphate → glucose 6-phosphate	−7.3
fructose 6-phosphate → glucose 6-phosphate	−1.7
malate → fumarate + H_2O	3.1
glucose + $6O_2$ → $6CO_2$ + $6H_2O$	−2,840
palmitate + $23O_2$ → $16CO_2$ + 16 H_2O	−9,770

I-9) Standard reduction potentials of some biochemical systems with biological conventions: E'°
(V) (according to "Lehninger Principles of biochemistry" see general bibliography)

$NO_3^- + 2H^+ + 2e^- → NO_2^- + H_2O$	0.421
cytochrome f (Fe^{3+}) + e^- → cytochrome f (Fe^{2+})	0.365
cytochrome a_3 (Fe^{3+}) + e^- → cytochrome a_3 (Fe^{2+})	0.35
$O_2 + 2H^+ + 2e^- → H_2O_2$	0.295
cytochrome c_1 (Fe^{3+}) + e^- → cytochrome c_1 (Fe^{2+})	0.22
cytochrome b (Fe^{3+}) + e^- → cytochrome b (Fe^{2+})	0.077
ubiquinone + $2H^+ + 2e^-$ → ubiquinol + H_2	0.045
crotonyl-CoA + $2H^+ + 2e^-$ → butyryl-CoA	−0.015
glutathione + $2H^+ + 2e^-$ → 2 reduced glutathione	−0.23
lipoic acid + $2H^+ + 2e^-$ → dihydrolipoic acid	−0.29
$NADP^+ + H^+ + 2e^-$ → NADPH	−0.324
acetoacetate + $2H^+ + 2e^-$ → β-hydroxybutyrate	−0.346
α-ketoglutarate + $CO_2 + 2H^+ + 2e^-$ → isocitrate	−0,38
$2H^+ + 2e^- → H_2$	−0,414 (pH = 7)
ferredoxin (Fe^{3+}) + $1e^-$ → ferredoxin (Fe^{2+})	−0,432

I-10) Listing of the 20 common amino acids of proteins

Glycine-alanine-proline-valine-leucine-isoleucine-methionine-serine-threonine-cysteine-asparagine-glutamine-phenylalanine-tyrosine-tryptophan-lysine-arginine-histidine-aspartate-glutamate.

(concerning their structure as a function of pH see Chapter 27).

II) Mathematical Appendices

II-1) Derivative of a function

   1-1) Derivative of a function

   Let us consider the function y = f(x). We know that its derivative y' with respect to x, at any point of the curve representing it, is the slope of its geometrical tangent at this point, that is to say (Figure II-1 ap):

   y' = tg α

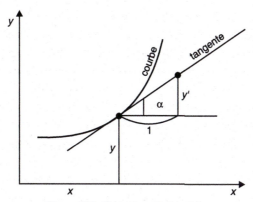

Figure II-1. Derivative of a function.

   1-2) Differential of a function

   Now, let us consider the Figure II-2.

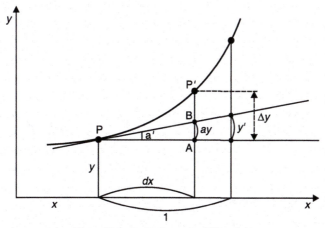

Figure II-2. Derivative and a differential.

Let us give a very small constant change dx of the variable x. dx is conceivably as small as possible. It is called its differential. The corresponding change in the function y is dy. Δy is the result of the variation dx. As other result, there is the lowering dy of the tangent of the curve at the considered point. Both rectangular triangles PAB and PA'B' being similar, one can write:

y'/1 = dy/dx

or

dy = y'dx   and

dy/dx = y'

dy is the differential of y. The derivative is hence the ratio of both differentials. It is the ratio of two very small, but fixed quantities.

It appears that the differential dy of the function y is equal to the product of its derivative y' with the differential of the variable. As a very simple example, the differential of x is:

dx = 1dx

It can be demonstrated that, since dx is very small, BP' becomes negligible with respect to AB (Figure II-2) and dy is a good approximation of the actual change of the function Δy.

II-2)   One meaning of an integral

It is sufficient, within the framework of this book, to know that an integral is a sum of infinitely small quantities, sum consisting of an infinitely great number of terms.

Let us draw the curve f(x) (Figure II-3), take any abscisse x and divide x in n equal parts Δx.

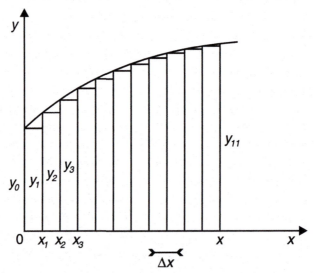

Figure II-3. One meaning of an integral.

Let us represent the different corresponding ordinates $y_0, ..y_n$ and draw the steps of a ladder at each step such as it is represented on the figure. These steps are of changing heights depending on the form of the curve. Hence, the rectangles of eras $y_0\Delta x$, $y_1\Delta x$,.......$y_n\Delta x$ are defined.

The sum of all these surfaces is not still the era S located between the curve and the absissa between the values 0 and x. In order to get the exact era S, we must take an infinite number of such rectangles of infinitely small widths, that is to say of widths equal to the differential dx. When this is the case, the height of each small rectangle becomes equal to the value y of the function and each rectangle to a vertical line of height y.

This explanation may be justified by the symbolism:

$$S = \lim_{\substack{i \to \infty \\ \Delta x \to dx}} \Sigma\, y_i\, \Delta x$$

and by definition:

$$\lim_{\substack{i \to \infty \\ \Delta x \to dx}} \Sigma\, y_i\, \Delta x = \int y\, dx$$

Of course, the limits of the abscissa must be noticed. ($\int y\, dx$ must be pronounced "sum of ydx").

Recall for our purpose that:

$$\int x^m dx = x^{m+1}/(m+1) + Cte \qquad (m \neq -1)$$

$$\int dx/x = \ln x + Cte$$

II-3)   Gradient (of concentration)

The following explanations are sufficient for our purpose.

Think of the following situation in mechanics as an example. Let us study the work done to lift a mass from an initial height x_i to a final height x_f. One knows that it is equal to the difference in gravitational potential (i.e., in gravitational energies) ΔU at the two positions (Figure II-4):

$$W = \Delta U$$

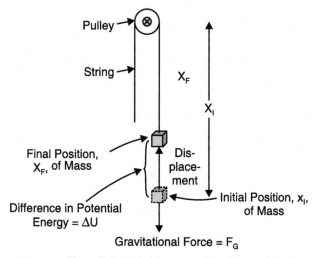

Figure II-4. Potential energy and gradient.

A work W has to be done because the gravitational force F_G acts on the body and:

$$W = -F_G (x_i - x_f)$$

$$W = -F_G \Delta x$$

$$-F_G \Delta x = \Delta U$$

(The minus sign arises from the fact that the displacement Δx is upward whereas the force acts downward. Without the minus sign inserted, the product of both forces would be negative. It must be positive because of the convention that the work done on a system must be positive).

In this example, the gravitational force can be defined by:

$$F_G = -\Delta U / \Delta x$$

More generally, there are numerous cases in which the potential energy does not vary linearly with distance. Then, the ratio $\Delta U / \Delta x$ is no longer a constant. Thus, it is better to adopt the definition:

$$F_G = -dU / dx$$

It is said that the gravitational force F_G is given by the *gradient* $-dU/dx$ of the gravitational potential energy U. This example is particularly simple because the force is unidirectional. But a gradient may be a directional derivative and it is a vector.

II-4) Partial derivatives—Total differential—State functions and total exact differentials

4-1) Partial derivatives

Up to now, we considered functions of only one variable x. Most often, we are faced with functions of several variables, one independent from the other. (For example, it is the case of the volume of a cylinder which depends both on the rayon r of its base and on its height h, variables which are independent of each other. The function is:

$$V = f(r, h)$$

and more generally:

$$z = f(x, y)$$

Variables x and y (r and h) being independent, one can change the value of one of them without changing the other (Figure II-5).

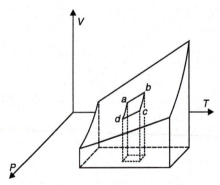

Figure II-5. A function of two variables.

The quantities:

$$(\partial z/\partial x)_y \, (\partial z/\partial y)_x$$

are respectively named "partial derivatives" of the function z with respect to x and with respect to y. They are simply calculated by considering one of the variables as being held constant and by calculating the derivative with respect to the remaining variable as usual. It is done in the case for which only one variable would exist. For example, let us consider the function:

$$z = x^3 y - e^{xy}$$

Since, alternatively in the operations of partial differentiations, y and x are considered as being constants, we find (given, of course, the facts that derivatives of functions $y = ax^n$ and e^{ax}, where a is a constant, are respectively nax^{n-1} and ae^{ax}):

$$(\partial z/\partial x)_y = 3x^2 y - ye^{xy} \quad \text{and} \quad (\partial z/\partial y)_x = x^3 - xe^{xy}$$

(Symbols ∂ of the partial derivatives must be pronounced "round d" and subscripts y and x indicate the variable being held constant in the indicated partial differentiation).

Remark: writing partial derivatives with their subscripts is essential because derivatives of the kinds, for example, $(\partial L/\partial m)n,p..)$ are in principle different from the following $(\partial L/\partial m)n,y..)$ in which the subscripts are not strictly the same.

– total differentials

Let us consider the function $z = f(x, y)$. This function is represented by a curve in the three directions z, x, y. More precisely, Figure II-5 (reinforced curves) represents a portion of the surface $z = f(x, y)$ (replacing coordinates x, y, z by the more thermodynamic coordinates P, V, T). By definition, its total differential is given by the equation:

$$dz = (\partial z/\partial x)_y \, dx + (\partial z/\partial y)_x \, dy$$

z changes with x and with y. As previously, since the variables x and y are independent, we can deal separately with the changes of z with x and with y. They are geometrically represented by the slopes of the tangents to the surface drawn in the x and y directions.

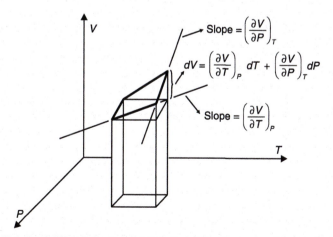

Figure II-6. Total differential and partial derivatives of the function $z = f(x, y)$ or $V = f(P, T)$.

The slopes are purely and simply the partial derivatives involved in the equation of the total differential dz. As the differentials dx and dy are chosen as being very small (but constant), we can therefore reasonably expect dz to be a good approximation of the change in the function Δz.

These considerations can be generalized to a function of several variables such as L= f (x,z,y,...), its total differential being given by the equation:

$$dL(x,y,z,..) = (\partial L/\partial x)_{y,z} \, dx + (\partial L/\partial y)_{x,z} \, dy + (\partial L/\partial z)_{y,x} \, dz +.....$$

So far the differentials are very small, dL is a good approximation of ΔL.

4-2) State functions and total exact differentials

Physics and especially thermodynamics tell us that there exist functions such that their changes from a state A to a state B are independent from the way along which the process is carried out. In this case:

$$\Delta L = L_B - L_A$$

$$\Delta L = constant$$

L_B and L_A are the values of the function L in states B and A. Such functions are named state functions.

From the mathematical standpoint, in order for a function L to be a state function, its total differential must be exact. A convenient criterion of exactness of a total differential is that the partial derivatives related to this function obey the equation given below. For the sake of simplification, let us suppose that L is a function of only two variables. Its total differential is:

$$dL(x,y) = (\partial L/\partial x)_y \, dx + (\partial L/\partial y)_x \, dy$$

Most often, both partial derivatives are themselves functions of x and y, that is to say:

$$(\partial L/\partial x)_y = M(x,y) \text{ and } (\partial L/\partial y)_x = N(x,y)$$

The total differential can be written:

$$dL(x,y) = M(x,y) \, dx + N(x,y)dy$$

The condition, so that the total differential dL(x,y) be an exact one and, hence, L(x,y) be a state function, is the following equality:

$$[\partial M(x,y)/\partial y]_x = [\partial N(x,y)/\partial x]_y$$

II-5) Handling the internal energy and other state functions of thermodynamics depending on two independent variables

The demonstration involves several steps.

– Given the functions linking the quantities U, V, T, p together, the total differential dV can be written:

$$dV = (\partial V/\partial p)_T dp + (\partial V/\partial T)_p dT$$

Its replacement in Equation (19) in the book gives:

$$dU = (\partial U/\partial V)_T [(\partial V/\partial p)_T dp + (\partial V/\partial T)_p dT] + (\partial U/\partial T)_V dT$$

After grouping the coefficients of the same differentials dp and dT together, we obtain:

$$dU = (\partial U/\partial V)_T (\partial V/\partial P)_T dp + [(\partial U/\partial V)_T (\partial V/\partial T)_p + (\partial U/\partial T)_V] dT \qquad (1')$$

The comparison of the latter equation with (20) in the text permits the identifications immediately:

$$(\partial U/\partial p)_T = (\partial U/\partial V)_T (\partial V/\partial p)_T \qquad (2')$$

$$(\partial U/\partial T)_p = (\partial U/\partial V)_T (\partial V/\partial T)_p + (\partial U/\partial T)_V \qquad (3')$$

– An analogous reasoning permits to obtain:

$$(\partial U/\partial T)_V = (\partial U/\partial p)_V (\partial p/\partial T)_V \qquad (4')$$

$$(\partial U/\partial V)_T = (\partial U/\partial p)_V (\partial p/\partial V)_T + (\partial U/\partial V)_p \qquad (5')$$

– We can note that in equations (15)(8) (2'), (16)(9) (3'), (17)(10) (4') and (18)(11) (5'), the coefficients $(\partial V/\partial p)_T$, $(\partial V/\partial T)_p$, $(\partial p/\partial T)_V$, $(\partial p/\partial V)_T$ (which do not involve U) are known because of the occurrence of the characteristic equation or if two of these coefficients have experimentally been determined. The remaining of the reasoning is straightforward if we recall that:

$$1/(\partial V/\partial p)_T = (\partial p/\partial V)_T \quad \text{and} \quad 1/(\partial p/\partial T)_V = (\partial T/\partial p)_V$$

– Another interesting expression of the internal energy is:

$$dU = TdS - pdV$$

where dS is the change of entropy accompanying the process. It appears immediately that (see Chapter 12):

$$T = (\partial U/\partial S)_V \quad \text{and} \quad p = -(\partial U/\partial V)_S$$

These reasonings are general and they can also be followed with other thermodynamic state functions.

II-6) Schwartz's theorem

The Schwartz's theorem stipulates that for a function of two independent variables x and z, the derivation order in order to obtain the cross derivative is of no importance. Hence for the function:

$$y = f(x, z) \quad (x \text{ and } z \text{ independent variables})$$

$$\partial^2 f/\partial x \partial z = \partial^2 f/\partial z \partial x$$

The second mixed derivatives are equal.

General Bibliography

Alberty, R.A. 2005. *Thermodynamics of Biochemical Reactions* edn Wiley-Intersciences. John Wiley, New York.

Atkins, P.W. 1990. *Physical Chemistry.* 4th edn Oxford Unjversity Press; Oxford.

Barrow, G.W. 2000. *Physical Chemistry for the Life Sciences.* 2nd edn Custom series, McGraw Hill Companies, New York.

Burgot, J.-L. 2010. *Ionic Equilibria in Analytical Chemistry.* Springer New York.

Burgot, J.-L. 2017. *The Notion of Activity in Chemistry.* Springer New York.

Denbigh, K. 1989. *The Principles of Chemical Equilibrium.* 4th edn Cambridge University Press, Cambridge.

Glasstone, S. 1960. *Thermodynamics for Chemists.* 11th edn D van Nostrand, Princeton.

Haynie, D.T. 2008. *Biological Thermodynamics.* 2 edn Cambridge University Press, Cambridge.

Hill, T.L. 1986. *An Introduction of Statistical Thermodynamics.* Dover, New York.

Klotz, I.M. 1964. *Chemical Thermodynamics: Basic Theory and Methods.* W.A. Benjamin, New York.

Lehninger, A.L. 1965. Bioenergetics. W.A. Benjamin, New York.

Nelson, D.L. and M.M. Cox. 2013. *In Lehninger's Principles of Biochemistry.* 6th edn W.H. Freeman and Company, New York.

Prigogine, I. 1968. *Introduction to Thermodynamics of Irreversible Processes.* 3th edn, Dunod, Paris.

Stryer, L. 1992. *La biochimie de Lubert Stryer.* 3th edn Flammarion, Paris.

Roberts, J.D. and M.C. Caserio. 1964. *Basic Principles of Organic Chemistry.* edn W.A. Benjamin, New York.

Waley, S.G. 1962. *Mechanisms of Organic and Enzymic Reactions.* edn. Oxford University Press, London.

Index